AF722526

Psychosomatic Medicine: Theory and Practice

Psychosomatic Medicine: Theory and Practice

Editor: Linda Easton

AMERICAN
MEDICAL PUBLISHERS
www.americanmedicalpublishers.com

AMERICAN
MEDICAL PUBLISHERS
www.americanmedicalpublishers.com

Cataloging-in-publication Data

Psychosomatic medicine : theory and practice / edited by Linda Easton.
p. cm.
Includes bibliographical references and index.
ISBN 979-8-88740-408-0
1. Medicine, Psychosomatic. 2. Psychology, Pathological.
3. Medicine and psychology. I. Easton, Linda.
RC49 .P79 2023
616.08--dc23

© American Medical Publishers, 2023

American Medical Publishers,
41 Flatbush Avenue,
1st Floor, New York,
NY 11217, USA

ISBN 979-8-88740-408-0 (Hardback)

This book contains information obtained from authentic and highly regarded sources. Copyright for all individual chapters remain with the respective authors as indicated. All chapters are published with permission under the Creative Commons Attribution License or equivalent. A wide variety of references are listed. Permission and sources are indicated; for detailed attributions, please refer to the permissions page and list of contributors. Reasonable efforts have been made to publish reliable data and information, but the authors, editors and publisher cannot assume any responsibility for the validity of all materials or the consequences of their use.

Trademark Notice: Registered trademark of products or corporate names are used only for explanation and identification without intent to infringe.

Contents

Preface

Psychosomatic medicine refers to an interdisciplinary medical specialty that studies the effects of behavioral, social and psychological factors on bodily functions and quality of life in both animals and human beings. Two distinguishing characteristics of psychosomatic practice are the clinical model of thinking and the holistic approach to patient management. The primary aim of psychosomatic medicine is to address the shortcomings in medical care, through the integration of novel operational tactics into clinical practice. Medical assessment and treatment can be enhanced through employment of psychosomatic medicine techniques, particularly with regard to lifestyle modification, medically unexplained symptoms and chronic diseases. Psychosomatic medicine is significant in clinical settings, where mental processes play a significant role in the medical results. It oversees the emotional and mental states as having the capability to affect the course of an illness. This book will provide in-depth knowledge about the theory and practice of psychosomatic medicine. Those with an interest in this field would find it helpful.

This book is the end result of constructive efforts and intensive research done by experts in this field. The aim of this book is to enlighten the readers with recent information in this area of research. The information provided in this profound book would serve as a valuable reference to students and researchers in this field.

At the end, I would like to thank all the authors for devoting their precious time and providing their valuable contribution to this book. I would also like to express my gratitude to my fellow colleagues who encouraged me throughout the process.

Editor

1

Psychosomatic Medicine and Palliative Care

Manuel Mejías-Estévez, Rocio Dominguez Álvarez and Ignacio Jauregi Lobera

"In psychosomatic diseases the body takes the voice so that the emotions tell stories through their words that are the symptoms".

Mejias [1]

Abstract

Psychosomatic medicine (MP) and palliative care are disciplines with history and both are based in the scientific world. Although the psychosomatic diagnosis is exclusionary, it can help palliative care to be more effective. The influence of the psychosomatic in the palliative exists. According to all the bibliography available in the electronic databases, psychosomatic medicine is a biopsychosocial model related to both physical and psychosocial factors, which helps improve the care of patients with advanced cancer in palliative care (improved survival, quality of life, reduces the burden on caregivers). It helps analyze and address psychiatric disorders, as well as in the control of complex symptoms such as life-threatening anxiety, depression or delirium. Therefore, both medical disciplines are related from the beginning and help to the quality of life of terminally ill patients.

Keywords: palliative care, physical factors, quality of life, medical discipline, terminal illness

1. Introduction

The first great historical relationship between both disciplines is referenced by the Paracelsus himself who could inspire centuries later the great Professor Sigmund Freud, since he was the promater of psychotherapy as a science: psychoanalysis, as a part of the birth of medicine itself psychosomatic (MP). This conclusion is understood when reading Dr. Freud's own words about his own condition, that of an oncological disease for 26 years, caused by his smoking habit, of a squamous cell carcinoma of the palate and jaw, which led him to numerous interventions surgical and painful conditions [2, 3]. Although the breaking news pointed to morphine overdose as the immediate cause of death, the fundamental cause was that terminal tumor, which turned off the light of genius in London on 23 September 1939. If palliative care, a later discipline, had been able to intervene, they would have allowed relief from his suffering, from the symptoms that tormented him, and, consequently, a dignified, natural and not accelerated death.

Psychosomatic medicine (PM), coined in 1818 by Heinroth, sought to relate psychosocial variables to psychophysiological changes. Although the first great evolution came from psychoanalysis, from 1965 this orientation changed towards other explanatory theoretical models based on the temporal and evolutionary analysis of the underlying disorder, somatic syndrome, pathogenesis, conflict, neurosis, personality, reliability of the signs, gains (primary and secondary) ..., and thus reach from psychosomatic factors (alexithymia, demoralization, irritability, behavior A), to psychosomatic diseases (according to the Chicago school, chronic with outbreaks) such as high blood pressure, bronchial asthma, peptic ulcer, ulcer-ative colitis, rheumatoid arthritis, thyrotoxicosis, neurodermatitis.

This medicine "is not a specialty but rather a point of view that applies to all aspects of Medicine and Surgery. It does not mean studying the body less; it means studying the psyche more. It is a reaffirmation of the old principle that the mind and body are one, that they function as interactive and interdependent organs, a principle that has always guided the intelligent practical physician. As a science, psychosomatic medicine aims to discover the precise nature of the relationship between emotions and bodily function. Research in this field is based on the con-vergence of modern physiological research, as developed by laboratory science and animal experimentation, as well as the discoveries of psychoanalysis, as previously mentioned, both dynamic developments in medicine [4]. It is established from the 1960s of the twentieth century as a multifactorial biopsychosocial model for all disease processes and not only for a group of diseases [5, 6].

The American Board of Medical Specialties recognizes it as the subspecialty of Psychiatry that is dedicated to the diagnosis, treatment and prevention of psychiat-ric morbidity in medical patients, through psychiatric counseling and the training of health professionals, especially in the hospital context [7]. However, in essence, psychosomatic medicine is multidisciplinary for the evaluation of psychosocial factors involved in individual vulnerability within the disease, holistic clinical care and the integration of psychological interventions with therapeutic, preventive and rehabilitative functions of medical diseases [8].

There are various theories that guide the psychosomatic model in our times, highlighting the complexity of the reality of the problems and the need for an interdisciplinary and multidisciplinary vision. Although it is a way of understanding medicine referring to the concept of disease, it is usually associated in a restricted way with a group of diseases that are variable but superimposable according to many tendencies to the somatoform disorders of DSM-IV-TR, the result of the influence of American origins, where it is equated with the somatopsychic, defined as a psychic alteration that causes organic symptoms through the somatic nervous system (mainly vegetative). The DSM-V criteria for the diagnosis of disorders with somatic symptoms continue to be incomplete because they do not take into account disease behaviors, such as denial of disease or experimental avoidance, which can be very important in the effect on quality of life of patients, for example, in pain, or in palliative care [5, 9].

Circumscribing the psychosomatic as a psychological disorder that generates a physical effect, causing some consequence in the body, although practical, would limit our analysis, since psychosomatic medicine as an integrative science, always tries to overcome itself, fleeing from partial or reductionist visions for integrate the manifestations of the biological, psychological, social world in the understanding of the human being, that is, the support of the good doctor or health professional, whose objective is to help the sick person, integrating the humanistic essence. Possibly for this reason, Laín Entralgo, already defined it as *"an orientation of Medicine that is characterized by including in each medical act and in each clinical judgment, the consider-ation of unconscious emotions that contribute to each patient configuring a sick person in a situation different"*.

Palliative care (PC) is a relatively new field with which a good part of the health system professionals are not familiar, despite its importance. Callahan reminds us in a paradigmatic article in the New England Journal of Medicine, that the main goals of today's medicine are not only to diagnose and treat diseases, but also, and equally important, to help die in peace. The English word "care" has its root in the goth term "Kara", which means to grieve, suffer, cry out in pain. The one who really cares must join the other person in his suffering (caring is assisting). Paliar derives from "pallium" (from the Latin "under the Canopy") which means mitigating the violence of certain diseases by making them more bearable. Palliative care is to attend, with the intention of making the patient's coexistence with their disease more comfortable.

Palliative care or "Hospice" care, as they were called from their origin in the fifth century, since they were carried out in hospices, led to the great modern movement in the United Kingdom in the 1960s–1970s of the twentieth century with Cicely Saunders as main figure and after expand to the rest of Europe, North America. The Hospice concept refers more to the physical structure of an organization, and PC would be a special type of care designed to provide well-being and support to patients and their families, in the final stages of a terminal illness (currently called advanced disease). Palliative Medicine from its first steps highlights two important aspects of medical ethics: respect for the weak and evicted, and recognition of the finite nature of curative medicine.

Emphasize that palliative care offers the most basic of the concept of caring, covering the needs of the patient and their family regardless of where they are being cared for or the evolutionary stage of the underlying disease. They affirm life considering death as a normal biological process, that is, the final part of the life process (biography of the subject). Therefore, they seek to preserve the best possible quality of life to the end without accelerating or delaying death. This improvement in the quality of life of patients and their families is achieved by facing the many problems associated with a fatal disease through the prevention and relief of suffering, identifying early, assessing and using adequate treatments for pain and other physical, psychological, social and spritual problems. Its application, when necessary, ranges from the diagnosis of the disease to the death of the patient, continuing with the care of the family in mourning [10, 11].

Determining which diseases are subsidiary to PC is complex, although it is currently based on the well-known McNamara list, the recommendations of the National Hospice Organization (NHO) of 1996 and the NECPAL CCOMS-ICO© instrument, which basically includes the following diseases [12–15]:

- Cancer.
- Advanced chronic heart disease.
- Advanced chronic kidney failure.
- Advanced liver failure (liver cirrhosis).
- Advanced lung disease.
- Chronic neurological disease. Highlight:
  - Advanced chronic cerebrovascular disease.
  - Motor neuron disease: amyotrophic lateral sclerosis (ALS).
  - Dementia.

  - Advanced Parkinson's disease.
  - Advanced Huntington's disease.
  - Advanced Alzheimer's disease.
  - Persistent vegetative states.
- Geriatric patient with advanced frailty.
- Advanced AIDS.

It is estimated that the need for PC varies between 50 and 90% of patients who die, being higher during the last year of life. In absolute numbers, cases of non-oncology are much more frequent, although the complexity of the cancer is usually greater, which explains at least in part that the scientific experience and clinical practice of tumor-related PC is greater. All health professionals must possess basic knowledge to care for these individuals and families, and in the most complex cases, it is when the Specific Palliative Care Teams or Units must intervene.

A disease is terminal if it has the following criteria:

1. Advanced and incurable and progressive disease, without reasonable possibilities of response to its specific treatment, and with a limited prognosis for life.
2. Presence of intense and changing multifactorial symptoms.
3. Great emotional impact on patients, families and professionals, which gener-ates a great demand for care.
4. Implicit or explicit presence of death.

So what criteria can we use to establish terminality or advanced disease?. Two types of criteria [1]:

1. General.
   a. Advanced age.
   b. Comorbidity versus vulnerability.
   c. Well-documented disease progression that has generated an increasing need for healthcare. It is established according to:
      i. Clinical criteria.
         - Independently include advanced cognitive decline.
      ii. Lab tests.
      iii. Supplementary tests.
   d. Emergencies or hospital admissions in the last 6 months, associated with:
      i. Recent functional impairment.
      ii. Dependency for at least three basic activities of daily life.

e. Nutritional impairment or malnutrition:

i. Weight loss >10% in the last 6 months.

ii. Serum albumin <2.5 g/dl.

2. Specific to the disease. Two subgroups:

a. Cancer: They are mainly based on the histology and staging of the tumor.

b. No cancer:

i. Advanced organic insufficiencies.

ii. Advanced degenerative diseases of the central nervous system.

In the case of children, terminality is grouped into four groups:

1. Serious potentially curable diseases, such as cancer.

2. Progressive diseases without cure such as muscular dystrophy.

3. Diseases with premature death with long periods of treatment to promote a normal life, such as cystic fibrosis.

4. Non-progressive irreversible diseases, which cause great disability and vulnerability, such as cerebral palsy.

There is an instrument that helps to identify advanced terminal disease and the need for PC, which is the NECPAL CCOMS-ICO© instrument for the identification of people in a situation of advanced or terminal chronic disease (oncological or non-oncological) and need for care palliative in Health and Social Services. Its application is aimed at the subsidiary diseases of PC referred to above. Thanks to it, it is possible to detect at a certain moment if the person with an advanced disease requires palliative care, that is, to have quality of life and comfort as a fundamental objective, without ruling out other curative therapeutic measures provided for the clinical and evolutionary state of the subject. Such care is normally welcomed by conventional health resources, and in the most difficult or complex cases, a Specialized Palliative Care Team will intervene [13, 16, 17].

The question in its three aspects: *how much do I have left to live?; How much does my loved one have left?; how much does my patient have left?*. These are constant questions when faced with a terminal illness in the final phase of life. But this issue is also fundamental for the health professional, since life estimation is fundamental for clinical decision-making and for the proper management of therapies, including communicative ones, such as giving bad news. The possible answer would be made as three questions to answer reflected in **Figure 1** [1, 18, 19]:

1. Presence of terminal illness.

2. Estimation of life prognosis. There is no single standard method for this due to its complexity. From the study of a multitude of variables, especially in the terminal cancer patient, a multitude of prognostic indices have been designed

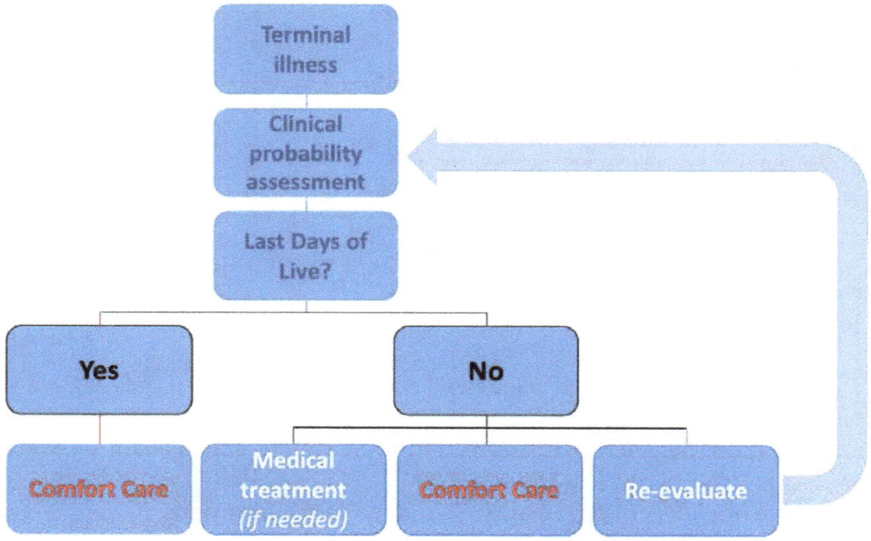

Figure 1.
Algorithm for the management of terminal illness, prognosis and last days of life (authorized by the author [1]).

based on laboratory tests, functional status, symptoms, signs and subjective clinical impression of the prognosis. The vital prognosis in non-oncological disease is more difficult to determine, so the need for palliative care will be given by the presence of organic failure and irreversible progressive deterioration with unrelieved suffering. It will be based on the analysis of the functionality of the patient, clinical estimation of the expert professional, present symptoms and laboratory analysis.

3. The third question is the culmination of the person's end of life, in which death comes progressively (as opposed to sudden death). It is the situation of the last days of life or state of pre-agony or agony, which indicates that death is next (between hours and a few days). It would be the last stage of a terminal illness known as the End of Life Phase (FFV). Therefore, it is a phase that precedes death when it occurs gradually (hours, days) with signs that begin with severe asthenia associated with bedriddenness, loss of interest in the surroundings, development of a semi-comatose state, intake limited to liquids or small sips (including total dysphagia), with the inability to take oral medication, it is establishing a very short life prognosis. The treatment is supportive, aimed at intensifying comfort and reducing suffering as much as possible, given that symptoms that cause discomfort to the dying person are frequent, for which fortunately we have effective medications, usually administered subcutaneously (more frequent at home) or intravenous (most often used in hospitals). In the necessary cases, palliative sedation will be ap-plied in order to control the refractory symptoms and alleviate the suffering of the patient.

The great contributions of Palliative Care to Medicine are [1, 10, 19–22]:

1. Accept death as a biological and natural process.

2. Give quality of life to life, helping the patient and the family in their suffering.

3. To confront the symptoms from a practical and decisive point of view so that their control allows helping the patient to have the greatest possible well-being, regardless of the evolutionary stage of their disease. It is common to confuse pain (*"Unpleasant sensory and emotional experience, associated with actual or potential tissue damage, or described in terms of such damage"*, defined in 1979 by the International Association for the study of pain or IASP) and suffering (grief). In Palliative Care there are 56 definitions of suffering, showing that although there are deficiencies in its definition, its relevance in the deep personal anguish it causes, especially in the last year of life, makes the person more vulnerable. Its most frequent causes are pain, dyspnea, delirium and depression.

4. Communication and emotional coping skills (especially for bad news, trustworthy therapeutic relationship acquisition or emotional ventilation).

Psycho-oncology (term that is related to Psychosomatic Medicine and Palliative Care) studies the impact of cancer on the psychological function of patients and their families. It arises, among other influences, from the PM as a need to respond to the needs of the cancer patient, from which the PC has tried to benefit. Its evolution has been possible thanks to the sustained advancement of multiple disciplines such as Oncology (Medical and Radiotherapy), Epidemiology, Surgery, Immunology, Genetics, Endocrinology, Sociology and Bioethics, among others, providing updated assistance protocols comprehensive for terminally ill patients in the Palliative Care Units. This development has clearly contributed to the development of the psychological and psychiatric aspects linked to cancer. Thus, as we have reiterated, it contributes to a better quality of life for cancer patients from the initial impact of the diagnosis. Adjustment disorders, related major depressive disorder, and acute confusional syndrome (delirium) are com-mon. There are effective treatment protocols for such adapted pathologies in each region [23, 24].

Psychosomatic physicians can play an important role in the field of cancer treatment through psycho-oncological activities such as psychological support after receiving bad news, before and/or after surgery and in chemotherapy cycles to control delirium associate [25].

Within the biopsychosocial framework and from the knowledge coming from the Psycho-oncology and the PC, one of the great problems is addressed which is the *Pact or Conspiracy of Silence*. This is usually defined as an agreement, implicit or explicit, between family members, relatives and health professionals, to hide or distort information about the patient's diagnostic, prognostic and/or therapeutic situation, in order to avoid the suffering of facing the end of your own life. This information deficit is regarding not only the diagnosis, but also and above all the prognosis. Only between 15 and 21% of people at the end of their lives know their diagnosis and prognosis, being the most important factor when communicating the diagnosis the fear of negative repercussions that may result from the communication of the real state of the patient [11, 26].

The idea behind this chapter is that PM and PC are related disciplines. I am pleased to find, albeit to a much lesser extent than we would like, that there is an attempt to verify this interrelation. For example, in Romania, how life experiences imprint the possible relationship of somatic effects in terminal diseases, espe-cially cancer [27] or as a professional paradigm of life, represented in Dr. Arthur H. Schmale, who advocated the relationship between PC, PM, and Psychosocial Oncology [28].

2. Relationship study (PM and PC)

The first known article that related both concepts in an indirect way was van der Valk [29], since he commented on the psychological aspects of palliative treatment of malignant tumors with a small psychosomatic veneer. In that same year, H. Zalce in the medical journal Gaceta de México, spoke in a shallow way when referring to the scarce training of doctors in the therapeutic management of advanced cancer. Geriatrician Dr. A. Verwoerdt, from the Southern American Medical Association, began to relate a little more, almost unintentionally, the importance of both, in reference to palliative care in the communication process, especially the bad news, becoming from the early 70s, a promoter of Counseling and of the psychologi-cal stress responses of physical illnesses, that is, he traveled from palliative to Psychosomatic Medicine, to finish the last third of his career focusing on study of sexual behavior [30–32].

It is in May 1965, when the German B. Staehelin, deals specifically with Psychosomatic Medicine (PM) and Palliative Care (CP) in a German magazine [33]. It showed that an adequate psychosomatic approach helped physicians to better treat patients with advanced cancer, subsidiaries of Palliative Care (PC).

The relevant aspects of this research that show the concern of Psychosomatic Medicine in Palliative Care and its interrelation, contain the following eight thematic pillars (summarized in **Table 1**):

1. Psychosomatic medicine is based on a biopsychosocial model related to physical and psychosocial factors, with many similar points of view in General Medicine, Psychosomatic Medicine and Palliative Care [35]. Thus, the PM also helps cancer survivors as psychosocial support services [34].

2. Psychosomatic medicine helps physicians to improve the care of patients with advanced cancer in palliative care [33], to get better the satisfaction of their own illness and at the same time helps to reduce the overload of professionals in palliative care that cares for patients and their families [35].

   Psychosomatic medicine deals with relevant aspects in improving the survival of cancer patients. An aging population, advances in diagnosis and treatment, have led to a rapidly growing population of people affected by cancer. People live longer after a cancer diagnosis, tolerating more advanced and even aggressive treatments more and better than in times past. In the evolution of tumors, there is an impact on the quality of life, with a psychological repercussion, where Psychiatry, Psychology, Psychotherapy, Mental Health Services, in short, provide tools to all professionals (doctors, nurses, social workers, physiotherapists, psychologists, trained volunteers, etc.), who have contact with these patients and their families, many medical specialties: Medical Oncology, Radiation Oncology, Internal Medicine, Primary Care, Psychiatry, Pediatric, Emergency Medicine, other medical and/or surgical specialties (Cardiology, Dermatology, Endocrine, Nephrology, Pulmonology, Neurology, Rheumatology, Gynecology, General, Digestive, Cardiovascular, Neurosurgery, Traumatology, Maxillo-facial, Otorhinolaryngology, Ophthalmology, Urology). Therefore, the increase in life expectancy in cancer has increased interest for its impact on psychosocial problems and quality of life, rather than just focusing on longevity [37].

   Psychiatry has been collaborating more and more with the above all hospitable services of palliative care, although there is much to improve because it is not a general trend [36].

Thematic area	**Relevant ideas**	Featured authors
1. Biopsychosocial model	• Psychosocial support	[34] [35]
2. Improved care in PC (especially advanced cancer)	• Decreased load • Improved survival • Impact on quality of life • Psychiatry (area of work to be developed)	[33] [35] [36] [37]
3. Analysis of psychiatric disorders in cancer patients in PC	• Early detection • Specific derivation • Psychosocial suffering • Psychosocial interview • Disorders: ○ Adaptive (anxiety, depression) ○ Delirium	[38] [39] [37] [40]
4. Bad news communication	• Kübler-Ross phases • Psychosomatic symptoms • Denial, anger, negotiation, depression, acceptance	[41] [37]
5. Symptom control (especially in terminal cancer)	• Life distress • Cancer as a stressful life event • Impaired quality of life • Fatigue by compassion of professionals • Depression in cancer • Anorexia in cancer	[42] [37] [43] [44] [45]
6. Psychotherapy to patients and family (basic concepts)	• Anxiety before death • Chronic pain	[46] [47] [48] [49] [50]
7. Psychotherapeutic interventions	• Emotional Support • Psychoeducation • Cognitive-behavioral (self-regulation) • Individual ○ Mindfulness ○ Counseling ○ Meditation and hypnosis ○ Others • Group • Specific	[51] [52] [37] [53] [54]

Thematic area	Relevant ideas	Featured authors
8. Others aspects of interest	• Non-cancer PC • Pediatric PC • Caregivers (overload) • Anxiety about death and relationships • Assessment and perception of health care received • Place of exitus • Attention to grief	[55] [49] [56] [57] [58] [59] [50] [50] [60] [61] [62]

Table 1.
Thematic summary of Psychosomatic Medicine in Palliative Care.

3. The psychosomatic spectrum analyzes psychiatric disorders in cancer pa-tients and very sensitively when they are also subsidiaries of palliative care. A double operational advantage is provided: teaching professionals to detect the most common problems in order to address them and specifically refer experts (psychiatrists, physiotherapists, psychologists,...) when it'd been necessary [37, 38].

A fundamental question is to measure the presence of mental disorders. There are many different variables that act as factors on individual vulnerability (for example, life events, chronic stress, well-being and health attitudes) and the psychosocial correlates of medical illness (for example, psychiatric disorders, psychological symptoms, disease behavior, quality of life,...), which are possibly involved not only in classic psychiatric disorders, but more broadly in psycho-social suffering in cancer and in Palliative Care. There are many studies, so we summarize the highlights of this analysis [37–40]:

- The specific psychosocial interview with diagnostic criteria for psychoso-matic research (known as Diagnostic Criteria for Psychosomatic Research or DCPR) represents a way to detect and evaluate emotional distress, anxiety, depression, wrong coping, dysfunctional attachment and other dimensions psychosocial. Intercultural problems, such as language, ethnicity, race, and religion, are also discussed as possible factors influencing perception of the disease in patients and families (another important aspects may be survival mechanisms and the psychological response to cancer diagnosis).

- Psychiatric disorders can be found in up to 47% of cancer patients. In some cases they are direct responses to this disease, in others it acts as a trigger or enhancer.

- Psychiatric disorders depend mainly on individual factors. In cancer the most frequent are:

  - Adaptive disorder (68%) with depressed and/or anxious mood. It's a response to a vital stressor that produces harmful interference in the social role. It requires a follow-up to differentiate it from depressive or anxiety disorders.

  - Others (10–34%): major depression, anxiety disorders, delirium or acute confusional syndrome (more frequent in the last days of life).

- In specific types of cancer, for example prostate cancer, depression is more frequent in the elderly and anxiety in young adults.

4. People diagnosed with cancer, their families and close friends experience normalized responses, such as those derived from the impact as bad news of having a tumor (knowledge of diagnosis and/or prognosis), initially described by Elizabeth Kübler-Ross in 1969, in the following phases where psychosomatic phenomenology stands out [37, 41]:

- *Denial (Phase I)*. It's an isolation phase as a defense mechanism against the perception of the disease and its consequences. The information received produces an emotional impact, which requires progressive and usually adaptive elaboration. Therefore, if it's maintained throughout the disease process, it becomes a difficult pathology to treat. The most convenient attitude on the part of professionals is respect, trying to combat it with patience and delicacy, without reinforcing denial with lies. Communication skills are essential.

- *Fury or anger (Phase II)*. It's characterized by outrage and the fight against the inevitable, looking for guilty people. Anger is a feeling that appears at the perception of injustice due to illness. It's important that this fury directed at oneself, the family for not having cared for the patient, friends, work environ-ment, superior forces (like God), but especially towards the health workers, the doctor who did not detect the pathology, the tests that took time to carry out, the medication that was not effective,... It's essential to know that this is not a personal attack, so the professional should not judge or participate in the confrontation. Self-blame involves extra suffering.

- *Negotiation (looking for a pact: Phase III)*. It's a pact that faces reality but looks for the possibility of improvement, cure or even miracle. Pacts are made with a supreme being (in our culture it would be God), others and oneself. The attitude towards this phase will have to be formed by tolerance, respect, without prejudices. The patient can seek relief in other complementary or less conventional therapies, so an integrative and communicative medicine should be promoted. Dialog is specially important to face this phase.

- *Depression (Phase IV)*. The disease progresses and cannot escape from reality, adopting different attitudes: crying, sadness, indifference, isolation,... Although it's a very hard phase for the family and the health workers, it can be an adaptive mechanism and the beginning of acceptance. That is why we must maximize communication skills, knowing how to be active listening, managing silences and promoting emotional expression.

- *Acceptance (Phase V)*. After the depression phase, the inevitability progression of the disease and the physical-psychological exhaustion, can reach a degree of acceptance of reality, entering a state of serenity, tranquility and inner peace that's always recommended, although not always possible. Spiritual needs take on greater importance at this time, and farewells are important to close life cycles and unfinished situations.

These phases do not always appear all of them nor do they have to be consecutive. Each person has a phase rhythm, so that for example one person can be angry (Phase II) throughout the disease process and another can come directly to acceptance.

5. The importance of recognizing and addressing symptoms is the principle on which PC are based. PM brings its vision to some of the more complex symptoms to treat.

  - In the process of oncological disease, psychological or vital anguish (valued through emotional reactions, physical restrictions, communication deficits, negative social reactions, pain and gastrointestinal symptoms) has a prominent psychosomatic role, the origin of which emanates from the four main actors involved in the palliative disease process [37, 42]:

    - Patient.

    - Family.

    - Health professionals.

    - Society and culture.

  Understanding these factors allows professionals involved in cancer to better assess the patient and adapt therapies in a more personalized way, also helping their families, because cancer is a stressful life event (SLE), tumor pathology involves a change of life throughout the family, especially when the patient is a child, in addition to developmental problems and cognitive disor-ders, behavioral changes (including schooling), financial difficulties... Young adults fight especially for the changes that the disease implies in the work and in their social or personal relationships. The elderly focus on the challenge of aging and cancer.

  Therefore, the psychological and social care of cancer patients is part of quality medical care, and training professionals in diagnostic (test, questionnaires...) and therapeutic techniques (psychotherapy, pharmacology...) are priority needs.

  - Burnout and compassion fatigue of health professionals who care for cancer patients can have two major problems for themselves: professional and personal damage and the negative repercussion on patient care and on the work environment in general [37].

  - Depression in cancer patients is a frequent symptom. PM tries to study its relationship with age, where it seems that there is an inverse relationship, improving depression with increasing age or senescence [43]. Likewise, it has helped to show the negative impact of depression on cancer, measured by quality-adjusted life year. That is, if depression exists, life is shorter and with loss of quality [44].

  - Anorexia is one of the most frequent symptoms in patients with terminal cancer. It's characterized by a lack of appetite, where treatment is very limited, especially with corticotherapy and antiestrogens [45].

6. The PM investigates relevant aspects of psychotherapy in Palliative Care.

  - It's common for the family to hide both what they know and their negative emotions (anxiety, fear, sadness ...) to the cancer patient's dying [49]. It's shown that this process also influences caregivers [50].

- The presence of chronic pain in general (whether oncological or non-oncological), and particularly in terminal illnesses, should benefit from psychological therapies applied, both for seniors, adults and children [46–48].

7. The types of recommended psychotherapeutic interventions that have shown improvement in the quality of life, anxiety and distress of cancer patients are short-term therapies, aimed at supporting and helping in their anxiety and stress crises. Obviously, these therapies often require psychotropic drugs to control symptoms, especially anxiety, depression, negative thoughts, conduct disorders, etc. Therefore, the following are included as types of recommended therapies [37, 51–54]:

- Emotional *support to the patient and caregivers* (essential treatment). Through like-minded thinking (empathy), a comprehensive and integrative vision of personal life can be provided, transferring a coherent, real and meaningful hope.

- *Psychoeducation.* It can be carried out by other members of the health team, and helps to know the disease, its natural evolution...

- *Cognitive and behavioral therapies,* especially self-regulation (for example, relax-ation exercises, distraction tools, rehearsal of dreaded events, suggestion ...). They are especially effective in pain, fatigue and post-chemotherapy emetic syndrome, especially if they are done preventively.

- *Individual psychotherapy*. Are included:

    - Mindfulness: effective technique especially for anxiety and depression. It's popular on PC because is widely used in professionals' self-care. It's a person-centered therapy, based on meditation and compassion, to reduce anxiety and strengthen resilience and motivation.

    - Counseling: therapy that helps especially in the existential crisis of a tumor, especially if it's advanced. It's about guiding and advising from empathetic listening to be able to handle negative thoughts and the emotions that are generated. It's a therapy frequently followed in PC, applicable to patients, family and health personnel.

    - Meditation and hypnosis: neuropsychobiological management of stress and anxiety, although it has also been used for difficult pain, nausea and vomiting.

    - Others: psychotherapy focused on meaning, therapy for preserving dignity ...

- *Group psychotherapy*. Its objective is to educate, guide and reduce social isola-tion. Couples and family therapy are included. A very important example is group therapy for caregirvers of patiente with long survival.

- *Specific treatment implemented by specialists in Mental Health Systems* (Psychotherapy, Psychopharmacology, other interventions such as psychological support, among others...). This type of intervention is formally requested in appropriate situations where patients face challenges, especially during active cancer treatment, survival, and in the worst case, end of life. However, there are disparities in criteria regarding these assumptions given that in clinical practice the cases are not always the same. Therefore, psychosomatic medicine tries to emphasize what are the most frequent stages in palliative care, in order to provide the best care for patients with severe cancer.

8. The PM has been concerned with other topics of interest in PC, less recognized but important, which would be:

- Palliative care in non-cancer patients, such as Phase IV and V advanced chronic kidney disease (end-stage renal disease). The stress of hemodialysis has a negative impact on the mental health of the patients. Spiritual well-being can be a great predictor of mental health, psychological distress, sleep disturbance, and psychosomatic complaints [63].

  ○ Palliative care in the pediatric age. Pathological behaviors produce symptoms, functional deterioration and difficulty in therapeutic coping. For this reason, integrated models of behavioral health care have been implemented to promote resilience (adaptability of a living being against a disturbing agent or an adverse state or situation) in: Oncology, PC, pain, Neuropsychiatry, Cystic Fibrosis and Transplants. This psychosomatic treatment helps the child comprehensively and effectively and reduces costs derived from tests and hospitalizations of pathologies such as asthma [58].

  ○ Caregivers and family. Throughout the chapter, we have emphasized the importance of the role of the family. We highlight the following studies:

    a. In relatives of patients with cerebral malignancy, it's found that financial support in most cases does not exist, and that there is an increased risk of psychosomatic problems such as anxiety or depression. Caregivers worsen care overload, quality of life and mental state [55].

    b. Caregiver burden is often a difficulty in increasing family satisfaction in end-of-life care at home. A caregiver burden-centered home care model could improve end-of-life experiences for patients and family caregivers [59].

    c. Death anxiety can produce negative emotions that hinder the search for meaning in family members and in dying patients themselves with advanced or metastatic cancer. A study qualitative to highlight on these aspects investigated the relationship of a couple of patients diagnosed with melanoma along 6 months, revealing how the image of the relationship and its nature changed in a complex way, especially in aspects of care patterns, closeness, distance regulation and the communica-tion process between each couple. Thus, 50% of the patients and their partners hid negative emotions to avoid worries in the other person (this phenomenon i more frequent in Latin and South American cultures). And yet in those who did not hide these emotions, changes continued to appear in the relationship. Using a scale such as the Death and Dying Distress Scale (DADDS) in the sessions, it was shown in this work how the score depended on the knowledge and reflective capacity of one's own death. Consequently, when anxiety is very high, high-intensity emotions dominate and hinder the search for meaning in their death process. On the contrary, if anxiety is low, there is more psychological preparation for death without the need to reflect on it. It's shown that this process influences both patients and their caregivers [49, 50, 56].

d. The majority of caregivers who lose loved ones in PC Units are satisfied with the behavior of doctors in the face of death, integrating professionalism and friendliness, being these factors most commonly associated with caregivers'satisfaction health care [60].

e. The place of exitus can have an effect on the grief of caregivers, where generally the quality of death is better at home or in Hospice compared to acute care hospitals. The most frequent causes of hospital admission are pain and dyspnea because they are the ones that generate the most stress in the whole family, including the dying sick [50, 57].

f. Family grief care is a reflection of the continuity of care before and after the death of the patient. After death (usually months and more in couples), depression, insufficient social support and decreased physical activity are frequent. Fluent communication, especially before death, helps reduce depression and complicated grief, improving coping and the quality of life of the dying person's death [61, 62].

3. Conclusions

1. In the last 15 years, there has been an increase in electronic literature on PM and PC (especially scientific books and papers). Even so, there is "a lot of bibliographic noise" as in any search for information (large number of duplica-tions, documents unrelated to search criteria, etc.), that make analysis of the relationship more difficult, in this case than usual of both medical disciplines. This is mainly due to the fact that the close relationship with the PM has not been accepted internationally in PC.

2. Currently, the psychosomatic diagnosis is by exclusion, largely because Evidence-Based Medicine is based on the need to explain the existence of a palpable or visible substrate of the disease. It's probable that functional imaging tests (nuclear magnetic resonance imaging and others), will demonstrate the organic substrate of many diseases understood today as "mental".

3. Mental illness is one of the most striking complications in terminal illnesses, which could have the same or greater prognostic impact than the tumor stage, the leukocyte formula, the presence of symptoms such as delirium, dyspnea or cachexia, among others.

4. The influence of the psychosomatic world is objectified in the increase of electronic scientific resources in recent years. It's striking how from the oriental culture, mainly from Japan, the largest studies in reference to both disciplines of knowledge have come in last years, although this phenomenon is increasing more and more in all areas of research in Medicine.

5. There is an influence of the PM on the PC, reflected to a lesser extent than the real one in the scientific literature, where Palliative Care in general as a

discipline has not recognized this contribution. In the most professional in PC the PM is applied, although its deep association is unknown. Many aspects collected in the research in this chapter support the experience of palliative care professionals (the suffering of patients and relatives, the concern to protect the other from the disease and its consequences ...). More research is needed to help patients, families and healthcare professionals.

6. The PM provides insight in Psychiatry for specific disorders, but also, in its breadth, it can be useful for any discipline such as cancer or PC.

7. To reach the soul of a person (understood as the essence that defines each person against the rest), according to their nature, the health professional must know how to be a psychotherapist. Because this way you will be able to treat from the symptoms of the body, the emotions or from the thought. Although these three structures are the great summary of what a human being can explain, the reality is always more complicated, where good human relations would be a great bridge with the person who suffers to help them.

Note

This chapter is based on research awarded "In Memoriam Juan Rof Carballo" by the Royal Academy of Medicine and Surgery of Cadiz (Spain), at the titled "Psychosomatic Medicine and Palliative Care in the scientific literature", whose author was Mejias MD.

Author details

Manuel Mejías-Estévez[1,2,3]*, Rocio Dominguez Álvarez[4] and Ignacio Jauregi Lobera[5]

1 Primary Care District of Seville, Clinic Historical Round, Seville, Spain

2 University of Pablo de Olavide, Seville, Spain

3 Training and Research Department of the Sant Ángela Institute (ISA) for Chronic Disease and Palliative Care, Seville, Spain

4 Internal Medicine Unit, Virgen Macarena University Hospital, Seville, Spain

5 Department of Molecular Biology and Biochemical Engineering, University of Pablo de Olavide of Seville, Seville, Spain

*Address all correspondence to: drmjme@hotmail.com

References

[1] Mejías MJ. Practical Guide to Home Management of Pain and Other Symptoms. 2nd ed. Editorial Sanaidea; 2016. ISBN: 978-84-617-5641-4

[2] Rosin U. Palliative psychosomatic medicine. Therapeutische Umschau. 2001;**58**(7):449-452

[3] Senn HJ. Paracelsus, scientific research and supportive care—500 years after! Supportive Care in Cancer. 1993;**1**(5):230-232

[4] Weiss E, English OE. Psychosomatic medicine. In: The Clinical Application of Psychopathology to General Medical Problems, w.b. Saunders Co. 2nd ed. Philadelphia and London; 1949

[5] Sirri L, Fava GA. Diagnostic criteria for psychosomatic research and somatic symptom disorders. International Review of Psychiatry. 2013;**25**:19-30

[6] Engel GL. The need for a new medical model: A challenge for bio-medicine. Science. 1977;**196**:129-136

[7] Lipowski ZJ. Current trends in consultation-liaison psychiatry. Canaidan Journal of Psychiatry. 1983;**28**:329-338

[8] Berrocal C, Fava GA, Sonino N. Contributions of psychosomatic medicine to clinical and preventive medicine. Annals of Psychology. 2016;**32**(3):828-836

[9] Bernini O et al. The psychometric properties of the CPAQ in Italian patients with chronic pain. Journal of Health Psychology. 2010;**5**:1-10

[10] Gawande A. Quantity and quality of life: Duties of care in life-limiting illness. JAMA. 2016;**315**(3):267-269. DOI: 10.1001/jama.2015.19206

[11] González J, Stablé M. Palliative care: Therapeutic recommendations for primary care. Panamericana Editorial. 2014

[12] Esteban M et al. Care complexity in end-of-life care: Criteria and levels of intervention in community health care. Med Pal. 2015;**22**(2):69-80

[13] Gómez X et al. Instrument for the Identification of People in Situation of Advanced Chronic Disease and Need for Palliative Care in Health and Social Services. Qualy Observatory, WHO Collaborating Center for Public Palliative Care Programs (CCOMS-ICO), Institut Català d'Oncologia; 2011

[14] Pastrana T et al. A matter of definition–Key elements identified in a discourse analysis of definition of palliative care. Palliative Medicine. 2008;**22**:222-232

[15] McNamara B, Rosenwax L, Holman DC. A method for defining and estimating the palliative care population. Journal of Pain and Symptom Management. 2006;**32**(1):5-12

[16] Mayo. White Paper on Quality Standards and Palliative Care Standards of the European Society for Palliative Care. Madrid: Spanish Society for Palliative Care; 2012

[17] Iwase S et al. Assessment of cancer-related fatigue, pain, and quality of life in cancer patients at palliative care team referral: A multicenter observational study (JORTC PAL-09). 2015;**10**(8):e0134022. DOI: 10.1371/journal.pone.0134022

[18] Beller E et al. Palliative pharma-cological sedation for terminally ill adults. Cochrane Database of Systematic Reviews. 2015;**1**:Art. No.: CD010206. DOI: 10.1002/14651858.CD010206

[19] Boston P, Bruce A, Schreiber R. Existential suffering in the palliative

care setting: An integrated literature review. Journal of Pain and Symptom Management. 2016;**41**(3):604-618

[20] Balaguer A et al. An International Consensus Definition of the wish to hasten death and its related factors. PLoS One. 2016;**11**(1):e0146184. DOI: 10.1371/journal.pone.0146184

[21] Porta J, Gómez X, Tuca A, et al. Symptom Control Manual in Patients with Advanced and Terminal Cancer. 3rd ed. Generalitat de Catalunya, Departament de Salut, Institut Català d'Oncologia, Editorial Focus S.C; 2013

[22] Anneser J et al. Needs, expectations, and concerns of medical students regarding end-of-life issues before the introduction of a mandatory undergraduate palliative care curriculum. Journal of Palliative Medicine. 2014;**17**(11):1201-1205

[23] Rojas O, Fuentes C, Robert V. Psycho-oncology in the general hospital. Approaches in cancer and depression. Las Condes Clinic Medical Magazine. 2017;**28**:450-459

[24] Holland JC. Improving the human side of cancer care: Psycho-oncology's contribution. The Cancer Journal. 2001;**7**(6):458-471

[25] Originals. The significance of a specific psycho-oncology outpatient service for cancer patients run by psychosomatic medical doctors. 2011. Disponible en: BASE

[26] De Lugo M, Coca M. The pact of silence in the relatives of terminal cancer patients. Psycho-oncology. 2008;**5**(1):53-69

[27] Macarie G, Filipescu R, Voichita A. Framing the cancer patients' life experiences and attitudes: A psychosomatic approach. Postmodern Openings. 2013;**4**(1):103-116

[28] Quill T, Holland J, Arthur H, Schmale MD. 14 March 1924-17 March 1993. Psycho-Oncology. 1994;**3**(1):77-78

[29] van der Valk JM. Psychological aspects in the palliative treatment of malignant tumors. Jaar Kankeronderz Kankerbestrijd. 1964;**14**:231-237

[30] Verwoerdt A. Communication with the fatally ill. Southern Medical Journal. 1964;**57**:787-795

[31] Verwoerdt A. Communication with the fatally ill. CA: A Cancer Journal for Clinicians. 1965;**15**:105-111

[32] Verwoerdt A. The physician's role in retirement counseling. Gerontologist. 1970;**10**(1):22-26

[33] Staehelein B. Some psychiatric and psychosomatic aspects of palliative treatment of advanced cancer. Therapeutische Umschau. 1965;**22**:218-222

[34] Matsui T, Tanimukai H. The use of psychosocial support services among Japanese breast cancer survivors. Japanese Journal of Clinical Oncology. 2017, 2017;**47**(8):743-748

[35] Matsuoka H et al. The role of psychosomatic medicine doctors in palliative care medicine: Two case reports. Gan To Kagaku Ryoho. 2010;**37**(2):359-362

[36] Ogawa A et al. Availability of psychiatric consultation-liaison services as an integral component of palliative care programs at Japanese cancer hospitals. Japanese Journal of Clinical Oncology. 2012;**42**(1):42-52

[37] Mehta RD, Roth AJ. Psychiatric considerations in the oncology setting. CA: A Cancer Journal for Clinicians. 2015;**65**:299-314

[38] Zabora J et al. The prevalence of psychological distress by cancer site. Psychooncology. 2001;**10**:19-28

[39] Rayner L et al. The clinical epidemiology of depression in palliative care and the predictive value of somatic symptoms: Cross-sectional survey with four-week follow-up. Palliative Medicine. 2011;**25**(3):229-241

[40] Grassi L et al. Psychosocial screening and assessment in oncology and palliative care settings. Frontiers in Psychology. 2015;**5**

[41] Kübler-Ross E. On death and dying. Macmilan Co. 1969

[42] Fischbeck S et al. Assessing somatic, psychosocial, and spiritual distress of patients with advanced cancer: Development of the Advanced Cancer Patients' Distress Scale. American Journal of Hospice and Palliative Care. 2013;**30**(4):339-346

[43] Wada S et al. The Association between depressive symptoms and age in cancer patients: A multicenter cross-sectional study. Journal of Pain and Symptom Management. 2015;**50**(6):768-777

[44] Fujisawa D et al. Impact of depression on health utility value in cancer patients. Psychooncology. 2016;**25**(5):491-495

[45] Matsuo N et al. Predictors of responses to corticosteroids for anorexia in advanced cancer patients: A multicenter prospective observational study. Supportive Care in Cancer. 2017;**25**(1):41-50

[46] Virizuela JA, Escobar Y, Casinello J, Borrega P. Treatment of cancer pain: Spanish Society of Medical Oncology (SEOM) recommendations for clinical practice. Clinical and Translational Oncology. 2012;**14**(7):499-504

[47] Eccleston C et al. Psychological therapies (through the internet) for the treatment of chronic pain in adults. Cochrane Database of Systematic Reviews. 2014;**2**:Art. No.: CD010152. DOI: 10.1002/14651858.CD010152

[48] Fisher E et al. Psychological (remote) therapies for the treatment of chronic and recurrent pain in children and adolescents. Cochrane Database of Systematic Reviews. 2015;**3**:Art. No.: CD011118. DOI: 10.1002/14651858. CD011118

[49] Drabe N et al. When cancer cannot be cured: A qualitative study on relationship changes in couples facing advanced melanoma. Palliative & Supportive Care. 2016:1-12

[50] Hatano Y et al. The relationship between cancer patients' place of death and bereaved caregivers' mental health status. Psycho-Oncology. 2017

[51] Iglesias A. Hypnosis and existential psychotherapy with end-stage terminally ill patients. American Journal of Clinical Hypnosis. 2004;**46**(3):201-213

[52] Ayers T. A partnership in like-minded thinking-generating hopefulness in persons with cancer. Med Health Care Philos. 2007;**10**(1):65-80

[53] Satsangi A, Brugnoli M. Anxiety and psychosomatic symptoms in palliative care: From neuro-psychobiological response to stress, to symptoms' management with clinical hypnosis and meditative states. Annals of Palliative Medicine. 2017

[54] Orellana-Ríos CL et al. Mindfulness and compassion-oriented practices at work reduce distress and enhance self-care of palliative care teams: A mixed-method evaluation of an "on the job" program. BMC Palliative Care. 2017;**17**(1):3

[55] Wasner M, Paal P, Borasio GD. Psychosocial care for the caregivers of primary malignant brain tumor patients. Journal of Social Work in End-of-Life & Palliative Care. 2013;**9**(1):74-95

[56] Tong E et al. The meaning of self-reported death anxiety in advanced cancer. Palliative Medicine. 2016;**30**(8):772-779

[57] Okamoto Y et al. Do symptoms among home palliative care patients with advanced cancer decide the place of death? Focusing on the presence or absence of symptoms during home care. Journal of Palliative Medicine. 2016;**19**(5):488-495

[58] Samsel C et al. Integrated behavioral health care in pediatric subspecialty clinics. Child and Adolescent Psychiatric Clinics of North America. 2017;**26**(Pediatric Integrated Care):785-794

[59] Naoki Y et al. Association between family satisfaction and caregiver burden in cancer patients receiving outreach palliative care at home. Palliative & Supportive Care. 2017:1-9

[60] Hatano Y et al. Physician behavior toward death pronouncement in palliative care units. Journal of Palliative Medicine. 2017

[61] Götze H et al. Anxiety, depression and quality of life in family caregivers of palliative cancer patients during home care and after the patient's death. European Journal of Cancer Care (England). 2016

[62] Yamaguchi T et al. Effects of end-of-life discussions on the mental health of bereaved family members and quality of patient death and care. Journal of Pain and Symptom Management. 2017;**54**(1):17-26

[63] Martínez BB, Custodio RP. Relationship between mental health and spiritual wellbeing among hemodialysis patients: A correlation study. São Paulo Medical Journal. 2014;**132**(1):23-27

2

The Network Paradigm: New Niches for Psychosomatic Medicine

Imre Lázár

Abstract

Psychosomatic medicine, as a philosophical frame and practical approach of the diagnostic and therapeutical agency, had been undergone several renewals and reframing in the past. We overview the history of psychosomatics and map its branches. Psychoanalytic and psychodynamic frameworks, the Engelian biopsychosocial concept, the paradigm of behavioral medicine, the clinical psychophysiological research background, the clinical fields of PNI, psychocardiology, biobehavioral oncology, the so-called mind-body medicine, and stress medicine frameworks reflect a converging pluralism. Psychoneuroimmunology offers a comprehensive framework to analyze key issues of psychosomatics in a social neuroscience framework and to demonstrate the significance of the network approach in bridging the gap between psychosomatics and biomedicine. Network medicine creates a shared denominator for analyzing socioeconomic, interpersonal, life event-based narra-tive factors together with psychophysiological features of the clinical and health psychological problems and promotes convergence of psychosomatics, biomedicine, and lifestyle medicine, too. On the other side, psychosomatic medicine as a particular professional medical specialization is not universal at all. In Europe, one can find such specialization only in Germany, while psychotherapy applied by somatic experts is practiced in wider circles. Finally, we explore the new niches for psychosomatic orientation offered by integrative frameworks like lifestyle medicine and network medicine.

Keywords: names and frames of psychosomatics, psychoneuroimmunology, network medicine, institutionalization

1. The network paradigm: new niches for psychosomatic medicine

> *Man is not an indifferent hanger for carrying the disease. Man is the larger part of the disease. Temperament affects even skull fractures. It affects the coloration of acute diseases and especially certain chronic and maybe non-exogenous disease types, which cannot be properly understood or judged unless we follow the internal and typically more significant threads of their etiology into the unique tangle of individual characteristics* (László Németh [1]).

1.1 Roots and branches, names and frames of psychosomatics: a historical analysis

Psychosomatic medicine, as a philosophical frame and practical approach of the diagnostic and therapeutical agency, had been undergone several renewals and reframing in the past. If we try to explore the archeology of psychosomatics, we can trace its orientation back to Galenus, Hippocrates, or the Chinese *The Yellow Emperor's Classic of Medicine*.

Galenus wrote about the connection between melancholy and mammary carcinoma following theories by Hippocrates, attributing the cause of breast cancer to an "excess of black bile," implying more than a disbalance of humor, and pointing to the habitus, the emotional and behavioral character. Emotional disorders and mental illnesses also had been considered to constitute a significant part of diseases in Chinese medicine, where such illnesses were classified as Qing Zhi disorders. The so-called emotion-wills implied the Qi Qing:-seven emotion, namely happi-ness, anger, anxiety, pensiveness, sorrow, fear, and fright and the Wu Zhi five wills: happiness, anger, thinking, sorrow, and fear. According to the ancient Chinese approach, they play a primary role in the onset, progress, and prognosis of most of the diseases.

As emotions are deep *human ecological representations* of the environment depending on perceptions, evaluation, and interpretation of the outer and internal environment, we can realize that psychosomatics is also a human ecological approach immersed into external and internal networks of social, psychological, neuroendocrine-immune and molecular layers.

The emotional response to environmental challenges depends on personality (A, C, D type) as a result of personal history (early mother–child attachment, adverse childhood experiences); personal development; Pavlov's, Skinner's, and Bandura's learning processes and system-like social influences (family relationships in frame of Milano School, worksite mental health issues); competition and frustration; domination and submission; social rank; and self-evaluation (shame, feeling guilty).

In an overview of the history of psychosomatic concepts regarding human suffering, we find changing frames for the connection between mind and body in a multilayered human ecological setting. The psychoanalytic and psychodynamic frameworks, the hypnotic phenomena, stress medicine based on Cannon's fight-or-flight reaction, Selye's stress, Lipowski's consultation-liaison medicine, the Engelian biopsychosocial concept, and the paradigm of behavioral medicine have network features in common.

In the background, the clinical psychophysiological research emerges with the clinical fields of psychoneuroimmunology, psychocardiology, and biobehavioral oncology. This way, the so-called mind-body medicine and stress medicine frameworks reflect a converging pluralism. The frames are diverse, and the foci are common. Information flow through the social, cognitive-emotional, psychological, neural, endocrine, and immune interfaces and the molecular transcriptomic interfaces and *backward*. These paths and regulative networks have shared evolutionary origins. These are the structural-functional, patterned heritage of ours, organizing biopsychosocial adaptation and the structural wisdom of the human body. Their adaptive/maladaptive potential depends on the changing environmental context.

Drawing a Venn diagram of different historical or competing schools of psychosomatic medical philosophy, we find many overlapping themes, which might also be considered as hubs of multilayered network organization of psychosomatic phenomena, working as a network of networks (**Figure 1**). The letters sign some of the evolutionary steps of psychosomatics without a claim for the whole picture (**Table 1**).

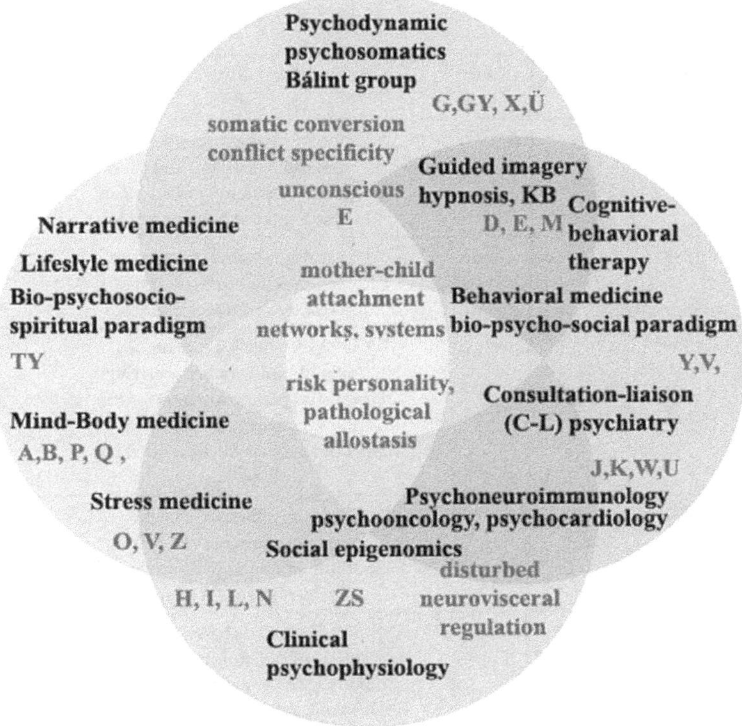

Figure 1.
Venn diagram of different psychosomatic discourses.

Contemporary psychosomatic medicine broke away from the psychoanalytic foundations, and its research directions reflected a turn toward networking with other disciplines, as an interdisciplinary approach named behavioral medicine. The behavioral medicine and the concept of consultation-liaison psychosomatics bound to Lipowski [2] brought psychosomatics closer to mainstream biomedicine, enhancing their collaboration. The Engelian turn of the biopsychosocial paradigm explicitly expressed the importance of information flow through the network of networks that built up dynamically connected social, psychological, somatic, and molecular-genetic layers.

In 1977, the Yale Conference on Behavioral Medicine had a strong impact to the history of psychosomatic medicine. The participants, like Joseph Matarazzo, Redford Williams, David Shapiro, and Gary Schwartz, defined a new framework for the former psychosomatic medicine, as the study and treatment of diseases, disorders, or abnormal states in which psychological processes and reactions are believed to play a prominent role. There were several opinions regarding the identification of psychosomatics with behavioral medicine. Some considered it identical; others expressed the opinion that behavioral medicine was only a fraction of psychosomatics, while others viewed behavioral medicine imply-ing psychosomatic medicine and additional areas of medical and psychological concern. The wider definition of behavioral medicine extended the former borders of psychosomatics, proposing *behavioral medicine as* "the field concerned with the development of behavioral-science knowledge and techniques relevant to the understanding of physical health and illness and the application of this knowledge and these techniques to prevention, diagnosis, treatment, and reha-bilitation. Psychosis, neurosis, and substance use are included only insofar as they contribute to physical disorders as an endpoint" [3]. Further extension of former

A	1818	Heinroth	The name "psychosomatics"	Mind-body network
B	1843	Le Cabanis	Relationship between body and spirit	Mind-body network
C	1880	Fabre	A nervous system disorder can cause organ damage, and the abnormal functioning of an organ always affects the nervous system	Neurovisceral network
D	1886	Bernheim	Physical symptoms of hypnotic suggestions are results of ideosensory and motoric reflexes	Neurovisceral network
E	1889	Janet	The block, the dissociation, and reversible amnesia between the conscious and unconscious results in several psychopathological phenomena that can be treated by hypnosis	Neurovisceral network
F	1892	Male	Pathology of emotions, the organ symptoms that result from emotions, is similar to those caused by physical factors	Neurovisceral network
G	1896	Freud	Psychoanalysis based on the theory of dynamic psychiatry, libido theory, conversion neurosis, hysteria, symbolic organ speech	Mind-body network
Gy	1905	Ferenczi	Short dynamic psychotherapy	Mind-body network
H	1905	Pavlov	Paradigm of conditioned reflexes providing a framework for neurobiological learning theory	Neurovisceral network
I	1909	Eppinger and Hess	Description of sympathicotony and vagotony	Neurovisceral network
J	1928	Heileg and Hoff	Relationship between environmental pressure and infection incidence	Neuroimmune network
K	1926–1935	Metalnikov and Chorin 1926 Speransky 1935	The conditioned neutral stimulus might provoke inflammation "immune conditioning"	Neuroimmune network
L	1932	Cannon	The alarm reaction Fight-or-flight versus tend or mend	Neurovisceral network
M	1932	Erickson M.H.	Traumatic amnesia and psychosomatic symptoms are psychoneuro-physiological dissociations that can be resolved by "internal resynthesis" using hypnotherapy	Neurovisceral network
N	1935	Breur	Relationships between tuberculosis relapses and life events	Neuroimmune network
O	1936	Selye	Designates the information pathways of HPA axis as mechanism of stress-related psychosomatic problems	Neuroimmune network Neuroendocrine network

P	1936	Bergmann	Pathology of functional internal medicine	Neurovisceral network
Q	1937	Hetényi	Autonomous nervous system-based diseases of internal medicine	Neurovisceral network
R	1937	Papez	Mental experience is transformed into the psychophysiological pattern of emotions by the limbic-hypothalamic system	Neurovisceral network
S	1940	Scharrer	The central nervous system controls the hormone production of the endocrine system through the hypothalamus	Neuroendocrine network
T	1942	Bykow	Corticovisceral pathology	Neurovisceral network
TY	1943	Dunbar	Relationship between personality and psychosomatic disease	Mind-body network
X	1950	Alexander	Psychosomatic medicine	Neuroimmune network
Y	1955	Charva	The system model of neurohumoral integration	Neurovisceral network Neuroendocrine network
U	1955	LeShan	Specific pattern of cancer risk based on a biographical history and personality survey of cancer patients	Neuroimmune network
Ü	1957	Bálint	Doctor-patient relationship and communication as a factor in healing. Bálint groups	Mind-body network
V	1972	Weiner	Psychosomatic problems as disorders of information transmission between the limbic-hypothalamic–pituitary system	Neuroendocrine network
W	1974	Ader	Psychoneuroimmunology	Neuroimmune network
Sz	1977 1978	Matarazzo Schwartz/Weiss	Behavioral medicine	Mind-body network
Z	1984	Caccioppo	Development of social neuroscience	Mind-body network
ZS	1995	Meaney	Social epigenomics	Mind-body network

Table 1.
Network features of psychosomatic models [4, 5].

psychosomatics included social and institutional spheres and deep biological system and network insights as well.

The disciplines contributing to the study of behavioral phenomena include psychology, sociology, anthropology, education, epidemiology, biostatistics, and psychiatry. These disciplines must be coupled with the biological and medical sciences relevant to understanding the disease processes under study. The networking posi-tion of behavioral medicine is apparent from epistemological perspective, too. The following matrix clarifies the deep connection with network medicine (**Figure 2**).

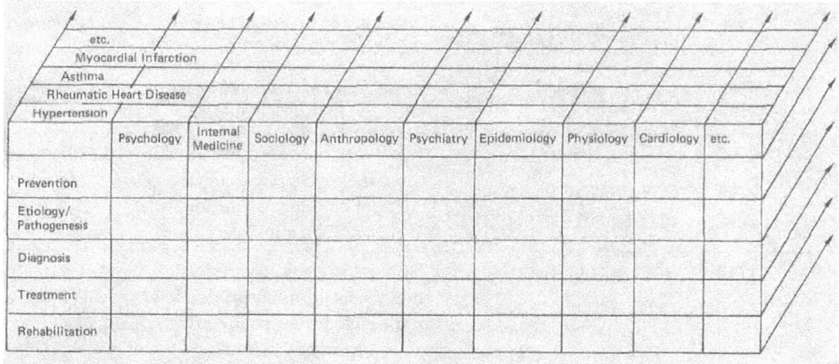

Figure 2.
Matrix of problems with which behavioral medicine is concerned [3].

In this matrix, a disease is indexed at the sociological, epidemiological, anthropological, psychological, biomedical, and physiological levels of networks, and this is a multidimensional analysis with reference to different times (risks, pathophysiology, prognosis, treatment, and rehabilitation) and agency.

While behavioral medicine extended the core psychosomatic view to the broadest hermeneutical frame, the consultation-liaison psychosomatic medicine was connected to the mainstream psychiatry, with the following scope of interest:

1. The role of *psychosocial variables* in the development of illness (etiology)

2. The examination of the *causative connections between the changes of psychosocial variables and physiological parameters* (psycho-endocrinology, psychoimmunol-ogy, psychocardiology)

3. The fundamental *psychological changes accompanying illness* (illness behavior)

4. The *psychological and mental concomitants* of specific somatic processes

5. The effect of *therapeutic methods affecting behavior on somatic conditions* and somatic variables

Research into neuroimmunomodulation in immune laboratories had an explosion in the 1970s, in addition to research into the physiology of stress, creating the basis for a new "network" field of psychosomatics, the psychoneuroimmunology.

1.2 Psychoneuroimmunology: a "network discipline"

The rise of psychoneuroimmunology is a typic example of behavioral and medical interpretation of human disease. Its core explanatory model is based on insights of neuroimmune modulation, the bidirectional communication between neuroendocrine and immune system enabled by shared receptors and cross talk of messengers, and their integrated neuroendocrine-immune information pathways consisting of neurotransmitters, interleukins, neuropeptides, and hormone, including even myokines and adipokines [6]. These evolutionary patterned communication networks create a *network of networks* throughout the whole body, including the brain and all the organs. In the social-psychological, cognitive-evaluative, emotional, neurovisceral associations, connections, and circles, regulative positive and negative feedback loops create unity of rational, emotive, visceral, molecular, receptoral, and transcriptomic-genetic levels. The prehistory of psychoimmunology is mostly shared with psychosomatics, and its hermeneutic and heuristic features are close to what network medicine offers [6].

As early as at the end of the nineteenth century, we see data about the effect of damaging the nervous system on the loss of protection against anthrax. At the beginning of the twentieth century, Salomondsen and Mandsen already connected vagotomy and the atopic and anaphylactic reactions, and Hatiegan first described the effect of adrenaline on increasing the amount of lymphocytes in 1925, which was confirmed by Frey and Tonietty in 1927.

In Metalnikov and Chorine's 1926 work, they already discussed the condition-ability of immune phenomena. The general immunological influence of emotions was described by Erich Wittkower, when he detected an increase in the number of white blood cells in the states of anxiety, anger, grief, and heightened mood. He coined the term "Affektleukocytose" to describe this phenomenon, which he explained with the stimulation of the sympathetic nervous system. A group of physiologists from Cluj-Napoca, Csaba Hadnagy and the Romanian Baciu, also joined this trend when they examined the effects of emotions and the autono-mous nervous system on the number of white blood cells at the beginning of the 1940s.

Locke had already prepared a bibliography of more than 1500 articles in 1983 under the title *Behavioral Immunology*. If we take into account the names given to the scientific field discussed in these articles, the first "christening" took place in 1974 and is connected to Robert Ader, who used the term psychoimmunology and in 1981 extended it as psychoneuroimmunology. The term of *neuroimmunomodula-tion* is connected to Herbert Spector, while Berczi and Szentiványi used the term *neuroimmune biology*. They all include the overlap of different networks thought to be autonomous.

Even in the comprehensive work of Franz Alexander, psychosomatic medicine includes also internal diseases which, some decades later, turned to be under-stood in psychoneuroimmune contexts, like IBD, bronchial asthma, rheumatoid arthritis, peptic ulcer, Graves disease, neurodermatitis, and, as recent data show, hypertension which is not an exception at all. Although Alexander did not realize the neuroimmune information pathways and the networked features behind these diseases, his "psychosomatic" internal medicine was strongly attached to psychoso-cial relationships and conflicts including clinical phenomena generated by neuro-immunobiological networks.

1.3 Hungarians' contributions to psychoneuroimmunology

Reviewing contributions to the prehistory of psychoimmunology, we can find the researchers' sensitivity toward the neuro-immunobiological network response to environmental challenges, as a shared feature in oeuvre of Hungarian scien-tists, like Selye, Berczi and Nagy, Bertók, Bohus, or Jancsó Jr. Selye presented the first neuroendocrine-immunological insight to human adaptation in 1936 when he proved the somatic triad of general adaptation syndrome, including peptic ulcer, adrenal hypertrophy (endocrine), and thymic and lymphoid atrophy. Selye confirmed the effect of the adrenocortical extract on inducing thymic atrophy in rats in 1943, and he called attention to the role of corticosteroids in regulating the inflammatory response in 1949. This research resulted in the development of the medication that is so important for autoimmune or allergic patients. However, Selye's Hungarian students also achieved important results in the field of endocrine immunology. István Berczi became a colleague of Selye in the 1960s, and he was exploring the immunological effects of hypophysis hormones together with Éva Nagy. They were among the first to confirm that not only cortisol but other stress hormones, such as the growth hormone or prolactin, also participate in the regula-tion of the hemo-lymphopoietic system and the immune functions. Lóránd Bertók, a guest researcher of Selye in the 1960s, can also be considered one of the pioneers of natural immunity research. He examined the protective role of bile acids against bacterial lipopolysaccharides. The toxic effect of the lipopolysaccharide endo-toxins released by bacteria is an essential promoter of inflammation since their membrane-disrupting, capillary-penetrating, shock-inducing, and fever-inducing effects provide dramatic components of the illness. During endotoxic shock, the levels of ACTH, corticoids, and beta-endorphin increase; however, the levels of prolactin, TSH, T3, and T4 are reduced. These effects are mediated by immune mediators such as IL-1, IL-6, and TNF, which are secreted by the macrophages acti-vated by endotoxins and monocytes. Lóránd Bertók's research also confirmed that the radiotherapeutic treatment of the endotoxins reduces their toxic effect and this harmless product, the so-called Tolerin, can increase the natural immune reaction and mobilize stem cells.

Hungarian researchers played a pioneering role in the discovery of another system of connections, the "neuroimmune network." Besides István Berczi, Andor Szentiványi also played a role in discovering the nature of the connections between neuroendocrine-immune networks when he prevented the anaphylactic response by lesions created in the tubular area of the hypothalamus. The work of Miklós Jancsó Jr. was also important. He investigated the effect of histamine on the endothelial vascular cells and the reticuloendothelial system as early as in the 1940s and identified histamine as the physiological activator of the reticuloendothelial system. However, he also identified another neuroimmune network, which played a large role in the understanding of the neuroimmune processes taking place on the internal and external surface of the body. Through research sensory neurons in the 1950s, Miklós Jancsó Jr. concluded for the first time that *a neuroimmune network must exist*, in which the sensory fibers play an important role. The antidromic electric excitation of the sensory nerves triggered an inflammatory response, which the researcher was able to prevent with capsaicin treatment and the selective destruction of C fibers. On the internal surfaces of the gut or joints, sensory fibers and the increase of substance P play an essential role in inflammatory processes. The discovery of Miklós Jancsó Jr. still provides a *paradigmatic network interpretation* framework for psycho-immune research today. This network might play a role in trigger point and referred pain theory of Janet Travell and other reflextherapy theories, too.

Béla Bohus and his colleagues also brought a new slice of reality into the range of interpretation of PNI, examining the correlations between social interactions, dominance, subordination, behavioral traits, and physiological indicators. Social hierarchy is a network structure at ethological/social levels, which is transferred to neuroendocrine-immune networks through cognitive behavioral networks.

We should mention further Hungarian think tanks as well, such as the works of Elemér Endrőczy Csaba Nyakas and Lajos Korányi, or the research group led by Szilveszter Vizy, among which Ilia Elenkov's or Judit Szelényi can be mentioned as outstanding representatives of the field. In the field of applied psychoimmunology, we have to mention the pioneering role of György Németh and András Guseo.

The turning points and parallel evolutionary pathways of psychosomatics and psychoneuroimmunology, listed in **Table 1**, share covert network logic.

2. The neuroimmune networks

Networks are stand-alone factors in themselves, displayed by graphs depicting symmetrical or asymmetrical relations between cells, molecules, organs, and social relationships and life events. The network-type depiction is also warranted by the need to present regulatory cycles in block schematics, system theory modeling, and the communication and information paths and logical relationships. The neuroimmune networks are graphs, and the task is to identify the nodes (sometimes hubs) connecting them and the system of relations between them. However, under the socio-psychoimmunological approach, the limits of the graph's validity exceed the levels of the systems of molecules, organs, and organ systems and bypass the individual and personal as well. Under this approach, partnerships, social support, control, power, the territorial principle, dominance and submission, and social ranking are all presented in a set of relationships that can be outlined by graphs, edges, and hubs. However, connections over time are also aligned to the psychoimmunological interpretation of diseases as a graph and network, in the narrative framework of psychosomatics. Therefore, the particular "metagraph network" of socio-psychoimmunology lies across several layers of graphs.

The anamnesis and history disclosed by the patient, the writing or conversation therapy for exploring and disclosing traumas, the research for early traumas, and the investigation of infection chains, learning about the dramatic dynam-ics underlying socio-somatic relations, are all possible using the toolset of this expanded, narrative network analysis.

This is the anatomy of experience embodied in text, the crystallography of the petrified personal suffering. Identifying the persons and events included in the fate-text and exploring the system of their relations pose the same kind of challenge for network theory as the exploring the "small-world" networks of relevant mediators, and comparison of the neural, endocrine, and immune networks, and locating the hubs that connect them and drawing the graph lines of the relationships in them.

The identification of key players, dominant communities, groups, and the system of relationships between them, based on the personal narrative, and the understanding of tensions of social rank are an inevitable part of "decoding" the socio-psycho-immune network. This is how actual *dramatic hubs* connect patterns of vulnerable personality reactions, traumatic life events, social rank, and dominance relations and neuroimmune stress networks. As it is the person who explores and reveals it in the therapeutic process, psychoimmunotherapy includes a rearrangement of the representations of the external set of relations
and the set of relations hidden by time generated in mind. This means a network analysis of social behavioral cognitive and clinical psychophysiological networks of relevance. This might offer revelatory rearrangements between the related set of life events, personality, and psychological network pattern and the narrative representation network, which may reach even the neuroimmune networks in the deep. This is why the social networks and their narrative reflection in life history should be analyzed together with biological networks of the socio-psychoimmu-nological network model.

Situation assessment, psychophysiological, and neuroendocrine networks make up such extended networks, and so do the neuroendocrine and neuropeptide patterns, cytokine networks, extracellular messengers, and intracellular molecular paths, genetic programs, and transcription processes. Overrepresented hubs and edges that determine the dynamics and types of physiological and pathological events, as well as possible therapies, are also outlined here.

2.1 Network features of Solomon postulates

George Freeman Solomon was one of those pioneers who established the scientific paradigm of psychoimmunology in the 1960s and 1970s, pointing to the connections between brain, behavior, and immunity. He gathered the psychoimmu-nological revelations in a corpus of postulates [7]. We can test these postulates from the network perspective.

Graph of neuroendocrine-immune networks might be seen as real *small-world networks* in which most nodes are not neighbors of one another, but the neighbors of any given node are likely to be neighbors of each other, and most nodes can be reached from every other node by a small number of hops or steps.

2.1.1 Neuroendocrine-immune chain

IL-1, paraventricular NA secretion- CRH-ACTH-adrenocortical cortisol/(sickness behavior, neuroendocrine-immune feedback, inflammation theory of depression based on depletion of dopamine, or diminishing serotonin secretion)

Immunological abnormalities may be accompanied by psychological or mental disorders.

Activation of the immune system can lead to changes in the activity of the central nervous system.

Immune signaling can also affect the central nervous system.

Cytokines of the immune system, as part of the neuroimmune endocrine axis, play a role in endocrine regulation, including stress-induced endocrine processes.

Cytokines influence psychological processes and cause psychiatric symptoms.
Immunity influences behavior, and behavior can aid in immune regulatory functions.

2.1.2 Psychoneuro-endocrine-immune chain

Psychological states/traits-neural networks-stress hormones-immune system (C-type personality, right frontal hemispherical dominance, chronic stress, depres-sion, shame, submissive status)

Adaptive coping styles and enduring characteristics can improve the prognosis of immune diseases and protect susceptible patients from the disease.

Stress coping and traits, including personality traits that influence stress management, may influence the immune response to exogenous antigenic stimuli.

Emotional changes and distress (state characteristics) can influence the onset, severity, and course of disorders controlled by immune processes or resulting from disturbed immune processes (allergies, autoimmune, diseases, AIDS).

Severe emotional and mental disorders can cause immunological disorders. Immune functions may also be affected by altered states of consciousness. Experimental behavioral effects may lead to immunological changes. Damage to and stimulation of some regions of the central nervous system may lead to immunological changes.

Substances produced and regulated by the central nervous system (neurotransmitters, neuropeptides, other neuroendocrine factors) must influence immune processes.

2.1.3 Social-psychoneuroimmune network chains (social rank, social evaluative theory, shame, bereavement, social losses, social exclusion, voodoo, cultural nocebos)

In extensive prospective studies, specific patterns of psychological risk should be associated with a higher incidence of immune disease.

Genetic, gender, and behavioral factors influence the immunological effects of stress.

In addition to the influence on the adult psyche, early injury and the traumatic mother-child relationship can affect the adult immune system.

Therapeutic influencing behavior (psychotherapy, relaxation, biofeedback, and hypnosis) may also affect immune function.

Positive emotions stimulate immune function.

2.2. Bridges in the network

Immunocompetent cells have receptors for receiving neuropeptides, neurotrans-mitters, and endocrine signals.

Central nervous and hormonal factors may play a role in the regulation of feedback processes in the immune system.

Lymphocyte receptors are also affected by changes in transducer sensitivities that are characteristic of mental disorders and cells of the central nervous system.

2.3 Hubs in the network

Thymic hormones that regulate immune function may be under central nervous system influence.

CRH plays a role in the processes and symptoms of depression and immunosuppression associated with depression.

Certain cell groups of the nervous and immune systems occur together.

The prenatal hormonal environment has an effect on CNS and the development of the immune system, which can have lasting effects on both behavioral and immune functions.

Sleep affects both CNS and immune processes.

Immunological processes and specific personality characteristics (coping style, "hardiness") may play a role in longevity.

Enzymes for the synthesis of brain neurotransmitters are found in immunocom-petent cells and neurons.

Melatonin, a neuronal hormone involved in the regulation of circadian rhythmicity and affected by stress, affects immune function.

Mitogens, potent, non-specific immunostimulants, also act on the nervous system.

Immune cells influence the development and function of the surrounding nervous system.

Lymphokines may affect pituitary hormones directly and via the central nervous system.

Some cells of the central nervous system are capable of lymphokine production.

Cytokines of the immune system, as part of the neuroimmune endocrine axis, play a role in endocrine regulation, including stress-induced endocrine processes.

These psychoimmunological facts support the profound relevance of social and psychological network changes exerting deep visceral influence through psychophysiological networks. It also supports the connection between psychosomatics and broad areas of internal medicine.

The network-based interpretation of crucial issues of psychosomatics mapped in **Table 1** follows the above principles. Social networks and neuro-immunobiological networks are linked with psycho developmental hubs. Common, hub-like narrative foci are the early mother–child relationships and the adverse childhood experiences, just like the syndrome of post-traumatic stress. Distorted early mother-child attachment organizations have an impact on the so-called internal working model and other personality features creating enhanced risks for some somatic diseases. A-type anxious avoidant secondary attachment organization might diminish empathy and hypothetically create a tendency toward A-type personality development, strive for dominance, competition, and hostility and tendencies for cardiovascular vulner-ability. In contrast, C-type secondary anxious/ambivalent attachment organization creates lower self-esteem, behavioral inhibition of aggression, and expression of emotions, high anxiety, and psychophysiological arousal [8, 9].

Epigenetic consequences of distorted mother-child attachment, like down-regulation of hippocampal GR receptors via histone methylation, distorted HPA feedback, and distorted estrogen regulation with consequences on adult maternal behavior also prove the hub-like role of the mother-child relationship between socio-psychological and developmental personality networks, stress physiological networks, and neuroimmune network.

Relations between transactional events, traumas, feelings of submission, and loss of control, just as chronic psychosocial stressors, that carry psychological meaning are explored in the networks of the socio-psychological layer. Alexithymia or social inhibition and the psychological network patterns of the C-type personal-ity convert all this into increased HPA activity, high arousal, and increased LC/NAerg activity, so that all this is eventually embodied in the disruptions of the immune cell network controlled by cytokines. Then, IL-1 and IL-6 as result of modified protein synthesis in the cell reach the central nervous system, and via modified dopaminerg and serotoninerg molecular network changes is transcribed into psychological network patterns and depression. The disturbances of the rank position experienced in social networks (reduced motivation, lack of adequacy in the workplace, family conflicts, loss of socioeconomic status) are also embodied this way (via neural networks and proinflammatory cytokines).

3. The psychoimmunology of social stress in the network context

Human social relationships might be occasionally the source of severe conflicts. In the light of social exchange theory, it is apparent that the individual is often exposed to severe distress in the high-cost medium of the temporal, monetary, and emotional strain of social interactions. Plenty of evidence is available for presenting the social-psychoimmune consequences of distorted human relationships.

The negative or ambivalent social relationships and the resulting conflicts and associated negative emotions can influence immune processes. Hostility, which we primarily know as a cardiovascular risk factor of psychosomatics, promotes inflam-matory processes as well, which is indicated by elevation of CRP and IL-6, accord-ing to the work of Suarez [10], and the increased level of the pro-inflammatory cytokines typical of depression as well.

Depression highlights a distinct area of research within social-psychoimmu-nology, taking the correlations between depression and social integration into account, as well as the relationship conflicts and its negative effect on social perception. Depression is proven to be a mediating factor between socioeconomic patterns (personal income) and physical consequences (number of sick days) in behavioral and epidemiological research called Hungarostudy, verified by route analysis [11]. Depression is proven to be also an independent risk factor of myocar-dial infarction [12].

The attitudes and emotions increasing the stress of social interaction and interpersonal emotional relationships, such as anger or the hardships caused by depression, are also reflected in the differences in the immune response. Social conflict influences the course of rheumatoid arthritis, in which case catecholamine plays an important role among the neurohormonal factors mediating psychosocial distress. In the social network of ambivalent individuals (those who exert positive and negative influence as well), the ambivalent persons cause increased adrenergic reactions based on the work of Uchino et al. [13], and the contact and conflict with ambivalent persons can provoke an increase in systolic blood pressure. Long-term tight ambivalent human relationships, rich in conflicts, are common in bad marriages, where worse health indicators are also often observed according to the findings of Kiecolt-Glaser and Newton [14]. The dissatisfaction indicator of marriage is accompanied by worse immune indicators, as seen in the case of the ratio of anti-EBV antibodies, CD4+, or CD8+ cells. The hostile behavior typical of bad marriage, impulsivity resulting in cutting each other off when speaking, as well as critical and judgmental impatience, can be indicators of physiological differences and increased blood pressure and endocrine values, based on the work of Malarkey et al. [15]. Among newlywed couples, those who are more prone to adverse, hostile reactions, and this is recalled during a short, 30-min discussion, suppressed immune function was shown in samples taken 24 h later. Kiecolt-Glaser et al. [16] stated that the discrepancy indicating dysfunction of the endocrine-immune regulation was true to older couples as well during discussions where they had to recall their conflicts. The amount of negativistic behavior was in direct correlation with the weakening of the immune response. Mayne et al. [17] confirmed that as much as 45 minutes of exploratory discussion of conflict was enough to reduce lymphocyte proliferation in the examined women. During prospective research, Levenstein et al. [18] found a connection between ulcerative inflammation of the oral cavity and marital stress, while Kiecolt-Glaser et al. observed significantly approximately 60% longer wound healing in the case of couples exhibiting hostile behavior.

Trait-like hostility, characterized by aggression, anger, and cynicism, causes an even more evident immune regulatory disorder in the event of family conflicts, according to Mayne et al. [17]. Miller et al. [19] found a distinct correlation between hostile and cynical attitudes and behavior during conflict manage-ment and the cardiovascular response, cortisol, and immune discrepancies. Social stressors induce a rise of pro-inflammatory mediators as well and cause systematic inflammation in the body, based on the work of Steptoe et al. [20]. Partnership conflicts, rejection, and exclusion have significant pro-inflammatory effects even compared to depression and various life events, according to the findings of Denson et al. [21].

4. Evolved network patterns in psychoimmunological risk situations

The neuroendocrine effects triggered in the brain by threatening environmental stimuli can create a preparatory pathogen-host defense effect on the native immune system, as a result of which the redistribution of the cells of the native immune system and their migration toward the exposed area are detected. All of this ensures the increased rate of healing after an injury. This response can be mobilized by both the presence of predators and the emergence of a significant conflict situation. In the opinion of Slavich and Cole [22], the mobilization of innate immunity is not only an evolutionary remnant but something that can be triggered by symbolic threats, social conflict, rejection, isolation, and exclusion as well. If we consider the genetic basis of the neuroendocrine and immune systems of mammals when investigating their immune system, we can identify a typical pro-inflammatory/anti-inflammatory response pattern by examining the transcriptome of the leukocytes circulated in the body that is the set of RNA typical of the cell.

Under normal circumstances, the activity of the sympathetic nervous system increases the conserved transcriptional response to adversity (CTRA) with the help of the adrenergic receptors, and the activity of the HPA axis reduces the CTRA-dependent inflammatory response as a result of the released cortisol.

However, in the case of chronic social isolation, the threat of grief, and post-traumatic stress, reduced activity of the anti-inflammatory glucocorticoid receptor (GR) can be detected. Therefore, the so-called conserved transcriptional response to adversity is triggered by threatening, stressful, or permanently uncertain adversity as well, as indicated in Antoni's report [23].

As mentioned above, the threat of grief, traumatic stress, social isolation, low socioeconomic status, or a cancer diagnosis all result in pro-inflammatory transcription disorders. In experimental animal models, social instability, low social rank, and repeated defeat also resulted in a CTRA. Such challenges increase the activity of the genes responsible for the inflammatory immune response to extracel-lular pathogens and bacterial infections and inhibit the genes responsible for the antiviral immune response to intracellular pathogens. The selective evolutionary advantage of all this is indicated by the fact that it increases the rate of CTRA, wound healing, and response to infection in the event of an actual physical threat. However, it is apparent from the observations that the CTRA is activated by several symbolic, social, anticipated, or imagined emergencies experienced in everyday life. In the event of prolonged perceived or real danger, social or physical threat, a glucocorticoid resistance might develop, which may lead to more severe inflamma-tion or depression.

These phenomena had evolved as a result of the coevolution of hierarchic layers of social, cognitive, neural, immune, and transcriptomic, genetic layers of this hierarchical construction of different networks linked to each other. The highly conserved biological response to adversity, described above, is crucial to overcome the physical threats or injury. Modern-day social, symbolic, or perceived, even imagined, threats might also lead to a pro-inflammatory phenotype of (mal) adaptive answer. The elevation of pro-inflammatory cytokines, such as IL-1 and IL-6, may contribute to elicit depressive symptoms. The overlap of depression with several physical conditions, including asthma, rheumatoid arthritis, chronic pain, metabolic syndrome, cardiovascular disease, obesity, and neurodegeneration, shows the psychosomatic significance and network character of this civilizational paradox. It is a central issue of psychosomatics and roots in the nonadaptive linking of different, environmental, social, cognitive-emotional, neuroimmune, and genetic networks. Psychosomatics deals with this network of networks, where the informational pathways are the edges between nodes, hubs, and the more extensive network "patches." The so-called social signal transduction theory of depression is a proper example to track how social-environmental information activate biological processes that lead to depression.

The hypothesis that experiences of social threat and adversity upregulate components of the immune system involved in inflammation is central to the social signal transduction theory of depression. The key mediators or messengers, called *pro-inflammatory cytokines*, play a hub-like role in the network, which might induce profound changes in behavior like psychomotor retardation and social behavioral withdrawal, and influencing immune networks, and neural regulations of mood, anhedonia, and fatigue as symptoms of depression. Self-perceived/perceived lower social status is associated with higher pro-inflamma-tory cytokines (IL-6) in the dorsomedial prefrontal cortex (DMPFC) activity. The DMPFC plays a crucial role in the so-called mentalizing network, which is active in brain processes that model the thoughts and feelings of others, as well as in evaluating the social status associated with this process. The ventromedial prefrontal cortex (VMPFC) plays an essential role in detecting and assessing signs of dominance. VMPFC damage leads to insensitivity to the social hierarchy and a lack of respect for age and gender. The amygdala plays an integrative role in the perception of dominance, learning processes are related to the social hierarchy, the perceived value of the individual within the group are linked to the amygdala, and its relationships with the hippocampus and striatum are produc-tive. The lateral prefrontal cortex (LPFC) integrates social hierarchy information from the intraparietal sulcus and hippocampus, while VMPFC is responsible for organizing adaptive behavior. The network approach gives these centers a real social-psychoneuroimmune "hub" position.

On the other hand, diverse anatomical connections connect it to the amygdala, hypothalamus, and periaqueductal gray matter, thus reaching the stress pathways affecting the immune processes. Beyond its role in empathy and mentalization, it is also part of the so-called "aversive amplification" subnetwork, which activates the appropriate limbic areas in the event of threatening stress. In this regard, it plays a role in the processing of social impulses, perceiving others' higher positions in social rank as a source of critical, negative, exclusionary, and punitive social impulses, as well as in their qualification of danger. The inferior social status presumption is associated with increased activity in this brain area.

The hypothesis of social signal transduction theory of depression regarding experiences of psychoimmunological effects of social threat and adversity is central in our network theory of psychosomatics.

5. Network medicine as a psychosomatic metamodel

In the network medicine, identification of networks, hubs, and edges represents a true "big data" challenge, as the protein synthesis is determined by nearly 25,000 genes and the network hubs of "interactomes" are created by numerous proteins and functional RNS molecules as cell builders, on a scale of thousands. The number of network interactions with functional relevance is even higher. Learning about these interactions and identifying biological networks are the tasks for network medicine. However, the logic of network pathology is followed by research on the connections between the brain, hormone organs, and the immune system, on physiological networks, exploration of which is also a mapping task for interactomes of different levels. Such a map, comprising nearly 7000 interactions, is drawn by the protein-protein interaction network map of Rual et al. [24], the metabolic network summary by Duarte et al. [25], as well as the cytokine maps. However, the concept of meaningful narratives, life events, personality types susceptible to disease, or Berne's transaction analysis also strives to draw up such maps. Exploring the connection between anamnesis and disease progression is also a similar effort at representation.

The task is to identify interactomes as networks, within which the network patterns and relevant connection paths associated with the disease should be identified. Probably, the analysis of the socio-psychoimmunology paths is necessary as well, given that the "interactomes" of this mappable system of network relations can be identified. It is possible to explore the relationships between these factors, causal relations, and multidirectional pathways of influence, the network characteristics of the personality and the body, and the dynamics of the evolution and progression of diseases. Low socioeconomic status, discrimination, and subordination are accompanied by an increased level of pro-inflammatory cytokines, with the mediation of neurohumoral pathways, as demonstrated by Dickerson et al. [26], for instance. Anxiety, depression, and post-traumatic stress disease, along with the accompanying social and behavioral phenomena, are connected to neurohumoral and immune network anomalies, such as increased pro-inflammatory cytokines (e.g., IL-6) or the activation of the NF-kappa B path, which has central significance in the activity of inflammatory networks, according to Haroon et al. [27].

Identifying the degree of distribution and identifying the hubs characterized by several connections are needed to find the characteristics of these networks. At a molecular level, these can be TLR4, NF-kappa B, caspase, or, at the cellular level, macrophages or the cellular elements of the HPA axis representing nodes of the network. More abstract network modeling makes neurological structures participating in the assessment of controllability, the psychological processes of social perception and assessment, and neurophysiological structures that organize the personality also such as hubs. This way, the early mother–child relationship, which is vital for the development of personality, in the evolution of neurobiological structures, and carries permanent immunobiological consequences, becomes a network hub, as described above. Similarly, several neural networks as centers might create a greater network system responsible for translating social events.

The network itself is held together by a few hubs that have many connections. This is why socio-psychoimmunology explores lifetime hubs pointing in so many directions (mother-child relationship, separation, loss of object, loss of control), positive or negative traits (pessimism, C-type personality, active or passive coping) that are sensitive in psychoimmunological terms, pathologic network patterns (blunted HPA activity, deregulation of glucocorticoid receptors, TH1/TH2 shift), and allergic or autoimmune disease patterns in patient narratives at the social level. (**Figure 3**). These various key "hubs" may connect several types of networks of correlations. These small worlds are features of complex networks. The interconnected molecular networks are surrounded by relatively short path connections where a large portion of the component proteins are responsible for a low number of interac-tions, while they may be along main routes affecting the entire body, influencing the entire network.

Therefore, the hubs responsible for specific local cellular processes may be deemed to be "party" hubs, while they may also be "date" hubs interconnecting processes and associating relationships that organize the interactome. Further char-acteristics of the network are the "subgraphs" having motif power and in charge of biological functions such as negative or positive feedback or the oscillator function. These subgraphs are the totality of the interconnected hubs that make up a subnet-work within the network. Most networks may be described by a substantial creation of beams and are accompanied by the generation of topology modules characterized by the emergence of a high local region with mutual connections. Hubs are charac-terized by a high *betweenness centrality that describes the number of the shortest paths running through the hub,* otherwise referred to as "bottleneck." This is the nature of regulatory networks with vector edges.

An essential part of network analysis is link analysis, which looks primarily at the relationships between factors, hubs, and objects. Psychoimmunology itself offers an excellent example for the analysis of key relationships and links between the various objects, as it identifies and maps relations between networks of different characters (wired neural, endocrine propagated by blood flow, immune cells and mediators moving through tissues). Socio-psychoimmunology allocates the anamnestic narrative network relations, life events, and the social and symbolic cultural hub networks, through personality patterns, social-neuroscientific insight to responsible neural circuits deep to the cellular transcriptomic level of neuro-endocrine-immune networks, exposing their mutual interactions. This network

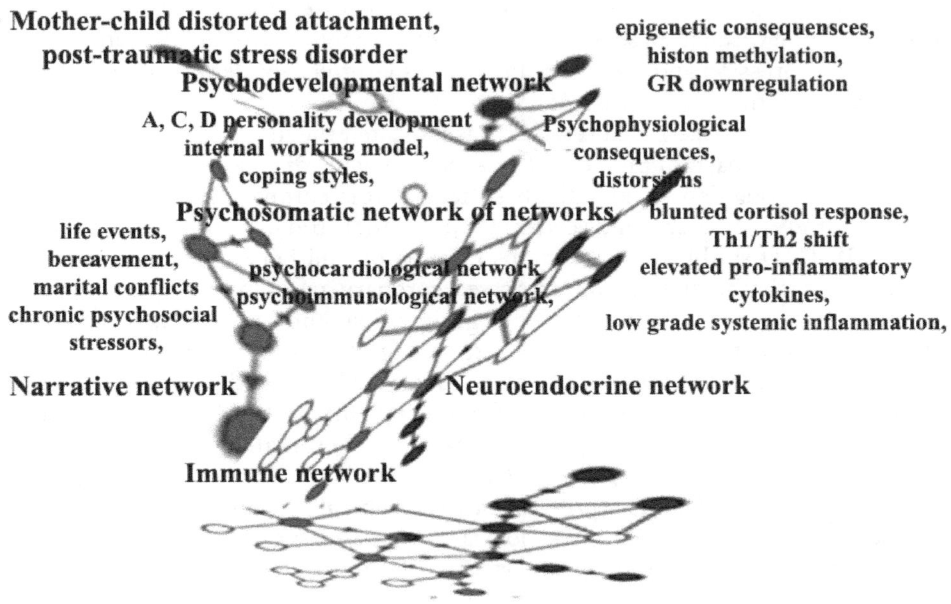

Figure 3.
Psychosomatic network of networks.

approach provides a new framework of cognitive mapping for anamnesis, diagnosis, and therapy. The result is a transversal metanetwork appearing through a series of information transcripts and translation mechanisms, which weaves a psychosomatic disease pattern through the network layers with its own heteronomous hubs.

6. Network framework as the common denominator of psychosomatics and internal medicine

The integrated internal medicine/psychosomatic/lifestyle medicine method is beneficial in improving the treatment of the disease, including the psychoso-cial factors to be taken into account [28]. Such are loneliness, chronic stress, the role of life events, the loss of object, and the personal characteristics of coping. Psychosomatic diagnosis is supported by the Diagnostic Criteria for Psychosomatic Research (DCPR), which incorporates relevant psychological variables into the diagnostic system along the lines of the most important psychosomatic syndromes, like anxiety, functional physical and conversion symptoms, somatic symptom formation of psychiatric origin, somatic and hypochondriac perceptions and fears (disease phobia and fear of death), and suppression of the disease that refers to psychosomatically colored disease behavior. In contrast, alexithymia; risk patterns of A-, C-, and D-type personality; and behavior patterns include trait and state features of personality characteristics that affect the patient's condition, including psychophysiological risks [29, 30]. Patients may require appropriate anxiety-reducing therapeutic support or cognitive behavioral therapy for psychophysiological involvement of chronic diseases. Clinical psychoimmunology offers new explanatory model and therapeutic framework for bronchial asthma, inflammatory bowel diseases, rheumatoid arthritis, specific autoimmune endocrine pathologies, and psychosomatic skin diseases. It is crucial if 25% of cardiovascular patients suffer from untreated depression, and the chronic inflammational process fed by depression, or similar psychoimmunological processes might contribute to the atherosclerotic vascular processes. Oncological patients have similar problems with untreated depression and the immunosuppressive effects of depression (in the case of NK cells) on the disease process.

Significant evidence-based research has indicated the increasing importance of a psychosocial approach in the field of internal medicine diseases, such as the SPIRR-CAD study among depressed patients suffering from coronary arterial disease [31]; the PISO study, somatoform disorders [32]; or DAD study, diabetes [33]. Although the SPIRR-CAD study did not demonstrate the overall benefit of cascading interventional psychotherapy among depressed coronary artery patients, it showed the success of therapy in a "bond-damaged" group of patients and among adult bypass-linked ISB patients [34]. Katon et al. [35] integrated "behavioral medicine" and psychosomatic approach to primary care. Lower HbA1c, blood pressure, and serum cholesterol was demonstrated among diabetic patients in the TEAM-care program than the control group receiving average care. Psychosomatics is not an alternative but an extension of the perspective of internal medicine. Lipowski [2] emphasizes that "psychosomatics" is an expression of the inseparability and interdependence of psychosocial and biological (physiological, somatic) aspects of human existence. This extension includes the extension of networks, too.

7. Risk factors and lifestyle risks of internal medicine diseases

Independent risk factors that increase the risk of internal medical diseases are also objects of a separate discipline, lifestyle medicine, addressing the relation-ship between avoidable risk factors and lifestyle. However, lifestyle medicine links biomedicine and psychosomatics, also. Obesity; distorted coping that escalates into addictions (smoking, alcohol, drugs, sedatives, chemical comforters); sedentary lifestyle, or, on the contrary, overtraining due to a distorted body image; eating disorders; and high carbohydrate and fat intake may affect the risk of developing cardiovascular and metabolic disorders.

The Framingham study was one of the early follow-up studies that demonstrated the role of hypertension, smoking, and high blood fats among independent risk factors for coronary sclerosis. Today, depression and anxiety must also be considered an independent risk factor for coronary artery disease [12].

Life events can also affect the development and course of the disease. Bereavement, divorce with high values in the Holmes-Rahe scale, and common everyday stress experience called daily hassles all might play a role. For example, in respiratory diseases, a correlation is observed between stressful life events, perceived stress, and upper respiratory symptoms. The risk of provoking asthma is known for severe adverse life events. Rheumatoid arthritis often flares up after bereavement, divorce, and job loss. Serious conflict, divorce, bereavement, or love disappointment might induce or worsen course of ulcerative colitis.

Lifestyle medicine offers network-like interventions along with behavioral modification. One of these is regular exercise. In a plague of sedentarism, physical exercise might be a panacea for many lifestyle problems. The active muscles are part of the neuroendocrine-immune network of the human organism and exert significant influence on the metabolic system, the immune system, the brain, and the abdominal fat, which is also part of the complex informational network. Exercise induces endorphin secretion. Myokines exert their influence by the presence of their receptors on muscle, fat, liver, pancreatic, bone, heart, immune, and brain cells. Myokines like myostatin, IL-6, IL-8, IL-15, FGF21, follistatin-like 1, brain-derived neurotrophic factor (BDNF), hepatocyte growth factor, fibroblast growth factor, and insulin-like growth factor play role in metabolism and tissue regeneration. IL-15 reduces abdominal adipose tissue, while in heavy physical exercise, the secreted IL-6 as myokine rises to 100-fold of resting level and increases IL-1 and IL-10 as an anti-inflammatory mediator. Brain-derived neurotrophic factor might be secreted as a myokine, and muscle-derived BDNF enhances fat oxidation.

8. Discourses and institutions: networks of psychosomatic agency

On the other side, psychosomatic medicine as a unique professional medical specialization is not universal at all. In Europe, one can find such psychosomatic professional specialization only in Germany, while psychotherapy applied by somatic experts is practiced in many other countries. The new niches for psychosomatic ori-entation offered by integrative frameworks of stress medicine, mind-body medicine, or lifestyle medicine and network medicine are based on the above insights of linked biopsychosocial networks. Is this a trans/interdisciplinary challenge or a constraint for networking of different disciplines? If we compare the definition of behavioral medicine by Schwartz and Weiss in 1978 [36] and the 2019 proposal for its renewal by the ISBM consensus boards, we find meaningful shifts. The "interdisciplinary field" was exchanged to "field characterized by the collaboration among multiple disciplines" with the meaning of networking of disciplines instead of filling the intermediary disciplinal gaps.

This way, network medicine means double challenge, to see the patient as socio-psycho-biological "network of networks" and organize his/her healing in networks of disciplines, discourses, and institutions.

Psychosomatic medicine has its permanent revival fed by new findings in social neuroscience, clinical psychophysiology, or the new public health; nevertheless, its institutional network shows a narrow picture. Mental disorders (depression, chronic stress) proved to be independent risk factors in the development of auto-immune, allergic and neoplastic diseases, and myocardial infarction. It has been confirmed by evidence-based basic research (social neuroscience, psychoneuroim-munology, psychocardiology) and epidemiological analyses.

However, the institutionalization of psychosomatic clinical discourse showed a rather marginal status in the shadow zone of the high-tech, evidence-based practi-cal development of biomedicine in the frontline. The discourse dynamics reflects the power inequities of health economic, academic, educational, and clinical health service networks.

In some countries (e.g., Germany, Japan), psychosomatic medicine can be practiced as a specialist field, with specialized psychosomatic clinical depart-ments, separate institutes, and somatic and psychotherapeutic care in a joint framework, in teamwork. In Germany, there are over 5000 specialist physicians with psychosomatic and psychotherapist certifications. Outpatient care employs 3058 psychosomatic professionals, while 10,269 physicians hold the title of the psychotherapist, and a total of 21,312 physicians with somatic background have the title of psychotherapist. There are 120 psychosomatic institutions in Germany with a total of approx. 20,000 beds (Statistik-Portal, 2014). Institutional care is also highly developed, and psychosomatic wards providing regional care in regional central hospitals provide patient care. Although the number of hospital beds is limited (9 to 36 beds), the units also provide consultation-liaison psychosomatic care for other clinical departments. The university and teaching hospitals (20–70 beds) have a higher supply capacity, where in addition to healing, there is research and education.

In March 2016, the Japanese Psychosomatic Society had 3300 members, 71.6% of whom were physicians (general practitioners, psychiatrists, pediatricians, obstetricians-gynecologists, dentists, and dermatologists). Psychosomatic internal therapists also formed a separate association with 1200 members (Japanese Society of Psychosomatic Internal Medicine) [37].

Although there are widespread organized discourse communities, academic associations of psychosomatic experts from gynecology and obstetrics, internal medicine, cardiology, and gastroenterology, just as numerous clinical departments all around the medical world, one can find significant disproportion between psychosomatic *medical specialization* and mainstream organized health care in most of the contemporary medical systems.

Psychosomatics might be absorbed by psychiatry, as C-L psychiatry might be seen as a branch of mainstream psychiatry. It shows the significant disciplinary distance from internal medicine and other disciplines, while issues of psychoimmunology and psychocardiology are deeply embedded in the health-care system of internal medicine. This way, the emerging network centered renewal of behavioral medicine remains only an ideology than everyday clinical practice.

If clinical practice incorporates psychosomatics as part of mainstream medical discourse, guaranteeing the possibility of specialist examinations and special-ized care and creating such specialist care units and scenes, the institutional and economic "emancipation" of the field is assured. In 2004, the so-called DAK/AHG study weighed the cost/benefit of long-term institutional psychosomatic treatment burdened with costly hotel services in 338 insured persons treated in psychosomatic hospital wards between January 1999 and February 2000. The results supported its "raison d'etre" and profitable values for *health economic* point of view [38].

One might see the reason of these contradictions even in nature of psychosomatic disease, as a patient complaining of somatic symptoms used to be reluctant to classify his or her complaints as psychiatric. One can overcome this situation by an invited consultation-liaison psychiatrist, as the patient is not seeking psychological treatment but a somatic care provider for his/her psychosomatic disorders. All of this requires collaboration, a psychosomatically informed professional organi-zational culture, and a genuinely competent psychosomatic therapeutic delivery environment for the other treatments offered. Psychosomatic patients travel through routes of somatic care with their symptoms because of their interpretation. Once treated in a somatic ward, they are strongly attached to the physical origin of their complaints based on their explanatory model. Psychological assessment of symptoms is often considered offensive. Therefore, psychosomatic care is highly dependent on patient choice. If the primary and specialist care systems do not offer this type of care, the patient will not make such a decision either. Few people turn to psychiatric care providers for physical complaints of psychological origin, and the fear of stigmatization is a barrier, too. It follows that the internal structural features of institutionalized discourse impede the proper care of a large group of patients. Whereas in general medical practice, about one-third of patients suffer from psychiatric symptoms, and 23% of patients in primary care experience depression, 22% with anxiety, and 20% with somatization, it may be relevant for primary care physicians to have additional psychosomatic licensure training. One-third of cardiological patients have mild depression without treatment; oncological patients have a similar situation, frequently. Beyond these institutional difficulties, there is a great need for integrating psychosomatic to biomedicine, as argued above.

Katon et al. [35] also demonstrated that the so-called TEAM-care program, integrating behavioral and psychosomatic approaches with the somatic practice of primary care, lowered HbA1c, blood pressure, and serum cholesterol levels. Psychosomatic patients also increase the costs of somatic care because of hotel costs and ineffective, sometimes unnecessary diagnostics efforts. This costly, unnecessary "evidence-driven" defensive medical practice consumes energy, time, and space in patients requiring care. Specified psychosomatic care is mostly related/ reducted to clinical "elite institutions" and does not form part of general public hospital and outpatient practice. A few psychosomatic centers are connected to the university education (e.g., like the Psychosomatic Outpatient Department at the Institute of Behavioral Sciences, Semmelweis University) or occasionally as a department of the psychiatry clinic or elements of hospital psychiatric wards.

The concept of networked medicine in medical systems can also create new theoretical "niches" for psychosomatic clinical thinking. All of this may be important to connect biomedicine with social neuroscience, clinical psychophysiology (e.g., psychoimmunology), stress medicine, or mind-body medicine. All these conceptual spaces, theoretical niches, also designate real institutional niches. There are vacant clinical spaces that can be filled with training, a new competent work-force, and purely organizational innovation. As the affected patient population is unaware of the psychological roots or modifiers of their complaints, and even this non-knowledge often forms the mechanics of symptom formation (suppression, complexation, alexithymia, traumatic learning,), therefore their care is closely linked to extension of somatic specialists' competence toward the psychosomatic horizon (specialist exam, license exam). On the other hand, the involvement of highly trained psychologists with clinical psychology specialization might also have an essential part of this organizational change. Such psychosomatic development can also affect oncology, dermatology, rheumatology, cardiology, and gastroenter-ology networks.

The occupational health services offer a wide surface for preventive network medicine, too. Occupational health might have an important priority area for psychosomatic preventive work and early disease detection. Recognizing the increasing work-related stress in the industrial space of globalization and the consequent economic loss of nearly EUR 40 billion to European Member States' budgets has prompted European Union decision-makers to do the management of work-related stress management and mental health support, as a Member State's duty from 2007. Preventive stress management can be part of health promotion and may be of interest to both the employee and the employer in health psychological and psycho-somatic practice, linked to screening and other public health preventive practices. The use of de-*medicalized* cognitive behavioral elements of mind-body preventive agency might be applied as worksite stress management training (like in case of Williams Life Skills training), new screening ways of psychophysiological risks, and available psychometric methods might help to implement worksite and community-based prevention and intervention.

Psychologists with such skills, and occupational health practitioners sensitized in this regard, would achieve economically demonstrable results. Occupational health is the apparent scene for preventive and early psychosomatic intervention, as such screening of employees is easy to do and suits to the personal and corporate interest.

Psychosomatic diagnostic and counseling work or psychosomatic "lifestyle medicine" might have their niches in spa health, wellness network. They are, like the occupational health or specialist network, empty niches to fill with psychosomatics. The map of diverse, nevertheless, coherent discourses of psychosomatics can be reframed by the network medicine concept, a common denominator. If clinical practice incorporates psychosomatics as part of mainstream medical discourse, guaranteeing the possibility of specialist examinations and specialized care and creating such specialist care units and scenes, the institutional and economic "emancipation" of the field is assured. The hermeneutic bridge, which had been already established in the biopsychosocial framework, did not lead to closer hybridization. The neuroimmune biological network frame might help the social and psychological aspects join to the evidence-based biomedical disciplines including the molecular and genomic transcriptomic level.

9. Conclusion

Steps in the history of psychosomatics share common heuristics in connecting different levels of environmental, psychological, neural, and visceral phenomena. This "multilayer" approach reflects the scientific will to follow the information flow from the social through the psychoneural and the visceral down to the molecular and genetic sphere and back. The psychophysiological core of psychosomatics has a human ecological context and deals with regulative network patterns of evolutionary roots. Concept of behavioral medicine shifted psychosomatics from a comprehensive psychodynamic explanatory model toward an integrative, multidisciplinary framework including levels of social, psychological, and somatic networks. Specific subfields of behavioral medicine, like psychoneuroimmunology, offer insights to the multilayered network-based interpretation of diseases. Dysregulation of evolutionary-based adaptive network activities like *the conserved transcriptional response to adversity* or the *social signal transduction theory of depression* reflects the clinical significance of network approach.

Depression itself is proven to be a mediating element between SES and sick days, between social and somatic, just as between the immunological and the psychological networks. Network theory offers an inclusive metanarrative for the description of the different social, narrative, and psychosomatic network layers and their interconnections as well anamnestic, diagnostic, and therapeutic significance. Behavioral medicine has shifted from an "*interdisciplinary field*" to the promoter of the collaboration among multiple disciplines, so this collaboration might be reframed by the extended and comprehensive network approach. Network medi-cine [39] as shared conceptual explanatory frame might bring closer behavioral epidemiology, the preventive lifestyle medicine, behavioral medicine, and occupa-tional health and biomedicine. The exploring and implementing efforts based on the above defined "networks of networks" includes medical sociology, medical ecol-ogy, behavioral epidemiology, new public health, health promotion on the social side, and clinical psychophysiological depth of psychosomatic therapies including several cognitive behavioral approaches, hypnosis, psychodynamic approaches, and narrative medicine on the psychological side. Internal medicine, behavioral medi-cine, and psychosomatics with related disciplines overlap in the different social and psychophysiological network layers; network medicine might be the common denominator and the widest inclusive conceptual framework for collaboration.

Author details

Imre Lázár[1,2]

1 Head of Medical Humanities Research Group, Institute of Behavioral Sciences, Semmelweis University, Budapest, Hungary

2 Faculty of Humanities and Social Sciences, Károli Gáspár University, Institution of Social and Communication Sciences, Budapest, Hungary

*Address all correspondence to: lazar.imre@med.semmelweis-univ.hu

References

[1] Németh L. Új Szempontok a Status Praesens Felvételében Megmentett Gondolatok I. Budapest: Magvető Kiadó; 1968. pp. 29-62

[2] Lipowski ZJ. What does the word "psychosomatic" really mean? A historical and semantic inquiry. Psychosomatic Medicine. 1984;**46**(2):153-171

[3] Proceedings of Yale Conference on Behavioral Medicine Department of Health, Education and Welfare Public Health Service; 1977. pp 7

[4] Lázár I. Üres nichek évadján A pszichoszomatikus diskurzus intézményesülésének kérdései (Age of empty niches, questions of institutionalization of psychosomatic discourse). Mentálhigiéné és Pszichoszomatika. 2018;**19**:243-267

[5] Császár GY. Pszichoszomatikus Orvoslás. Budapest: Medicina; 1980

[6] Lázár I. Pszichoneuroimmunológia [Psychoneuroimmunology]. Budapest: Végeken ed; 1991

[7] Solomon GF. Psychoneuroimmunology: Interactions between central nervous system and immune system. Journal of Neuroscience Research. 1987;**18**(1):1-9

[8] Lázár I. At the cradle of psychobiological risks: Distorted attachment organizations in human ecological and evolutionary contexts. In: Watson P, editor. Social Behavior Evolutionary Pathways, Environmental Influences and Impairments. New York: Nova Publishers; 2013

[9] Lázár I. "Attached Files": Anthropological Essays on Body, Psyche, Attachment and Spirituality. Newcastle upon Tyne, UK: Cambridge Scholars Publishing; 2015. p. 304

[10] Suarez EC, Lewis JG, Krishnan RR, Young KH. Enhanced expression of cytokines and chemokines by blood monocytes to in vitro lipopolysaccharide stimulation are associated with hostility and severity of depressive symptoms in healthy women. Psychoneuroendocrinology. 2004;**29**:1119-1128

[11] Kopp MS, Réthelyi J. Where psychology meets physiology: Chronic stress and premature mortality—The Central-Eastern European Health Paradox. Brain Research Bulletin. 2004;**62**(5):351-367

[12] Hemingway H, Marmot M. Evidence-based cardiology: Psychosocial factors in the aetiology and prognosis of coronary heart disease: Systematic review of prospective cohort studies. British Medical Journal. 1999;**318**:1460-1467

[13] Uchino BN, Holt-Lunstad J, Uno D, Flinders JB. Heterogeneity in the social networks of young and older adults: Prediction of mental health and cardiovascular reactivity during acute stress. Journal of Behavioral Medicine. 2001;**24**:361-382

[14] Kiecolt-Glaser JK, Newton T. Marriage and health: His and hers. Psychological Bulletin. 2001;**127**:472-503

[15] Malarkey WB, Kiecolt-Glaser JK, Pearl D, Glaser R. Hostile behavior during marital conflict alters pituitary and adrenal hormones. Psychosomatic Medicine. 1994;**56**(1):41-51

[16] Kiecolt-Glaser JK, Glaser R, Cacioppo JT, MacCallum RC, Snydersmith M, Kim C, et al. Marital conflict in older adults: Endocrinological and immunological correlates. Psychosomatic Medicine. 1997;**59**:339-349

[17] Mayne TJ, O'Leary A, McCrady B, Contrada R, Labouvie E. The differential effects of acute marital distress on emotional, physiological and immune functions in maritally distressed men and women. Psychology & Health. 1997;**12**:277-288

[18] Levenstein S, Ackerman S, Kiecolt-Glaser JK, Dubois A. Stress and peptic ulcer disease. JAMA. 1999;**281**:10-11

[19] Miller TQ, Smith TW, Turner CW, Guijarro ML, Hallet AJ. A meta-analytic review of research on hostility and physical health. Psychological Bulletin. 1996;**119**(2):322-348

[20] Steptoe A, Hamer M, Chida Y. The effects of acute psychological stress on circulating inflammatory factors in humans: A review and meta-analysis. Brain, Behavior, and Immunity. 2007;**21**(7):901-912

[21] Denson THF, Spanovic M, Miller N. Cognitive appraisals and emotions predict cortisol and immune responses: A meta-analysis of acute laboratory social stressors and emotion inductions. Psychological Bulletin. 2009;**135**(6):823-853

[22] Slavich GM, Cole SW. The emerging field of human social genomics. Clinical Psychological Science. 2013;**1**:331-348

[23] Antoni MH, Lutgendorf SK, Blomberg B, Carver CS, Lechner S, Diaz A, et al. Cognitive-behavioral stress management reverses anxiety-related leukocyte transcriptional dynamics. Biological Psychiatry. 2012;**71**:366-372

[24] Rual Gibbons FD, Dreze M, Ayivi-Guedehoussou N, Klitgord N, Simon C, Boxem M, et al. Towards a proteome-scale map of the human protein-protein interaction network. Nature. 2005;**437**(7062):1173-1178

[25] Duarte NC, Becker SA, Jamshidi N, Thiele I, Mo ML, Vo TD, et al. Global reconstruction of the human metabolic network based on genomic and bibliomic data. Proceedings of the National Academy of Sciences of the United States of America. 2007;**104**(6):1777-1782

[26] Dickerson SS, Gable SL, Irwin MR, Aziz N, Kemeny ME, et al. Psychological Science. 2009;**20**(10):1237-1244

[27] Haroon F, Drögemüller K, Händel U, Brunn A, Reinhold D, Nishanth G, et al. Gp130-dependent astrocytic survival is critical for the control of autoimmune central nervous system inflammation. Journal of Immunology. 2011;**186**(11):6521-6531

[28] Schmeling-Kludas C, Fehrs H. Effects of integrated internal medicine-psychosomatic management on coping with illness by patients. Psychotherapie, Psychosomatik, Medizinische Psychologie. 1997;**47**(8):285-294

[29] Porcelli P, Rafanelli C. Criteria for psychosomatic research (DCPR) in the medical setting. Current Psychiatry Reports. 2010;**12**(3):246-254

[30] Sirri L, Fava GA. Diagnostic criteria for psychosomatic research and somatic symptom disorders. International Review of Psychiatry. 2013;**25**(1):19-30

[31] Herrmann-Lingen C, Beutel ME, Bosbach A, Deter HC, Fritzsche K, Hellmich M, et al. A stepwise psychotherapy intervention for reducing risk in coronary artery disease (SPIRR-CAD): Results of an observer-blinded, multicenter, randomized trial in depressed patients with coronary artery disease. SPIRR-CAD Study Group. Psychosomatic Medicine. 2016;**78**(6):704-715

[32] Sattel H, Lahmann C, Gündel H, Guthrie E, Kruse J, Noll-Hussong M, et al. Brief psychodynamic interpersonal

psychotherapy for patients with multisomatoform disorder: Randomised controlled trial. British Journal of Psychiatry. 2012;**200**(1):60-67

[33] Petrak F, Herpertz S, Albus C, Hermanns N, Hiemke C, Hiller W, et al. Cognitive behavioral therapy versus sertraline in patients with depression and poorly controlled diabetes: The Diabetes and Depression (DAD) study: A randomized controlled multicenter trial. Diabetes Care. 2007;**38**:767-775

[34] Söllner W, Müller MM, Albus C, Behnisch R, Beutel ME, de Zwaan M, et al. The relationship between attachment orientations and the course of depression in coronary artery disease patients: A secondary analysis of the SPIRR-CAD trial. Journal of Psychosomatic Research. 2018;**108**:39-46

[35] Katon WJ, Lin EH, Von Korff M, Ciechanowski P, Ludman EJ, Young B, et al. Collaborative care for patients with depression and chronic illness. New England Journal of Medicine. 2010;**363**(27):2611-2620

[36] Schwartz GE, Weiss SM. Behavioral medicine revisited: An amended definition. Journal of Behavioral Medicine. 1978;**1**(3):249-251

[37] Murakami M, Nakai Y. Current state and future prospects for psychosomatic medicine in Japan. BioPsychoSocial Medicine. 2017;**11**:1

[38] Zielke M, Limbacher K. Fehlversorgung bei psysychischen Erkrankungen: Studie im Auftrag der DAK. Verhaltentherapie und Psychosoziale Praxis. 2004; **36**(Suppl. 3):S.8-S.12

[39] Loscalzo J, Barabási A-L, Silverman EK, editors. Network Medicine: Complex Systems in Human Disease and Therapeutics. Harvard University Press; 2017

3

Psychosomatic Inpatient Rehabilitation for People with Depression in Germany

Ralf F. Tauber, Carola Nisch, Mutahira M. Qureshi, Olivia Patsalos and Hubertus Himmerich

Abstract

In Germany, inpatient therapy for depression mainly takes place in either health insurance-financed psychiatric hospitals, or in pension insurance-financed, psychotherapy-focused, psychosomatic rehabilitation hospitals. In psychiatric hospitals, the diagnosis is made according to the International Classification of Diseases (ICD), and therapeutic attempts are made to achieve remission, whereas in rehabilitation hospitals, the International Classification of Functioning, Disability and Health (ICF) plays an essential diagnostic role. Accordingly, the main German pension insurance, Deutsche Rentenversicherung, has developed a rehabilita-tion therapy standard for depressive disorders. In this chapter, we focus on the psychotherapeutic inpatient rehabilitation for patients with depression based on an example of a specialized psychotherapeutic hospital. This example illustrates how psychotherapeutic inpatient rehabilitation can be tailored to the individual's needs and may include any of the following therapeutic modalities: Cognitive Behavior Therapy (CBT), Schema Therapy, Cognitive Behavioral Analysis System of Psychotherapy (CBASP), pharmacotherapy, group therapy for comorbid condi-tions, skills training, psychoeducation, occupational therapy (OT), movement therapy, physiotherapy, music therapy, social work, family work, and self-help groups. People with depression may benefit from this service model of psychoso-matic inpatient rehabilitation beyond symptom remission, as it focuses on increas-ing people's functional level as well as their quality of life.

Keywords: inpatient therapy, psychosomatic therapy, psychotherapy, depression, rehabilitation

1. Introduction

Mental and substance use disorders are the leading cause of years lived with disability (YLD) worldwide, whereby depressive disorders account for 42.5% of YLDs caused by mental and substance use disorders [1]. The health report of the German technicians' health insurance in 2016 [2] found that the number of work absences due to a mental disorder has almost doubled from the year 2000, reaching its highest value in 2015 at 245 sick leave days per 100 insurance years. Patients with depressive illnesses represented the group with most sick days [2]. Cumulative data for all public and private health insurance companies in Germany are not available, but comparable reports of individual insurances show similar results.

Compared to other diseases whose number of hospital admissions has remained relatively constant over the past few years (e.g., diseases of the circulatory system, the musculoskeletal system, and cancer), the incidence of mental illnesses in the inpatient care system has steadily increased since 1990. While the number of admissions due to somatic diseases has tended to decrease, psychiatric diagnoses have risen from 175 to 350 days per 1000 insured years since 1990. Among these psychiatric diagnoses, substance misuse disorders as well as depressive disorders are by far the most frequent ones [3]. The Federal Health Care Report (Gesundheitsberichterstattung des Bundes) estimates an increase in the direct cost of mental illness from €219 million in 2002 to about €254 million in 2008 [4]. Beyond the financial cost, mental illnesses, and specifically depression, are accompanied by severe suffering, considerable impairment of work performance, and reduced quality of life (QoL) [5].

2. The significance of mental disorders for German pension insurances

In contrast to other health systems such as the public National Health Service (NHS) in the United Kingdom, which is funded by the state, health care in Germany is mainly funded by either public or private health insurances, as well as by pension insurance, taxes, and out-of-pocket co-payments. Public and private health insurances as well as pension insurances are financed by contributions from both the employer and the employee; a percentage of the employee's gross income is transferred to the individual's health and pension scheme. Whereas health care in general is funded by public or private health care insurances, rehabilitation and work reintegration is funded by pension insurances, which also cover the costs of treatment in rehabilitation hospitals.

As a result, mental illnesses are placing an increasingly heavy burden on pension insurance schemes such as the German Statutory Pension Insurance (Deutschen Rentenversicherung; DRV). While only 6.6% of all occupational disability-related illnesses were of a mental nature in 1982, their incidence rose to 42% by 2012. Among women, almost half (48.5%) of sickness leave was due to a mental disorder [6]. In addition, the average age of retirement in patients with mental illness is lower as compared to other diagnostic groups (48.1 vs. 50.4 years) [6]. Consequently, fewer social insurance contributions are generated by patients and their employers (since they are no longer working), and the duration of pension payments increases (since patients retire earlier).

The amount of DRV reimbursement for medical rehabilitation of mental disorders in 2012 was €716 million as reported in their 2016 position paper of the DRV on the Significance of Mental Illnesses in Rehabilitation and Disability Reduction [7]. Against this background, the DRV has a pressing need to reduce the incapacity to work that results from depressive or other psychological disorders.

3. A disease model for the rehabilitative treatment of depressed patients

Acute and long-term treatments of mental illnesses are either directed at the assumed causes of a certain disorder or the presenting symptoms. They are primarily centered on the clinical picture as a manifestation of the disease or injury and are aimed at treatment response or remission. In the case of disorders with a tendency toward chronicity, prevention of episode aggravation or precipitation of another episode is crucial. The conceptual framework of acute and long-term psychiatric disorders is frequently based on a medical disease model that corresponds to the classification according to the International Classification of Diseases (ICD) of the World Health Organization (WHO) [8]. For example, in Germany a patient with a severe third episode of depressive symptoms is seen by a psychiatrist in their practice, referred and admitted to a psychiatric hospital, diagnosed with recurrent major depressive disorder (ICD-10 code: F33.2) [8], and treated by the multidisciplinary team on the psychiatric ward according to the German national guidelines for the treatment of unipolar depression [9], which advise psychopharmacological treatment with an antidepressant that will con-tinue after discharge. The costs of admission are incurred by the private or public health insurance.

In contrast, medical rehabilitation as practiced in rehabilitation hospitals in Germany is based on the biopsychosocial model of functioning, disability and health. This model has also been introduced by the WHO [10] in their International Classification of Functioning, Disability and Health (ICF) framework. While ICD-10 gives users an etiological or symptom-based framework for the classification, that is, the diagnosis of a disease, disorder, or health condition, the ICF classifies functioning and disability as associated with health conditions. The ICD-10 and ICF are therefore seen as complementary to one another [10, 11].

In the biopsychosocial model of functioning, disability and health, impairments take place on three levels: (1) body structures and functions, (2) activity, and (3) participation. Health is seen as embedded in the context of "functioning." A person is therefore "functionally healthy" when:

- Their physical functions including that of the mind and body are of accepted standards,
- They can perform all levels of activities that are expected of a person without a health problem, and
- They are able to develop their participation in all areas of life that are important to them, in the manner and extent that is expected of a person without impairment of body structures, functions, or activities (i.e., a level of participation in all spheres of life).

This model conceptualizes health and disease as a result of the interlocking of physiological, psychological, and social processes (see **Figure 1**). The type and extent of functional health of a person are therefore also dependent on the circumstances or the background of the person's life. These contextual factors consist of personal factors (e.g., age, sex, and lifestyle) and environmental factors (e.g., family, residential situation, and work situation). These factors can either exert a favorable influence (positive context factors) or have a detrimental influence (negative context factors or barriers) on the overall prognosis, recovery, and reintegration into work and society. **Figure 2** gives an example of how this model can be applied in the case of a patient with a depressive episode. By considering these context factors, it is ensured that in addition to any medical diagnoses, personal and/or social conditions, the patients' experience is part of the rehabilitative treatment [11].

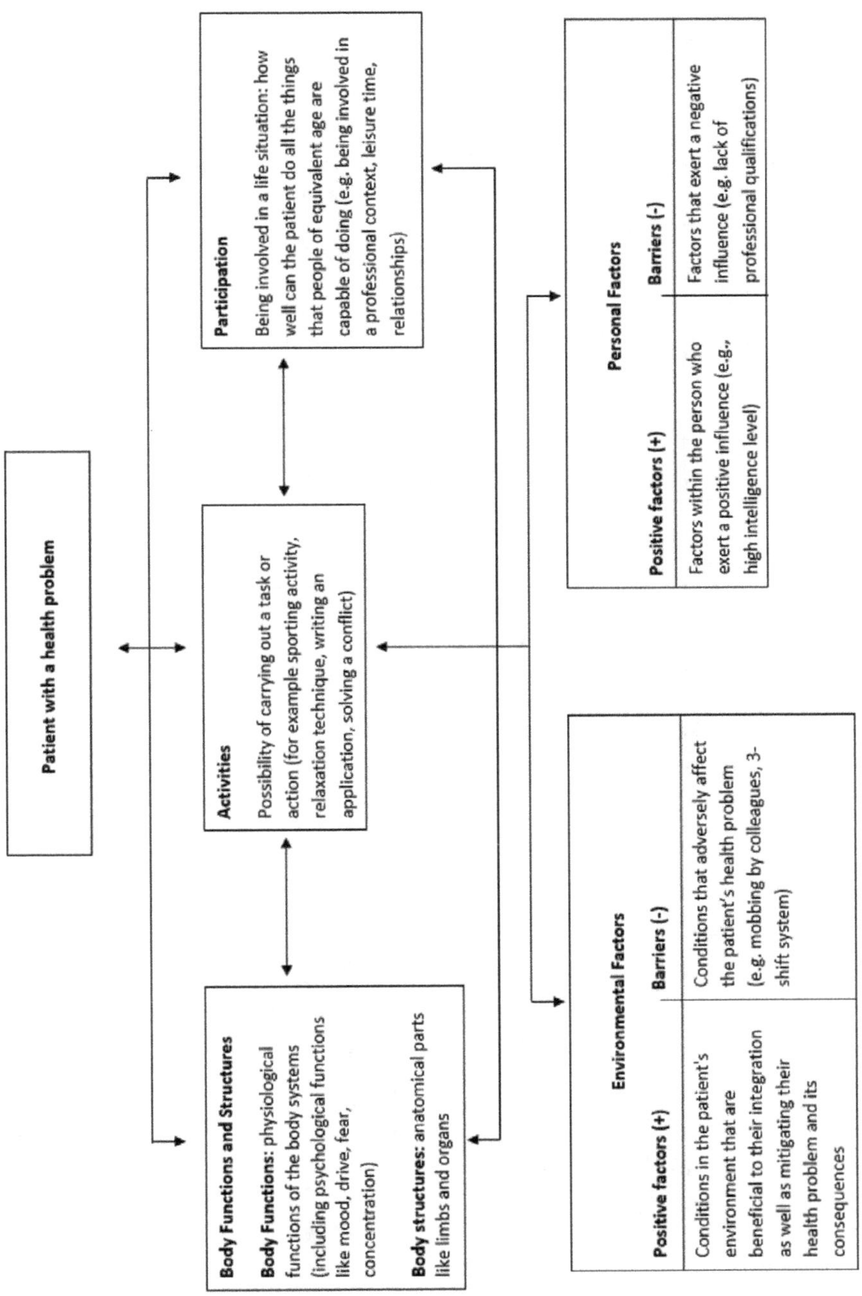

Figure 1.
ICF model with definitions of the terms used.

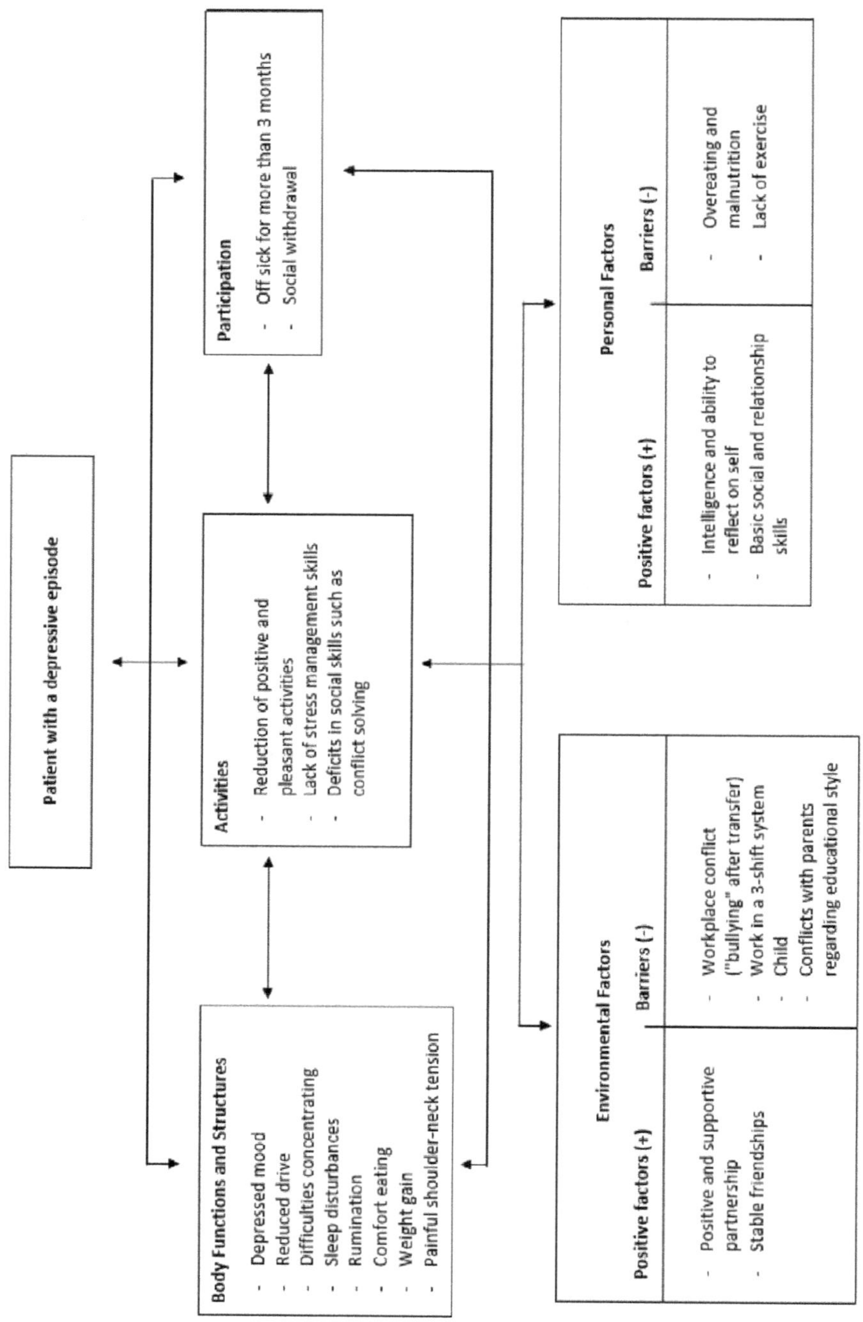

Figure 2.
Example of applying the ICF model to a sample patient with depression.

4. The goal of rehabilitative treatment of depressed patients

Against the background of the biopsychosocial model of functional health, the rehabilitation goals of each of three levels of functioning are specified taking into account their respective context factors (**Figure 3** exemplifies these goals for the patient described in **Figure 2**). The aim is to remove or reduce the impending or already manifest impairments of participation or prevent their exacerbation and worsening. The patient is ultimately to be enabled or re-enabled by the rehabilitation to spend their life in a way that is normal within their personal life context.

Participation in their professional life may be of specific interest, even if their job has not been the trigger of a depressive episode. For example, a depressive episode following the death of a close relative may require psychosomatic rehabilitation, because it may impact on the capacity to work and subsequent disability. Therefore, it is in the interest of the cost-bearers such as the pension insurance to prevent such depressive disorders at an early stage.

In psychosomatic rehabilitation for depression, the acute psychiatric treat-ment is usually not yet completed by the time of discharge from hospital. In some cases, the rehabilitation hospitals are the first treatment providers and thus must provide acute care including psychoeducation, psychopharmacological and psychological therapy. Thus, good psychosomatic rehabilitation encompasses elements of acute psychiatric treatment in addition to the core rehabilitation goals of enhancing the individual's resources, removing barriers, and improv-ing the overall performance to compensate for remaining restrictions and disabilities.

5. The therapeutic standard for rehabilitation in depressive disorders

In recent years, several national and international clinical guidelines have been developed, which provide an optimal, up-to-date therapy or action algorithm as a guidance for the practicing physician. In Germany, the national guidelines for the treatment of unipolar depression [9] constitute the central systematic summary of the current scientific status on the acute treatment and care for people with depression. In addition to this guideline, the DRV has developed a therapeutic standard for rehabilitation (RTS) of depressive disorder [12]. In this standard, the so-called "evidence-based therapy modules" (ETMs) derived from rehabilitation research are defined. The RTS clarifies the specific therapies that constitute an ETM, as well as their duration and frequency. In turn, the therapies provided by the psychosomatic rehabilitation hospital are listed, described, and coded in the German Classification of Therapeutic Procedures [13].

The documentation of applied therapies according to the KTL system is regu-larly communicated to the funders, for example, a pension insurance, for each patient individually. This can then be used to determine annually to what extent the RTS was implemented by the hospital. We will depict the practicalities of rehabili-tative treatment of depressive illnesses in psychosomatic hospitals by using our own hospital, the Psychosomatic Department of the Sachsenklinik Bad Lausick, as an example. This will illustrate not only the application of the aforementioned guidelines, but also the freedom that exists within this framework to implement hospital-specific cognitive-behavioral approaches or novel concepts such as schema therapy [14] or Cognitive Behavioral Analysis System of Psychotherapy (CBASP) [15].

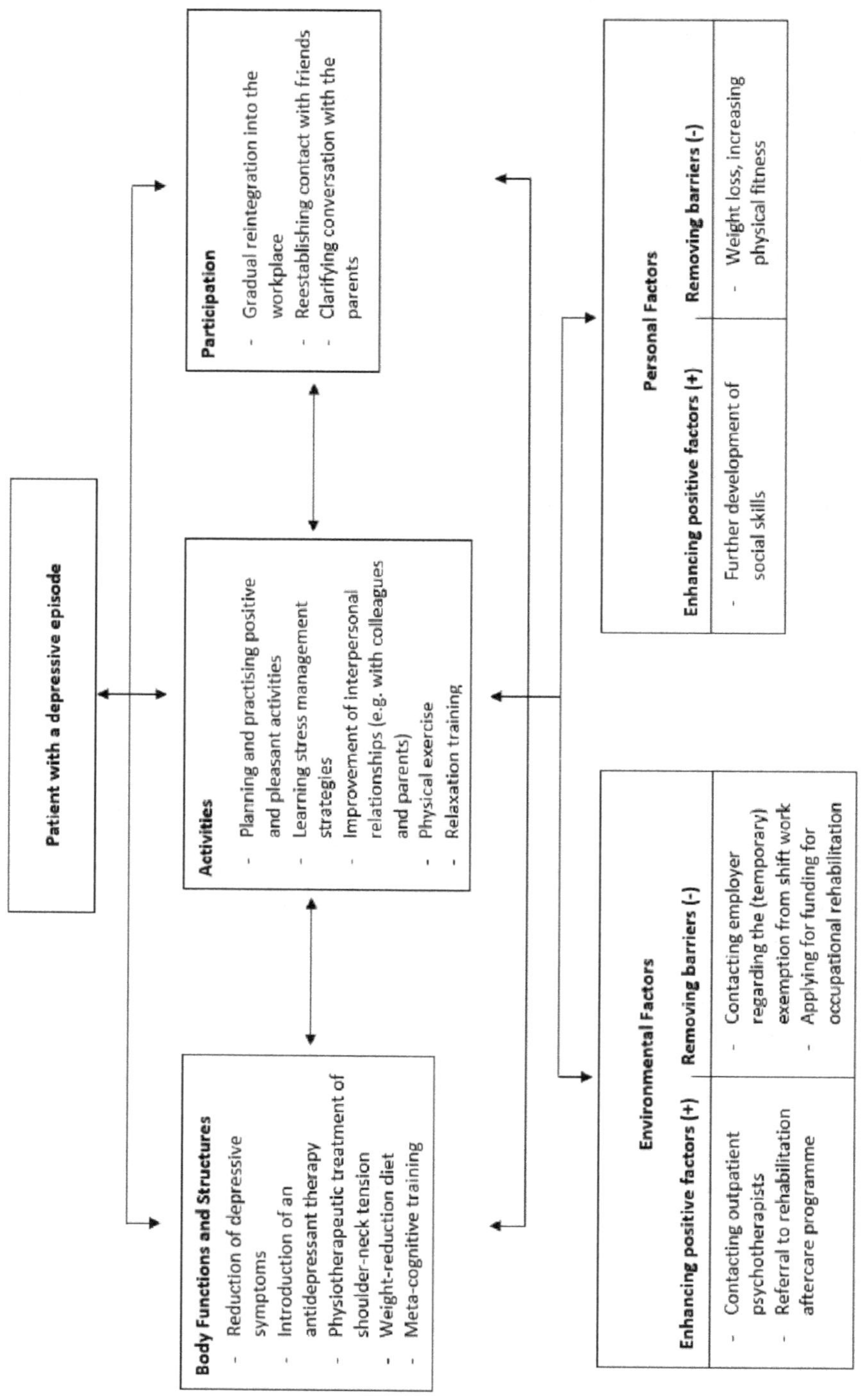

Figure 3.
Rehabilitation goals and therapeutic measures according to the ICF model for a patient with depression.

6. Example of psychosomatic inpatient treatment for depression

Psychotherapeutic and medical treatment: In the Psychosomatic Department of the Sachsenklinik Bad Lausick, a treatment concept is applied that places special emphasis on the high quality and density of specific psychotherapeutic interventions. The clinic currently comprises of 100 beds, which are allocated to six wards with multidisciplinary teams (MDT). Each MDT is divided into two thematically specialized sub-teams. Psychological and medical staff are permanently assigned to these sub-teams. **Table 1** depicts the structure of the Psychosomatic Department of the Sachsenklinik Bad Lausic in more detail. In each sub-team, approximately eight to nine patients are assigned and treated by their reference therapists within this family-like group. This allows frequent patient-centered contacts with the reference therapists. There are, in principle, three disorder-specific group therapies (90 min each) as well as at least one individual interview. Thus, the patients are guaranteed a total of at least 20 psychotherapeutic contacts with their reference therapist within a 5-week stay. Nine of the sub-teams of this department are specialized in treating depressive patients. However, there are conceptual differences between the sub-teams (see below).

For patients with psychiatric comorbidities, disorder-specific group therapies are offered, which are applied across all the teams and can thus be attended by those patients referred to by their sub-teams. According to cognitive-behavioral treatment principles, manualized group therapies are facilitated for people with anxiety disorders, pain disorders, obesity, binge eating disorder, obsessive-compulsive disorder, and tinnitus. In addition to these symptom-oriented skills, training is also offered according to the Dialectic Behavioral Therapy (DBT) created by Linehan [16]. These groups take place once or twice a week and each has a duration of 90–120 min per week.

In addition to the groups for the treatment of existing mental illnesses, further non-disorder-specific group therapy is offered. In these groups, patients are trained in general life skills (which are relevant at the ICF level of activities) geared toward coping with difficulties and not necessarily related to a specific psychiatric disorder. Examples include stress management, enjoyment training, social competences training, and imagination groups. In addition, there is a metacognitive training (MCT) group based on metacognitive therapy techniques, in which patients learn a new way of dealing with rumination or worrying thoughts.

Within this context, two separate groups are offered, which have a special working reference within the framework of medical-occupational rehabilitation (medizinisch-berufliche rehabilitation). One group, the so-called professional competence group, is designed to recognize, solve, and avoid workplace conflicts and interpersonal problems, such as bullying. The other group is known as the work-related motivation group. In this group, special focus is given to building up the systematic motivation necessary to take a proactive position and to (re-)enter professional life. Above all, the therapeutic community with other affected people can also be used as a resource to reduce the often-present despair or the sometimes-exaggerated concerns of returning to the workplace. The disorder-specific groups each have a timeframe of about 60–120 min per week.

In addition to goal-oriented therapeutic interventions for the reduction of unhelpful behavior and symptoms, resource-oriented approaches are also used to tap into previously unused potential and abilities of the patient. These well-prepared, high-quality, therapeutically guided cognitive-behavioral group therapies are not simply about psychoeducation or group participant interaction. Instead, in these groups, the therapeutic process between the individual participants and the therapist can be advanced and expanded, especially after appropriate preparation

Medical Director											
Consultant Psychiatrist 1						Consultant Psychiatrist 2					
Consultant Psychologist											
TEAM 1		**TEAM 2**		**TEAM 3**		**TEAM 4**		**TEAM 5**		**TEAM 6**	
Team 1A	Team 1B	Team 2A	Team 2B	Team 3A	Team 3B	Team 4A	Team 4B	Team 5A	Team 5B	Team 6A	Team 6B
Medical Indication: Depressive disorders Old-age depression	**Medical Indication:** Recurrent depressive disorders Personality disorders	**Medical Indication:** Somatic symptom disorders Pain disorders Migraine and chronic headache	**Medical Indication:** Somatic symptom disorders	**Medical Indication:** Anxiety Disorders Somatic symptom disorders Trauma-related disorders	**Medical Indication:** Obsessive-compulsive disorders Eating disorders Dissociative disorders	**Medical Indication:** Burnout-type depression Disorders related to conflicts at the workplace	**Medical Indication:** Burnout-type depression in workers	**Medical Indication:** Bereavement - and loss-type depression Adaptation disorder	**Medical Indication:** Chronic depressive disorder	**Medical Indication:** Burnout-type depression in managers	**Medical Indication:** Burnout-type depression in academics and helping professions
Therapeutic concept: Cognitive behaviour therapy for depression	**Therapeutic concept:** Schema therapy	**Therapeutic concept:** Cognitive behaviour therapy for pain disorders	**Therapeutic concept:** Cognitive behaviour therapy for depression and pain disorders	**Therapeutic concept:** Cognitive behaviour therapy for depression and pain disorders	**Therapeutic concept:** Exposition-focussed cognitive behaviour therapy	**Therapeutic concept:** Cognitive behaviour therapy plus stress training Social competences training	**Therapeutic concept:** Cognitive behaviour therapy plus stress training	**Therapeutic concept:** Cognitive behaviour therapy for depression plus interventions for anxiety and bereavement	**Therapeutic concept:** Cognitive Behavioural Analysis System of Psychotherap y	**Therapeutic concept:** Cognitive behaviour therapy plus stress training and coaching	**Therapeutic concept:** Cognitive behaviour therapy plus stress training
Psychologist 1	**Psychologist 2**	**Psychologist 1**	**Psychologist 2**	**Psychologist 1**	**Psychologist 2**	**Psychologist 1**	**Psychologist 2**	**Psychologist 1**	**Psychologist 2**	**Psychologist 1**	**Psychologist 2**
Ward Doctor		**Ward Doctor**		**Ward Doctor**		**Ward Doctor**		**Ward Doctor**		**Ward Doctor**	

Table 1.
Structure of the Psychosomatic Department of the Sachsenklinik Bad Lausick, Germany.

during individual therapy. Furthermore, these therapies provide opportunities to exchange experiences, to learn from other patients as well as the group leader, and test new behaviors in a protected environment, guided by the group therapist. Group psychotherapy is particularly well suited for the treatment of disorders that manifest predominantly in a group context [17, 18]. The experience gained in the group, the acquired knowledge, and the acquired abilities can be further strengthened in individual therapy. Overall, patients receive an average of 40–50 psychotherapy hours during their stay.

Although the main emphasis is on psychotherapy, drug treatment is also an important part of the overall treatment. As the name would suggest, in the bio-psycho-social approach, drug therapy is seen as an equally important treatment modality. Based on the latest evidence available, a combination of psychotherapy and antidepressant medication seems to be of most benefit for patients with depres-sive disorders [19], specifically with regard to QoL.

Another treatment modality available to medical professionals is light therapy. This treatment has been successfully used in seasonal depression and is scientifically recognized as an effective biological treatment methodology. Given its successful application in SAD, light therapy can also be utilized for other types of depression, where indications that this type of chronobiologic therapy could be beneficial are present [20].

Ultimately, the use of biofeedback is a treatment approach worthy of consideration. Patients could greatly benefit from being trained in this domain as disorder symptoms could potentially be reduced via feedback of otherwise unconsciously running processes controlled by the autonomic nervous system [21].

Complementary therapies: Occupational therapy (OT) includes classic OT, project-oriented OT, and expression-centered OT, within which patients learn different creative techniques. Thusly, patient resources and capabilities are rediscovered or reactivated. Participation in OT is thought to help in building up positive activities and lead to further insights that may be important for psychotherapy such as realizing one's own perfectionism.

In addition to this, specific measures of the medical-occupational rehabilitation are assessed using standardized tests. These could include workplace and concentration training, stress tests in the artisan or office work area, as well as targeted work-related skills tests. Examples of these are the "Diagnostic Instrument to Assess Work Skills" (IDA—Instrumentarium zur Diagnostik von Arbeitsfähigkeiten) and the "Psychological Traits Profiles for the Integration of Disabled People to Work" (MELBA—Psychologische Merkmalsprofile zur Eingliederung Behinderter in Arbeit). For patients with office jobs, workplace training is also offered for ergo-nomic sitting and working.

Art therapy, a predominantly non-linguistic therapeutic method, is a suitable open and direct emotional approach, which can be very beneficial to patients who have very limited contact with their emotions. In the Psychosomatic Department, art therapy is based on the concept of schema therapy.

Physiotherapy and sports therapy offer a wide range of therapeutic measures ranging from active sports therapy, to specific individual physiotherapy, to interaction-centered groups and, to medical training. The medical-occupational rehabilitation model also utilizes body-oriented workplace training along with problem-specific function-related physiotherapeutic tests and assessments. Furthermore, passive and relieving therapy measures, such as relaxation baths and massages, are also used where necessary, especially at the beginning of the therapeutic process.

The main relaxation technique, which is taught and practiced in our department is Progressive Muscle Relaxation (PMR) as described by Jacobson [22].

Alternatively, the Autogenic Training according to Schultz [23] is used. In addition, as a further relaxation measure, mindfulness and body-centered procedures such as yoga, TaiChi, QiGong, and specific exercises focusing on body perception are offered.

Dietary and nutritional therapy is an integral part of the therapeutic concept in patients with comorbid problematic eating behaviors. A dietary consultation is offered to all patients who have experienced nutritional or weight-related problems such as obesity or binge eating disorder.

Social therapy, which is usually facilitated by a social worker, consists of counseling on various issues relating to social law and participation in working life. This may include getting in contact with external institutions such as integration services, employment or pension agencies, as well as other appropriate services. In addition, social services also provide support with contacting the employer to plan a stepwise return to work, or to adjust the work plan or job description so that reintegration into the workplace can be as smooth as possible. Additionally, within this framework of the medical-occupational rehabilitation approach, social services can organize and support external stress tests in either a simulated or the actual working environment of the patient.

Special consideration of clinical subtypes of depression: Depressive disorders can show a variety of symptom clusters. Thus, it makes sense to have sub-teams that can offer more tailored approaches for each of the following specific symptom clusters:

- Chronic forms of affective disorders like dysthymia, chronic depression, and double depression.

- Depressive forms with predominant exhaustion and, in some cases, workplace-related conflict situations, which are often also referred to as "burnout syndrome."

- Depressive disorders after loss and death, which may be similar to the symptom pattern of stress-related disorders or grief disorder.

- Depressive forms complicated by specific personality traits, the so-called maladaptive schemata [14].

- Chronic or ever-flaring depressive pictures that can be described as post-traumatic embitterment [24], where there is a strong correlation between the individual's biography and certain traumatic experiences or failed adaptive performance.

In the context of psychosomatic medicine, therapies can be individually tailored with the intention of improving their effectiveness and generating a better subjec-tive understanding among patients. The assumptions and techniques of classic cognitive behavioral therapy (especially the development of activities and cognitive restructuring) form the basis of these therapies, since CBT has shown the most efficacy in these disorders, and its high efficiency and long-term effects are empiri-cally well documented [25, 26].

Through the systematic development of positive activities, which, in addition to leisure activities and enjoyment, can also include duties, work or other tasks, the patients are brought back into a more proactive position, thereby reducing "learned helplessness" as described by Alloy and Seligman [27]. For many patients, positive activities must be discovered or rediscovered and systematically practiced. As part of further treatment, the focus is on emotional perception and cognitive acceptance of the positive activities, which can be promoted by additional use of "mindfulness" and mindfulness techniques (according to Linehan [16]). Furthermore, a so-called "euthymic therapy," also referred to as genus training, is deemed to be very useful in this context [28].

In cognitive therapy, patients are guided toward dealing with negative cognitions in a systematic manner. The depressed and exaggerated negative character of the thoughts is examined against reality, and an attempt into modifying these thoughts into more helpful ones is made [29–31]. In addition, according to Wells, metacognitive therapy can also be used to improve mood and cognitive processes [32]. This is deemed to be particularly helpful in patients with constant negative thoughts and rumination. In the following paragraphs, we will explain the therapeutic focus relevant to each sub-team.

Focus on "Burnout" type: Burnout had originally been characterized by a pronounced physical, mental, and emotional exhaustion due to occupational stress and repeated frustration in caring professions. Over the years, the concept has expanded to include depressive syndromes, which are closely related to occupational or private stress [33]. Important therapeutic aims for these patients (treated by a specialist sub-team) could be to rediscover the positive aspects that originally gave meaning and pleasure to their work, to learn how to deal with frustrations, to clarify responsibilities at work, to identify stress-aggravating thoughts, to identify resources available to them, and to formulate achievable goals.

Focus on loss, grief, and adjustment processes: Patients whose depressive symptoms are related to a loss are allocated to a specific sub-team. This includes patients who are bereaved, those who have experienced separation or divorce, loss of home or property as well as those who are suffering from a physical illness. For all these situations, the common thread is the necessity for fundamental reorientation. Typical dysfunctional assumptions must be addressed (e.g., "If I stop mourning, it means that it (the loss) did not mean anything to me." or "The more you have loved a person, the longer you mourn"). Thus, patients need guidance to develop new and more realistic beliefs that enable them to view their life in a positive light. The specialized sub-team endeavors to achieve this by applying wisdom therapy [34] and Worden's Tasks of Mourning [35]. It also considers the role of avoidance or excessive work engagement as being a potentially unhealthy and harmful coping strategy (according to Rosner et al. [36]).

Focus on personality traits: Recurrent depressive disorders are frequently accompanied by unhelpful personality traits or personality disorders, which contribute significantly to the maintenance of the depressive disorder and therapy resistance [37]. These disturbances are treated in the Department of Psychosomatic Medicine using schema therapy developed by Jeffrey Young.

Using the Young Schema Questionnaire (YSQ) [38], the maladaptive cogni-tive and emotional schemata of the patient are identified, and personality-related problems are communicated to the patient in a transparent and friendly way that motivates the patient to cooperate [39]. Changes are achieved by imaginative, emotion- or relationship-oriented, or cognitive behavioral therapy [40]. In the Psychosomatic Department, weekly group exercises take place in the context of imagination exercises, in which the patient's injurious and traumatizing experiences of childhood are re-scripted by the introduction of a protective and helping person (in part the therapist, ideally the patient in the "healthy adult mode" themselves).

In addition, during weekly individual and group therapy sessions, specific exercises are employed. Any changes in the experience of the exercise and any accompanying behavior change are discussed, and appropriate responses are practiced. In this way, common, everyday scenarios are evaluated on memo cards and healthy adult behavior patterns are worked out and practiced.

Focus on chronic depression: Chronic forms of depression like persistent depressive disorder (formerly known as dysthymia), major depressive disorder (MDD), and double depression are a challenge to clinicians as these patients often do not respond to common psychotherapeutic or pharmacological treatment [41]. However, for patients with these presentations, a specialized psychotherapy treatment that shows satisfactory response rates is available. The Cognitive Behavioral Analysis System of Psychotherapy (CBASP) developed by McCullough and Negt et al. [15, 42] postulate that chronically depressed patients remain at the stage of preoperational thinking (according to Piaget) due to their specific learning history that took place during their cognitive-emotional development. Thought is therefore characterized by a global, pre-linguistic style, a strongly egocentric view, and the inability to feel authentic interpersonal empathy [43]. Moreover, their ability to regulate their mood is severely restricted; they experience constant depressive mood independent of external factors or influence, which they perceive as com-pletely unchangeable. In the context of CBASP, these patients are guided to develop their thinking style from preoperational thinking to formal operational thinking, and to establish more appropriate responses to external influences, including the therapist. Hence, CBASP is a method used to teach patients how to gradually reach the formal operational stage of cognitive thinking and to break the psychic barrier between themselves and their environment.

In addition to individual therapy, there are two further core elements of CBASP: situational analysis (according to McCullough) as well as a social competence train-ing specifically tailored to the CBASP model. In situational analysis, real-life occur-rences on the ward are thought about and analyzed. This is an essential technique of CBASP that teaches patients to recognize their own impact on the course and quality of their life. The social competence training serves to make patients aware of the influence of their behavior on others by means of exercises in the group context, and to jointly work out the desirable behavior in role-play situations with the aid of video feedback.

7. Conclusion

Taken together, we have outlined how the increasing incidence and prevalence of mental disorders, and specifically depressive disorders in Germany, has led to an escalating burden on public and private health, and pension insurance.

Consequently, pension insurance companies, such as the German Statutory Pension Insurance, are supporting therapy and rehabilitation in psychotherapy-focused psychosomatic rehabilitation hospitals. We have further explained that in these rehabilitation hospitals, the ICF and rehabilitation therapy standards play an essential diagnostic and therapeutic role. To explain how medical-occupational rehabilitation works in practice, we have used the Psychosomatic Department of the Sachsenklinik Bad Lausick as an example to illustrate how patients are treated with medical-psychological and complementary therapies by taking their specific depressive subtype into account. This article raises further questions about how the care and rehabilitation of patients with depression should be financed and com-missioned, how diagnostic approaches can meet the needs of the patients, whether we can distinguish clinical subtypes of depression with certainty, and how much evidence we have for the specific therapies currently available.

In principle, there are four main ways to fund treatment for mental health problems. Patients can pay privately for their treatment, a public or private health insurance covers the cost of treatment, a pension insurance, or pension fund sponsor the treatment, or costs are covered by the state. To fund treatment for mental health issues such as depression privately can be difficult or impossible, if people are not wealthy, because low income and indebtedness may have already been a contributing factor for the development of depression [44], and depression might lead to further debts due to medical bill problems [45]. Additionally, one has to consider that treatment time for depression might be unforeseeably long, especially in the case of a recurring or chronic depressive disorder. Public or private health insurances will provide the funding, if they cover mental health. However, they are only obligated to cover treatment costs where the patient has a formal diagnosis according to the ICD-10 [8] or the DSM-5 [46] and where the treatment is proposed according to national guidelines, such as the German national guide-lines for the treatment of depression (S3-Leitlinie/Nationale VersorgungsLeitlinie Unipolare Depression) [9]. Consequently, rehabilitation in which the main aim is increasing people's functional level as well as their quality of life, is usually not covered by health insurance. In Germany, this is paid for by pension insurance, if approved. Having different insurance providers dealing with different aspects of the same disorder can be quite challenging. For clinicians, it is sometimes tricky to decide whether the patient needs acute hospital treatment or medical-occupational rehabilitation, since treatment approaches often overlap. At first glance, it might seem more practical and efficient for the state to fund treatment, as is the case in the UK. However, at a closer look one can discern that even in the case of the UK, one has to apply for funding to different funding streams within the NHS (e.g., NHS England, Clinical Commissioning Groups, etc.). Hence, there does not seem to be a funding system to cover mental health costs in place that is generally agreed upon. Nevertheless, from the insurer's, the patients', and certainly the employers' perspective, a pension insurance-funded rehabilitation makes particularly good sense for those with depression who need and want support in order to resume working activities.

Accurately diagnosing mental disorders has always been a challenge, hence the constant revision of diagnostic entities and criteria; the 5th edition of the DSM and the soon to be 11th edition of ICD are a case in point. However, these diagnostic classifications base diagnoses mainly on acute symptoms, and less so on the level of functioning and QoL. As such, the WHO's ICF [10] complements the ICD, providing a more holistic diagnosis. Thus, the emphasis on ICF by pension insurance-financed psychosomatic hospitals for medical-occupational rehabilita-tion indicates their commitment to a comprehensive assessment of depressed patients.

A perhaps more controversial point worthy of discussion is the decision-making process by which patients are allocated to certain sub-teams in the Psychosomatic Department of the Sachsenklinik Bad Lausick, the case presented. The procedure suggests that certain subtypes of depression are assumed: the burnout, the loss and grief, the complicated personality, and the chronic subtype. However, there is currently no scientific evidence that supports the existence of these subtypes. In fact, diagnostic and genetic research has recently come up with two main subtypes of depression, an anxious subtype that is characterized by decreased appetite and body weight, and insomnia and suicidal ideation, and a metabolic subtype show-ing increased appetite and weight, low energy, hypersomnia, leaden paralysis, and a poor metabolic profile [47–49]. Despite the research evidence for these subtypes, they seem to be irrelevant for the purposes of treatment, since there are no subtype-specific treatment algorithms available. Another approach would be to define subtypes according to treatment response. This approach has been used in psychiatry since the development of tricyclic antidepressants, and subtypes were suggested according to whether patients responded or not respond to tricyclic antidepressant treatment [50]. This strategy seems natural from a practical point of view, and this line of thinking is the basis of how patients are assigned to specialized sub-teams who offer a specific psychotherapeutic focus. The question whether wisdom therapy [34] and the Worden's Tasks of Mourning model [35] are the best approach for people suffering from bereavement and loss, whether schema therapy according to Jeffrey Young [39] is most effective to treat patients with personality difficulties, whether CBASP is most efficient in patients with chronic depression, and—last but not least—whether inpatient rehabilitation is necessary and superior to outpatient rehabilitation and treatment, however, is beyond the scope of this article.

In summary, this article provides a review of the literature on rehabilitation for depression in psychosomatic hospitals in Germany. It highlights the importance of thinking beyond the clinical diagnosis by taking the level of functioning and QoL into account during assessment and therapeutic goal setting. It also explains the practicalities of medical-occupational inpatient rehabilitation for depression by reference to the Psychosomatic Department of the Sachsenklinik Bad Lausick. Questions which remain unanswered are how to fund rehabilitation for depressed patients in the best way possible, how to define subtypes of depression in order to provide an individually tailored therapy for people with depression, and what therapies and in what settings they are most effective.

Based on the example of how psychosomatic inpatient rehabilitation for people with depression is delivered at the Sachsenklinik Bad Lausick, this article reflected on the following principal ideas about psychosomatic and psychiatric diagnoses, individually tailored care as well as care provision and funding.

- Disease models can be based on the etiology, the pathophysiology, symptoms or symptom clusters, diagnoses, the level of functioning, activities and partici-pation, and QoL. Thus, in practice, a holistic diagnostic approach should not only make use of a disease classification but should also comprise an assess-ment of functioning, disability, and overall health.

- Therapies should be individually tailored; this can be achieved taking patient characteristics, personal and environmental factors, the diagnostic subtype, the profile of symptoms and impairments, the availability of therapies, and individual preferences of the patients and their therapists into account.

- Psychosomatic medicine aspires to holistic treatment approaches that consider a variety of therapeutic modalities such as psychoeducation, psychotherapy, pharmacotherapy and other biological therapies, OT, art and music therapy, skills training, movement therapy and physiotherapy, social work, family work, and self-help.

- Potential sources of funding for psychosomatic treatment include public institutions, private assets, and public or private health or pension insurances.

Funding statement

Hubertus Himmerich has received salary support from the National Institute for Health Research (NIHR) Biomedical Research Centre (BRC) at South London and Maudsley NHS Foundation Trust (SLaM) and King's College London. Olivia Patsalos is funded by OBELIX (Obesity, Lifestyle and Learning from Extreme Phenotypes), a research framework within the Biomedical Research Centre (BRC) of the South London and Maudsley NHS Foundation Trust (SLaM) and the IoPPN.

Declaration of interest

The authors declare no conflict of interest.

Author details

Ralf F. Tauber[1], Carola Nisch[1], Mutahira M. Qureshi[2], Olivia Patsalos[2] and Hubertus Himmerich[2,3*]

1 Fachabteilung für Psychosomatik, Sachsenklinik, Bad Lausick, Germany

2 Department of Psychological Medicine, Institute of Psychiatry, Psychology and Neuroscience, King's College London, London, UK

3 South London and Maudsley NHS Foundation Trust, London, UK

*Address all correspondence to: hubertus.himmerich@kcl.ac.uk

References

[1] Whiteford HA, Degenhardt L, Rehm J, et al. Global burden of disease attributable to mental and substance use disorders: Findings from the global burden of disease study 2010. Lancet. 2013;**382**:1575-1586

[2] Krankenkasse T. Gesundheitsreport 2016-Veröffentlichungen zum Betrieblichen Gesundheitsmanagement der TK. Retrieved from: www.tk.de [Accessed: 13 February 2020]

[3] Augurzky B, Wübker A, Pilny A, et al. Barmer GEK Report Krankenhaus 2016. Schriftenreihe zur Gesundheitsanalyse Band 40. Available from: http://dnb.ddb.de [Accessed: 13 February 2020]

[4] Cost of illness—Statistisches Bundesamt. Available from: https://www.destatis.de/EN/Themes/Society-Environment/Health/Cost-Illness/_node.html. [Accessed: 13 February 2020]

[5] Sheehan D, Nakagome K, Asami Y, et al. Restoring function in major depressive disorder: A systematic review. Journal of Affective Disorders. 2017;**215**:299-313

[6] DRV. Statistiken und Berichte-Statistiken und Berichte. Available from: https://www.deutsche-rentenversicheru-ng.de/DRV/DE/Experten/Zahlen-und-Fakten/Statistiken-und-Berichte/statist-iken_ und_berichte.html?https=1&nn-=254258 [Accessed: 13 February 2020]

[7] DRV. Homepage-Positionspapier der Deutschen Rentenversicherung zur Bedeutung psychischer Erkrankungen in der Rehabilitation und bei Erwerbsminderung. Available from: https://deutsche-rentenversicherung.de/SharedDocs/Downloads/DE/Experten/infos_reha_einrichtungen/konzepte_systemfragen/positionspapiere/pospap_psych_Erkrankung.html;jsessionid=59BD594F6D21E986C221DFBD3928D4F8. delivery1-9-replication. [Accessed: 13 February 2020]

[8] World Health Organization. The ICD-10 Classification of Mental and Behavioral Disorders: Clinical Descriptions and Diagnostic Guidelines. Geneva PP, Geneva: World Health Organization. Available from: https://apps.who.int/iris/handle/10665/37958 [Accessed: 13 February 2020]

[9] DGPPN, Bäk, KBV, et al. S3-Leitlinie/Nationale VersorgungsLeitlinie Unipolare Depression-Langfassung. Available from: https://www.awmf.org/uploads/tx_szleitlinien/nvl-005l_S3_Unipolare_Depression_2017-05.pdf. [Accessed: 13 February 2020]

[10] Towards a Common Language for Functioning, Disability and The International Classification of Functioning, Disability and Health. Available from: https://www.who.int/classifications/icf/icfbeginnersguide.pdf [Accessed: 13 February 2020]

[11] Nisch C, Tauber RF, Himmerich H. Stationäre Psychotherapie der Depression: Kliniken, Leitlinien, Methoden und Herausforderungen. Die Psychiatrie. 2017;**14**:143-150

[12] Deutsche Rentenversicherung Bund. Reha-Therapiestandards Depressive Störungen. Berlin; 2016

[13] KTL Klassifikation therapeutischer Leistungen in der medizinischen Rehabilitation Deutsche Rentenversicherung. Available from: www.deutsche-rentenversicherung.de [Accessed: 13 February 2020]

[14] Kellogg SH, Young JE. Schema therapy for borderline personality disorder. Journal of Clinical Psychology. 2006;**62**:445-458

[15] McCullough JP. Treatment for chronic depression using cognitive behavioral analysis system of psychotherapy (CBASP). Journal of Clinical Psychology. 2019;**59**:833-846

[16] Linehan M. Dialektisch-behaviorale Therapie der Borderline-Persönlichkeitsstörung. CIP-Medien: München; 1996

[17] Grawe K, Donati R, Bernauer F. Psychotherapie im Wandel Von der Konfession zur Profession. Göttingen: Hogrefe; 1994

[18] Grawe K, Donati R, Bernauer F. Psychotherapie Im Wandel. 4th ed. Göttingen: Hogrefe; 2001

[19] Kamenov K, Twomey C, Cabello M, et al. The efficacy of psychotherapy, pharmacotherapy and their combination on functioning and quality of life in depression: A meta-analysis. Psychological Medicine. 2017;**47**:414-425

[20] Even C, Schröder CM, Friedman S, et al. Efficacy of light therapy in nonseasonal depression: A systematic review. Journal of Affective Disorders. 2008;**108**:11-23

[21] Blase KL, van Dijke A, Cluitmans PJM, et al. Efficacy of HRV-biofeedback as additional treatment of depression and PTSD. Tijdschrift voor Psychiatrie. 2016;**58**:292-300

[22] Jacobson E. Progressive Relaxation. 2nd ed. Oxford: University Chicago Press; 1938

[23] Schultz JH, Luthe W. Autogenic Training: A Psychophysiologic Approach to Psychotherapy. Oxford: Grune & Stratton; 1959

[24] Linden M, Baumann K, Rotter M, et al. The psychopathology of posttraumatic embitterment disorders. Psychopathology. 2007;**40**:159-165

[25] Lepping P, Whittington R, Sambhi RS, et al. Clinical relevance of findings in trials of CBT for depression. European Psychiatry. 2017;**45**:207-211

[26] Gloaguen V, Cottraux J, Cucherat M, et al. A meta-analysis of the effects of cognitive therapy in depressed patients. Journal of Affective Disorders. 1998;**49**:59-72

[27] Alloy LB, Seligman MEP. On the cognitive component of learned helplessness and depression. In: Bower G, editor. The Psychology of Learning and Motivation. Vol. 13. New York: Academic Press; 1979

[28] Koppenhofer E. Kleine Schule des Geniessens: Ein verhaltenstherapeutisch orientierter Behandlungsansatz zum Aufbau positiven Erlebens und Handelns. Lengerich: Pabst Science Publishers; 2004

[29] Beck AT, Rush AJ, Shaw BF, et al. Cognitive Therapy of Depression. New York: Guilford Press; 1979

[30] Beck AT. Prisoners of Hate: The Cognitive Basis of Anger, Hostility, and Violence. New York: Harper Collins; 1999

[31] Meichenbaum DH. Cognitive-behavioral therapy in historical perspective. In: Bongar BM, Beutler LE, editors. Oxford Textbooks in Clinical Psychology, Vol. 1. Comprehensive Textbook of Psychotherapy: Theory and Practice. New York: Oxford University Press; 1995

[32] Fisher P, Wells A. Metacognitive therapy: Distinctive features. Available from: https://content.taylorfrancis.com/books/download?dac=C2009-0-06548-X&isbn=9781134108688&format=googlePreviewPdf [Accessed: 13 February 2020]

[33] Von Känel R. Das Burnout-Syndrom: Eine medizinische perspektive. Praxis. 2008;**97**:477-487

[34] Baumann K, Linden M. Weisheitstherapie. Verhaltenstherapiemanual. Berlin, Heidelberg: Springer Berlin Heidelberg; 2008. Available from: http://link.springer.com/10.1007/978-3-540-75740-5_82 [Accessed: 13 February 2020]

[35] Worden JW. Grief Counseling and Grief Therapy: A Handbook for the Mental Health Practitioner. 4th ed. New York: Springer Publishing Company; 2009

[36] Rosner R, Pfoh G, Kotoučová M. Treatment of complicated grief. European Journal of Psychotraumatology. 2011;**2**:7995

[37] Young M. Treatment-resistant depression: The importance of identifying and treating co-occurring personality disorders. The Psychiatric Clinics of North America. 2018;**41**:249-261

[38] Young JE, Brown G. Young schema questionnaire. In: Young JE, editor. Cognitive therapy for personality disorders: A schema-focused approach. Sarasota: Professional Resource Press; 1994

[39] Young JE, Klosko JS, Weishaar ME. Schema Therapy: A practitioner's Guide. New York: Guilford Press; 2003

[40] Rafaeli E, Bernstein D, Young J. Schema therapy: Distinctive features. Available from: https://www.taylorfrancis.com/books/9780203841709 [Accessed: 13 February 2020]

[41] Schüle C. Chronische Depression - Epidemiologische Daten und therapeutische Möglichkeiten. Fortschritte der Neurologie Psychiatrie. 2014;**82**:155-173

[42] Negt P, Brakemeier EL, Michalak J, et al. The treatment of chronic depression with cognitive behavioral analysis system of psychotherapy: A systematic review and meta-analysis of randomized-controlled clinical trials. Brain and Behavior. 2016;**6**:e00486

[43] Piaget J. The Origins of Intelligence in Children. 2nd ed. New York: International Universities Press; 1952

[44] Turunen E, Hiilamo H. Health effects of indebtedness: A systematic review. BMC Public Health. 2014;**14**:489

[45] Tu HT. Rising health costs, medical debt and chronic conditions. Issue Brief (Center for Studying Health System Change). 2004;**88**:1-5

[46] American Psychiatric Association. Diagnostic and Statistical Manual of Mental Disorders. 5th ed. Arlington: APA Publishing; 2013

[47] Lamers F, De Jonge P, Nolen WA, et al. Identifying depressive subtypes in a large cohort study: Results from the Netherlands study of depression and anxiety (NESDA). Journal of Clinical Psychiatry. 2010;**71**:1582-1589

[48] Milaneschi Y, Lamers F, Peyrot WJ, et al. Polygenic dissection of major depression clinical heterogeneity. Molecular Psychiatry. 2016;**21**:516-522

[49] Penninx BWJH, Milaneschi Y, Lamers F, et al. Understanding the somatic consequences of depression: Biological mechanisms and the role of depression symptom profile. BMC Medicine. 2013;**11**:129

[50] Kupfer DJ, Pickar D, Himmelhoch JM, et al. Are there two types of unipolar depression? Archives of General Psychiatry. 1975;**32**:866-871

4

Psychosomatic Approach to Fibromyalgia Syndrome: Medical, Psychological and Social Aspects

José Vicente Martínez-Quiñones, Mar Martínez Gamarra and Ignacio Jáuregui-Lobera

Abstract

Management of patients who describe chronic pain all over the body, associated with a range of symptoms as sleep disturbance, overwhelming fatigue, alteration in mood, or psychological distress that worsens the quality of life, is often complex and challenging. This syndrome has been named by terms such as "neurasthenia," "fibrositis," and "fibromyalgia". At the present time, fibromyalgia is considered the most common central sensitivity syndrome, affecting over 5% of the population, being often observed in people with rheumatic conditions. While typically presenting in middle-aged women, fibromyalgia can affect both sexes at any age. The causes of fibromyalgia remain unknown. Significant research findings have focused on dysfunction of central pain processing, with defects in the ascending and descending pain pathways leading to increased pain perception. There are two methods used in the diagnosis of fibromyalgia: *criteria-based diagnosis* and *clinical diagnosis*. Although fibromyalgia defies definitively efficacious management, much evidence underlies the importance of treating the psychological factors that affect pain management process. The primary purpose of this paper is to provide a psychosomatic approach to fibromyalgia from three points of view of processing: the viewpoint of the medical profession, the position of the psychologist, and finally the way of thinking of people.

Keywords: fibromyalgia, psychosomatic, chronic pain, central sensitivity syndrome

1. Introduction

Under conditions of psychological dysregulation or disease, pain can lose its physiological role and take on an aberrant course, resulting in chronic pain syndromes [1].

As doctors, we often take care of patients who describe chronic pain all over the body, which is associated with a range of other symptoms including poor sleep, fatigue, and depression. This complex of symptoms is sometimes referred to as *functional somatic syndrome*, part of a *somatization disorder*, *idiopathic pain disorder*, or *psychosomatic syndrome*, dismissing the true suffering of the patients [2]. By reason of that, it is not unusual for patients to see at least four physicians before the diagnosis is made.

At the present time, we know that fibromyalgia (FM) is a nonprogressive and nondegenerative syndrome with a spectrum of symptoms that most commonly include generalized chronic pain. It affects 0.4–8.8% of the general population worldwide, with a global mean prevalence of 2.7%, with women outnumbering men by an average of 3:1 [3].

FM is defined as a central sensitization syndrome characterized by chronic extensive "centralized pain." Central sensitization, as well, is defined as the process of becoming susceptible to a given stimulus that previously had no effect or signif-icance (i.e., pressure, light, medication, temperature) [4]. This increased central responsiveness causes hyperalgesia, allodynia, and pain across multiple spinal segments, leading to chronic widespread pain [2].

Although FM is commonly classified as "functional," because its etiology, pathogenesis, and symptoms are not completely explained, rheumatologists, pain specialists, and increasingly primary care providers are gaining confidence in making this diagnosis and initiating treatment [5].

Historically, its definition and content have changed repeatedly in the more than 100 years of its existence. Different terms have been proposed by the medical science [6–14], which summarizes the lack of understanding of this argumentative condition, which has evolved from a regional pain disorder to a multiple symptoms disorder [15] (**Table 1**).

Nowadays the ICD-11 considers FM to be a form of chronic widespread pain (CWP) [16, 17], besides it considers CWP a form of chronic primary pain (MG30.0) and is present when:

A. Chronic pain (persistent or recurrent pain for longer than 3 months) is present in at least three body quadrants plus the axial skeleton (4 of 5 regions).

B. The pain is associated with at least one of the following:

1. Emotional distress due to pain is present.

2. The pain interferes with daily life activities and social participation.

Disorders	Features
Neurasthenia Nervous exhaustion	Pathological entity in which there is a functional nervous dysfunction manifested by marked fatigability and irritability affecting various organs and functions without any demonstrable pathological tissue changes [6]. This term was abandoned in the 1930s
Fibrositis	Inflammation of white fibrous tissue wherever situated (panniculitis, interstitial neuritis, myositis, bursitis, capsulitis, etc.). In this sense these terms merely indicate the position of the fibrous tissue which is implicated. Tenders point needed. Widespread aching. Fatigue [7–9]
Chronic fatigue syndrome Myalgic encephalomyelitis	Medical condition characterized by symptom clusters that include pathological fatigue and malaise that is worse after exertion, cognitive dysfunction, immune dysfunction, unrefreshing sleep, pain, autonomic dysfunction, neuroendocrine, and immune symptoms [10, 11]
Burn out	Represents the total depletion of one's physical and mental resources [12]
Chronic widespread pain (CWP)	A pain variable that would identify potential FM patients. It represents a categorical designation of musculoskeletal body pain defined by the location, distribution, and number of painful musculoskeletal body locations or sites [13, 14]

Table 1.
Fibromyalgia-like conditions.

C. The pain is not better accounted for by another chronic pain condition.

This definition seems to define a CWP as a disease or disorder. Neither FM nor CWP is obviously a distinct entity.

In addition to the direct physical suffering that patients experience, the biopsychosocial nature of chronic pain affects their social lives, ability to work, and psychological well-being. People with FM often reported dismissive attitudes from others, such as disbelief, stigmatization, lack of acceptance by their relatives, and friends, and doctors may consider them as *lazy* or *attention seeking* people, with their symptoms *all in their head* [2]. Such disdainfulness can have a substantial negative impact on patients, who are already distressed [18]. Furthermore, patients have an increased lifetime prevalence of many psychological disorders.

The primary purpose of this paper is to provide an approach to FM from three points of view of processing: the viewpoint of the medical profession, the position of the psychologist, and finally, social aspects.

1. The medical profession:
    a. Diagnostic criteria of FM
    b. Pathogenesis
    c. What causes FM? Predisposing factors
    d. Comorbidities:
        i. Other central sensitivity syndromes
        ii. Psychiatric
        iii. Nonpsychiatric: rheumatology
2. The position of the psychologist:
    a. Psychosomatic disease?
    b. Emotional dysregulation
    c. Address the psychological in FM:
        i. Our experience
        ii. The main topics from a psychological point of view
3. Social aspects. Impact at three levels:
    a. Family
    b. Labor
    c. Health system

2. The medical profession

2.1 Diagnostic criteria of fibromyalgia

Diagnosing FM is quite challenging because there is an absence of a univocal identified biological cause [19].

Although two methods are used in the diagnosis, criteria-based and clinical one, FM remains a controversial interpretation, with some studies suggesting that FM is overdiagnosed and other reporting that community physicians have limited knowledge of FM diagnosis and criteria:

2.1.1 Criteria-based diagnosis

FM became officially established by formal criteria in 1990 [20], after which a multiplicity of symptoms became a central component of the illness. Nowadays there is evidence in support of FM as a dimensional or continuum disorder [21, 22] which is included in the international list of diseases of the World Health Organization [17] (**Table 2**).

In 2016, the widespread pain criterion was reinstalled; thus FM diagnosis requires:

- Widespread pain index (WPI) ≥ 7 and symptom severity scale (SSS) ≥ 5 or a WPI of 4–6 and an SSS score ≥9
- Presence of widespread pain (pain in four or five body regions)
- Symptoms of at least 3 months of duration

Classification criteria may help guide a diagnosis but are primarily useful for research and epidemiological studies.

2.1.2 Clinical diagnosis

It is based on the physician/patient relationship. FM, because of symptoms' intensities (pervasive fatigue, abdominal cramps, headaches, disturbed sleep, muscle spasms, stiffness, tenderness, reduced physical, social and cognitive functioning, depressed mood, anxiety, and irritability), constitutes a heterogeneous disorder in which "chronic widespread pain" is dominant [23–28]. Moreover, FM differs from the "chronic widespread pain" by its inclusion of non-pain symptoms, including severity measures of fatigue, unrefreshed sleep, cognitive problems, and somatic symptoms [29].

Common manifestations in FM are *hyperalgesia* (excessive sensitivity to a normally painful stimulus, such as pressure), *allodynia* (painful sensation to a normally non-painful stimulus, e.g., touch and massage), expansion of the receptive field (pain beyond the area of peripheral nerve supply), prolonged electrophysiological discharge, an after-stimulus unpleasant quality of the pain (e.g., burning, throbbing, tingling, or numbness), and referred pain across multiple spinal segments, leading to chronic widespread pain [20]. The number of pain sites is strongly correlated with somatic and psychological symptom burden in the general population. An example of making a record of the pain sites is by the "Michigan body map" [30] (**Figure 1**).

American College of Rheumatology (ACR)	Criteria stablished	Clarification
1990 Wolfe et al. [20]	Chronic widespread pain (CWP) + Pain in 11 of 18 *tender point* sites on "digital palpation"	CWP: Simultaneous pain in the axial skeleton, in the left and the right side of the body, and above and below the waist, for at least 3 months "Digital palpation" should be performed with an approximate force of 4 Kg Tender point positive: the subject must state that the palpation was painful
2010 Wolfe et al. [21]	Widespread pain index (WPI) + Symptom severity scale (SSS): *Fatigue* *Waking unrefreshed* *Cognitive symptom*	WPI: areas with pain over the last week SSS: the sum of the severity of the three symptoms plus the extent (severity) of somatic symptoms in general "It does not require a tender point examination"
2011 Wolfe et al. [22]	Widespread pain index (WPI): Left *Shoulder* Right Lt. Upper *Arm* Rt. Lower Lt. *Hip* Rt. Lt. Upper *Leg* Rt. Lower Lt. *Jaw* Rt. *Chest* *Abdomen* *Upper Back Lower* *Neck* + Symptom severity (SS) score: *Fatigue* *Waking unrefreshed* *Cognitive symptom*	• WPI ≥ 7/19 and SS score ≥ 5/12 *or* WPI between 3–6/19 and SS score ≥ 9/12. • Symptoms have been present at a similar level for at least 3 months • The patient does not have a disorder that would otherwise sufficiently explain the pain WPI: In how many areas has the patient had pain?Score will be between 0 and 19 SS score: For the each of these three symptoms, indicate the level of severity over the past week using the following scale: 0 = no problem; 1 = slight or mild problems; generally mild or intermittent; 2 = moderate; considerable problems; often present and/or at a moderate level; 3 = severe: pervasive, continuous, life-disturbing problems The SS score is the sum of the severity of the three symptoms plus the sum of the number of the following symptoms occurring during the previous 6 months: headaches, pain or cramps in lower abdomen, and depression (0–3). The final score is between 0 and 12

Table 2.
Fibromyalgia criteria according to the American College of Rheumatology.

Quantitative sensory testing should be undertaken to determine if augmented response is present or absent, using pressure, pinprick, cold, heat, vibration, electricity, ischemia, and chemical (capsaicin, hypertonic saline) stimuli. Patients should be tested for allodynia (using cotton swab, brush, Von Frey filaments), temporal summation, conditioned pain modulation, and nociceptive flexion reflex.

All common conditions, like depression or FM, are caught in the dilemma of disease versus illness state (of health) versus trait (characteristic feature distinguishing a particular human being).

2.2 Pathogenesis

Given the high incidence of chronic pain, it is fundamental to understand basic processes underlying this kind of suffering: repeated stimulation of the centripetal

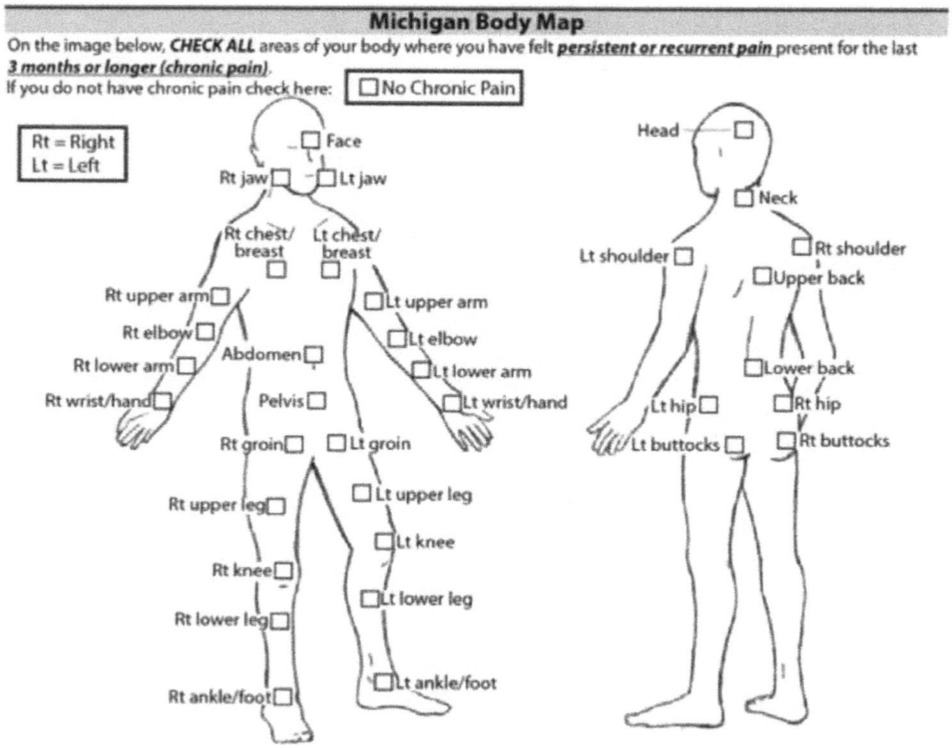

Figure 1.
The Michigan Body Map. ©2015 Regents of the University of Michigan (https://medicine.umich.edu/sites/default/files/content/downloads/MBM%202016.pdf).

nerves overtime causes changes to the way the pain signals are processed, leading to a pathophysiological state where the nervous system is sensitized and the perception of pain becomes heighten.

Both the peripheral and the central nervous system can become sensitize to pain signals in response to injury or inflammation nociceptors. The periphery can become more sensitive to painful stimuli, a process called "peripheral sensitization." These sensitize nociceptors and then send additional pain signals to the CNS which can lead to the overstimulation of the CNS.

"Central sensitization" is a proposed physiological phenomenon in which dysregulation in the central nervous system (imbalance between pain transmission and pain inhibition) causes neuronal dysregulation and hyperexcitability, resulting in hypersensitivity to both noxious and non-noxious stimuli and the perpetuation of pain [31] (**Figure 2**).

Central sensitization has been proposed as the root etiology for "central sensitivity syndromes" (CSS), which refer to a group of medically indistinct disorders for which no organic cause can be found. A number of authors state that the CSS symptoms are not medically explicable and are psychiatric, psychological, or psychosocial in nature [32–34]. Therefore, people with FM suffer from abnormalities in the central pain processing, what implies a lower threshold for interpreting sensory information as noxious, in addition to an increased excitation's mechanism or reduced inhibition's ones. This plays an important role in the development and maintenance of chronic pain.

On the other hand, some aberrations of the peripheral nervous system, as an antidromal axonal reflex of C fibers in response to a stimulus, may initialize

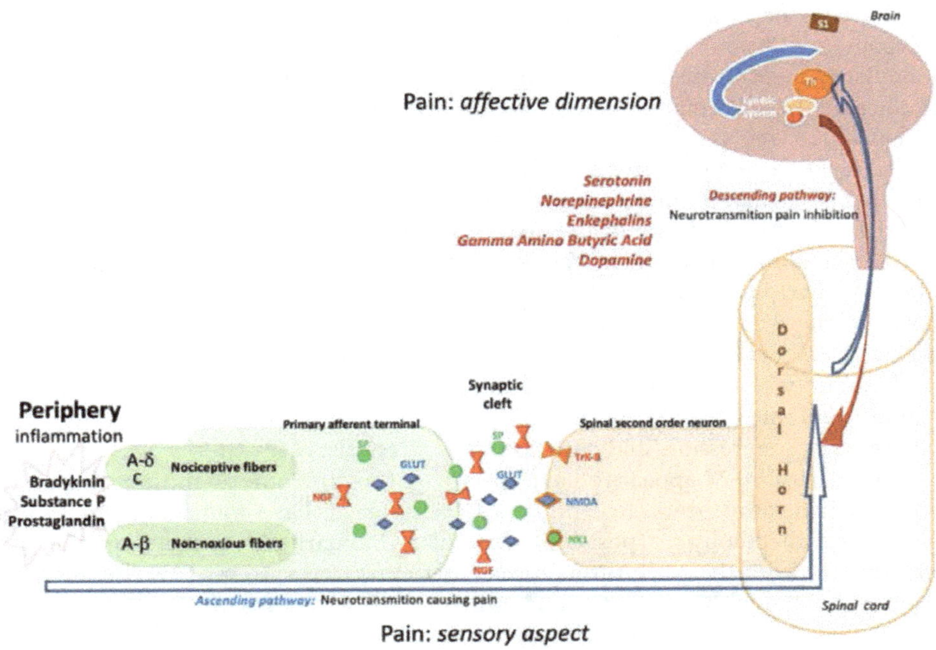

Figure 2.
Physiological pathways of pain. The activated C fibers express, at their nerve terminals, several neurotransmitters: Substance P (SP), nerve growth factor (NGF), calcitonin gene-related peptide, vasoactive intestinal peptide, glutamate (GLUT), aspartate, and brain-derived neurotrophic factor. These chemicals cause a barrage of impulses at the synapse that now hyperexcite the postsynaptic receptors: neurokinin1 (NK1), N-methyl-D-aspartate (NMDA), metabotropic glutamate, tyrosine kinase B (TrK-B), and protein kinase gamma. Activation of these receptors results in a remarkable physiologic change in the postsynaptic nerve cells, including membrane changes, intracellular influx of calcium, protein kinase activation, and expression of protein c-fos (marker for neuronal activity following peripheral stimulation). These changes cause an intensification of hyperexcitability of the second-order neurons, giving rise to hypersensitivity to various peripheral stimuli. "Central sensitivity": *perturbation in the central processing of sensory information that amplifies the response of the central nervous system to a peripheral input.*

neuroendocrine processes and vascular permeability. These processes encompass the phenomenon of neuro-inflammation, in which stress and other psychological factors induce these neural responses to amplify the pain perception.

Abnormal sensory and pain processing is the key factor in the pathophysiology of FM [35], and in addition, sensitization heightens the perception of pain.

2.3 What causes fibromyalgia? Predisposing factors

There is evidence for excessive pain-related neuronal activity at multiple levels of the central nervous system, structural and functional changes in the brain by imaging studies, and impaired function of normal descending inhibitory mechanisms [29].

Several factors, such as genetic predisposition or alteration in the expression of several genes (epigenetic mechanisms), deficiencies in neurotransmitter levels, biochemical changes in the body, endocrine dysfunction, certain types of infections (e.g., Epstein-Barr virus, Lyme disease, Q fever, viral hepatitis), mood states, sociocultural environment (early-life stress or adversity), psychological trauma, and past experiences in general (e.g., childhood or sexual abuse), have been pro-posed as explanatory mechanisms of patients' subjective experience of central sensitivity and subcortical nociceptive transmission [28, 36–43].

Genes associated with increased or decreased frequency of chronic pain states or pain sensitivity regulate the breakdown or binding of pain sensitivity-modulating neurotransmitters and other inflammatory pathways. Candidate genes implicated in FM include those controlling serotonin mechanisms, dopamine receptors, as well as metabolism of catecholamines [44, 45].

A recent review confirmed the key role of neurobiological substrates, including the hypothalamic-pituitary-adrenal (HPA) axis, monoaminergic, opioidergic, endocannabinoid, and immune systems, as well as some epigenetic mechanisms, in the association of early-life psychological stress and the risk of chronic pain in later life [40]. Early psychological trauma can alter the HPA axis response, which may result in the dysfunction of peripheral and spinal dorsal horn neurons, excitatory amino acids, and central neuropeptides that can lead to abnormal nociceptive input to the brain when there is no actual painful stimulus, resulting in a central sensitization syndrome [46, 47]. Similarly, many people with FM exposed to early abuse have anxiety, depression, and post-traumatic stress disorder [2].

Patients with FM appear to have specific gut microbiome alterations that differ from their healthy peers. Recently Clos-García et al. have found an alteration in glutamate metabolism (possible molecular biomarker) connecting the gut microbiome with the brain through the enteric nervous system. This alteration has been associated with psychiatric and gastrointestinal disorders [48].

Finally, there is no scientific support for the idea that physical trauma (e.g., motor vehicle accidents) causes FM [49].

2.4 Comorbidities

2.4.1 Other central sensitivity syndromes

Pain, fatigue and other distressing sensations, occurring in the absence of clinically obvious pathology are common health problems in medical practice. Such experiences are never uniform, yet symptoms often present together in stereotypically recognizable ways. Several criteria were suggested for classification of a disease as a member of the CSS group: (a) the presence of CS; (b) the absence of an underlying disease (primary conditions), and (c) mutual associations between the disorders.

Recently, Yunus proposed a number of ailments included in the list of CSS family: irritable bowel syndrome, primary (dysfunctional) dyspepsia, tension-type headache, migraine, myofascial pain syndrome, myofascial temporomandibular disorder, primary chronic neck pain, primary low back pain, restless legs syndrome, periodic limb movement disorder, and endometriosis, among others [42].

Because of the mutual associations between the disorders, the differential diagnosis of FM is difficult.

2.4.2 Psychiatric

Patients relate too many symptoms, and the symptoms appear too severe and too unusual, and the patients too healthy compared with patients with other pain disorders [15].

A recent clinical review summarized that 62% of FM patients showed major depressive disorder, 11% bipolar disorder, 29% panic disorder, and 29% social phobia [50].

Mental disorders, especially mood disorders, have been associated with a negative impact on pain, fatigue, sleep, physical functioning, and quality of life in FM [51].

2.4.3 Nonpsychiatric: rheumatology

It is said that non-arthritic rheumatism frequently covers anxiety states. The musculoskeletal pain or fatigue associated with other disorders may mimic those of FM and vice versa. Additionally, there are many similar disorders, which are not exclusive of FM, and will overlap concomitantly. The broad categories are the following [52]:

- Inflammatory and autoimmune disorders, including rheumatoid arthritis, systemic lupus erythematosus, Sjögren's syndrome, polymyalgia rheumatica, and spondyloarthritis
- Muscle disorders and myalgias
- Myofascial pain syndrome, temporomandibular joint dysfunction, lower back pain

3. The position of the psychologist

3.1 Psychosomatic disease

FM, as a paradigm of psychosomatic disorders, would have different repercussions:

a. Physical (inactivity, disability) that leads the person to a sick and invalid role

b. Psychological, resulting in emotional disturbances, vulnerability to substance abuse, etc.

c. Social, such as tendencies towards isolation, interpersonal conflicts, etc.

Sometimes pain becomes the center of life for the patients, leading to a successive demand for assistance, conflicts with professionals, etc.

Regarding the psychological point of view, pain has been approached from the theories of traits, psychodynamic thesis, behaviorism, neuropsychology, etc., since the cognitive perspective is one of the most relevant today, specifically the study of beliefs and internal language of the patients. Along with this, the study of the different styles in the locus of control is relevant and, from the constructivist perspective, the study of the meanings and the analysis of the narrations of pain by the patients. The study of personality traits and their link with pain would be the most basic psychological approach. The study of coping styles would be in an intermediate place. Finally, the most elaborate approach would be the study of meanings.

It is interesting to make it clear that among the very different styles of coping with pain (avoidance, ignoring, reinterpreting, giving self-instructions, etc.), the most negative, the one that makes the pain worse, is the catastrophic style.

In the well-known constructivist perspective, authors such as Walker, Holloway, and Sofaer [53] studied five sequential themes in the experience of pain:

- *The pain takes hold of me*
- *I lost something*

- *I feel lost in the system*
- *They do not understand me*
- *My situation is unacceptable, inexplicable, speechless*

3.2 Emotional dysregulation

In the psychosomatic field, stress has been a very studied element with respect to FM. When scales or questionnaires are applied, the stress scores in FM patients are higher than in the control groups. In addition, patients who score higher also show several psychological disorders. It has been postulated that chronic stress (but not acute stress) would contribute to the FM symptoms. It has also been noticed that specific situations of intense stress correlate with post-traumatic stress disorder and FM. Finally, among the patients with FM, a higher prevalence of experiences of victimization (abuse and sexual abuse), throughout the life, is detected. The intensity of the traumatic event correlates, in these cases, with pain and sleep disturbances.

Linked to this, it is worth noting the issue of social support, which is an issue usually over-mentioned by FM patients. Social support has three main functions:

a. Affective-emotional: intimacy, attachment, care, concern for the other, etc.

b. Material: provision of material assistance, assistance, etc., is an instrumental function.

c. Informative: advice, guide, education, etc.

The tendency to consider the first function as the most important is not correct. The key would be to give support based on the type of need that arises. Giving emotional support when the problem is strictly material, for example, may be tender, but it will not be effective. It must be noted that social support would lead to stress. Social relations imply obligations, and in turn, tensions can be derived from them. In short, stress can emerge. In fact, Helgeson [54], among others, points out that negative social interactions predict health- and well-being-related problems more than the positive ones do.

The differences between men and women in social support have not been studied much, although it is a simple fact that men and women differ in the way they participate in social relations. In this regard, it is necessary to mention something about gender roles. The traditional masculine role is associated with activity, the search for independence, competitiveness, objectives, assertiveness, self-confidence, etc., and within this role, it may be more difficult to seek and achieve social support. The role of women has been associated with expressiveness, emotions, intimacy, more ability to recognize difficulties (and with it to ask for help), cooperation, empathy, etc., thus giving and receiving social support seem to be easier tasks.

The association between social support, stress, and health has been studied without conclusive results due to serious methodological errors. Perhaps it would point out that the negative part of the social relations that we have already indicated is more relevant in the case of women. Why is it? Women tend to be a source of support more frequently and are more involved in socio-family networks. Belle already pointed out how support networks can create psychological distress: (a) for a lack of respect or disapproval of others; (b) for revealing confidences or not meeting the expectations of others; (c) when the support person is too demanding; and (d) when there is a sort of contagion of the stress from some members to others [55].

3.3 Address the psychological factors in fibromyalgia

Beyond works with quantitative methodology, we will focus this section on qualitative research. This way of approaching knowledge is interpretive. It would be the interpretative study of a particular problem in which the researcher is responsible for the production of meaning. Many times, we reach statistically significant results that are absolutely useless, that do not discover anything, and that do not tell us anything that we did not know from our conversations with patients, and that, simply, we did not care to measure in order to know. In a different way, qualitative methods study intersubjective meanings located and constructed rather than supposed objective facts. Observation and interview would be prioritized over the experiment and the standardized questionnaires. In the understanding of the meanings, one works with the narrative, being storytelling a good tool for it. The laws of physical objects imply that there is no history, which is something impossible for the person. Faced with paradigmatic, objectivist thinking, without a position on itself, narrative thinking poses positions depending on the context. The data is not the central element, but where the data comes from, the person is the starting point, the private representation of the person about the world or its disorder, the way the person lives reality. The subject is therefore interesting: how the person builds the own context and makes history. The narrative is the element to reach that meaning sought. It is a story, a story ordered in some way. The narratives are unique, individual, unrepeatable, and have an author. They provide, finally, a meaning.

3.4 Our experience

In order to research the experience of pain and its different repercussions in women diagnosed with FM, we performed individual in-depth interviews in a total of 15 patients. It is a semi-structured interview with some guide points but giving the patients the opportunity of a broad expression of their experiences. This way we tried to know the ideas that patients had about the disease but, above all, their experiences. The interviews lasted 50–60 min, were recorded in audio, and subsequently, transcribed with the collaboration of two psychologists. After the transcription, an analysis of the interviews was developed. For this purpose, in the clinical field, the methodology proposed by Weber for the analysis of content has been used [56]. It involves the following stages: (a) identifying common themes in the responses of patients and classifying them semantically, by their meaning; (b) grouping the themes of common meaning into categories; and (c) analyzing the frequency of each of the topics by watching its presence depending on the number of patients.

3.5 Our sample

Our patients had a mean age of 45 years (ranged 36–59), all of them were women and married. Regarding their training level, 46.46% had primary studies (7 out of 15), and the rest were divided between degree or diploma (26.66%) and professional training or baccalaureate (26.66%). Besides, 40% were housewives (6 out of 15), and the rest worked in extra domestic tasks (26.66% as administrative assistants, 13.33% as operators, one of them as a secondary school teacher, another as clerk, and one as head of section in the regional administration). Those who had extra domestic works said that they had in charge the housework with some help from their couples. Eight of the patients had two sons and daughters and seven of them only one son or daughter. In three cases (20%), in addition to the couple and the children, other family members lived at home and they needed care.

3.6 The main topics from a psychological point of view

As main concerns, patients referred the following:

a. The personal history of pain: time elapsed since the pain started, professionals consulted, treatments performed, time elapsed since the diagnosis of FM, biographical aspects at the onset of pain

b. The pain today: description (intensity, frequency, and duration) and treatment; what precipitates, worsens, or relieves

c. Thoughts regarding pain: what is attributed to, how to control it, what is thought when the pain appears

d. Feelings regarding pain: emotions that arise when facing pain

e. Behaviors as responses to pain: how the pain is faced

f. Repercussions of pain in daily life: functional impact on the patient (how pain limits life), impact on the family, social impact

g. Support against pain: what help do you have to deal with pain.

At this point, our focus was the personal history of pain. In this regard, it is worth noting some narratives of our patients:

> ***Patient A:*** *I was attended by several orthopedists and some of them gave me medication to the pain ... the problem is that when one has ... does not reach 30 years old and begins with continuous muscle contractures and without having a logical cause, well ... even while playing sports in those moments, well, you get annoyed, don't you? And then you go to one and the other, you even go to the neurosurgeon that the only thing he found was a minimal dehydration in ... a ... dorsal intervertebral disk ... and ... I think then it was progressively studied in case they found neck calcifications, they corrected them, they sent me to the rehabilitators ...*

> ***Patient B:*** *... It was mostly because of the birth of my daughter, well with ... my daughter is already 10 years old, perhaps was the upbringing of the girl and also my father was diagnosed with a retinal detachment from the second eye because I had already had one and had lost the other eye ... this brought me a lot of tension buildup ...*

> ***Patient C:*** *... When I was diagnosed with fibromyalgia I was suffering from pain for months, the pain started in the feet and hands, I had no strength in the hands, they became inflamed but I thought the housewives ... I thought it was from the mop, scrub ... always a blame for cleaning ... I said to me "today I'm more tired of cleaning," "today for ... " ... always blame until my husband told me to go to the*

> *doctor ... he has the consultation in ... and he made several medical checks, he gave me medications ... until I went to another doctor who finally diagnosed fibromyalgia ...*
>
> ***Patient D:*** *...The first symptoms were that I complained about my legs and I was said I had a column deviation; when I was 25 it hurts me a lot ... well with 25 ... no, with 23, my neck started to hurt me a lot and doctors told me that it was a cervical problem and they gave me laser ... well, I felt better, but pain remains, I always had pain and I continued with my medications ... I was bearing pain, it was easy when I was 23, but now ...*

From a psychological point of view, topics such as "personality and fibromyalgia," " emotional dysregulation," and "fibromyalgia as a psychosomatic disease (labeled as negative connotations)" would be the most relevant aspects to deep into the patients' thoughts, feelings, and behaviors.

FM is a disease with clear female predominance. Stress seems to be a highlighted element in its origin, especially chronic stress. Regarding social support, it is essential to mention that, in order to make it appropriate, the type of support (material, emotional, informative) must be in accordance with the needs that arise. Giving material support, when emotional support is necessary, is simply inefficient. We also said that social support can usually involve stress. Social relationships entail, for example, obligations from which tensions and stress may arise. It is also necessary to remember here that the traditional feminine role is associated with the expression of emotions and empathy.

In our patients we observe how they work mostly away from home, they bear the burden of homework, and in addition, one out of five not only takes care of their husbands and children but is in charge of some other relatives. And it is striking that 40% of these patients do not perceive any help to face their pain. *They work inside, they work outside, they take care of everyone, they have pain, and they have no help*. This is the reality of some women we interviewed. Chronic stress and FM? It does not seem to fit any doubt. And regarding the health of women, there is a chilling fact: patients usually take several drugs for more than 5 years, continuously, without a diagnosis of certainty. Some patients interviewed told us that the feeling that was seizing them on their pilgrimage from doctor to doctor was that they were labeled as hysterical or a merely storyteller and that they just told them to take a pain reliever when they had pain.

Some husbands, ratifying such clinical impressions, exclaim on more than one occasion: "Again, with your pain!" And since the traditional female role is designed to take care and not so much to receive care from others, to understand and not so much to be understood, in many cases it is hardly expected that, when a woman feels pain, the husband will give an adequate care. The trigger elements of pain are usually psychic tensions. There is nothing to add to it, chronic stress seems evident. Along with it there are thoughts of resignation not exempt of accompanying feelings of guilt. The random attribution of pain seems to be part of that female role of taking on loads ("this pain has also touched me!"). The feeling of guiltiness is strange. Facing pain limits the woman life, which prevents her to have a satisfying sex life, which keeps her at home, and which prevents her from performing her tasks. She feels guilty: guilty for not attending to her relatives and spoiling their vacations and guilty because she does not have sexual relations as often as she would wish and for not being able to enjoy them, for not having a clean house, etc. What makes her feel so guilty if it's not the assumption of a traditional role? We leave the answer for your own reflection [57].

4. Social aspects

By the time patients get to the FM treatment program at different health institutions, they typically have tried all the approved drugs for the disorder and are tired of the pain, the fatigue, the depression, and the skepticism. Many patients have been told for years (by friends, by family, by clinicians) that their symptoms are imaginary or that they are lazy or drug-seeking.

Above and beyond the specific impact on health, from a social perspective, FM contemplates an impact at three levels: (a) family, (b) labor, and (c) about the health system.

In the **family environment**, patients point to the existence of family imbalances, putting at risk the maintenance and quality of their relationships in that context. It seems that there are at least four aspects to highlight:

a. A certain family disruption from the psycho-affective point of view (before or after the onset of the disease)

b. Family loads secondary to fibromyalgia (change of roles in family components, redistribution of tasks, loss of role, etc.)

c. Family economic losses

d. Patterns of family behavior directly related to fibromyalgia and its repercussions

In the **work context**, fibromyalgia is an important cause of work hour lost. In Spain, for example, people with fibromyalgia have an annual average of 21 days of work lost, and approximately one third of patients (depending on their jobs) already have a disability pension before they reach the retirement age (in other diseases this figure is around 9–10%). And, in summary, the percentage of temporary leave and the number of sick leave days is 3–4 times higher than in the case of other workers. In addition, it is known that the occupational impact of fibromyalgia seems to be strongly influenced by psychopathological comorbidity (especially anxiety and depression).

The **impact on the health system** refers to the amount of resources that these patients use, with the consequent economic cost. The positive part is arriving at a diagnosis as soon as possible, these costs decrease as it stops the pilgrimage of patients in search of evidence that clarifies their health problem. Patients with fibromyalgia visit the primary care physician at an average of 8–13 times a year, with almost €1,000 annual cost for such visits, about €500 for testing, and another €1,500 for "nonmedical" therapies (e.g., physiotherapy or massages). We must add about €500 per year for the use of different medications.

Storytelling, as an instrument of communication in health context, can be used to create a story as a way to share or receive information as well as a way for us to understand our own lives and those of others around us [58]. In this case, one of the signatories (MG) has composed a narrative to make fibro**mya**lgia visible. **Mya**, the chief character of the play, wishes us to transmit the emotions and feelings of the people who bear patiently the illness. Sometimes, the lack of understanding or the disregard of those around them for the different aspect of their lives doesn't help them to make progress. Various conditions affecting fibromyalgia patients have been depicted in this story. A great help for patients would be an overall consider-ation of clinicians, relatives, friends, and coworkers. Let us go to the story: and who is **Mya** (see Appendix 1)?

5. About treatments

There is increasing recognition that multidisciplinary treatment models that address physical symptoms of the disease, as well as behavioral and psychological components, are effective, although total removal of symptoms is almost never achieved. The goal is improvement in health-related quality of life, function, and symptom burden. Patients should also know that symptoms will never kill them. The first step should be to address concerns, such as sleep or mood disorders. We are going to revise the different treatment options.

5.1 Psychoactive drugs

"Being on the hunt for the magic pill": drugs don't work very well with FM.

- **Antidepressants.** The three main antidepressants that have been studied through controlled clinical trials in FM are [59, 60]:
    - *Amitriptyline*. It reduces pain and fatigue, improves sleep, and produces a global feeling of improvement from the perspective of both the doctor and the patient. It is therefore highly recommended.
    - *Duloxetine*. It also reduces pain and improves sleep and mood and quality of life and functional capacity, so it is also equally recommended.
    - *Fluoxetine*. Its evidence on pain, sleep, and fatigue in FM patients is controversial, and it seems to be effective for depressive symptoms and functional limitation. I would not currently be at the forefront of the recommendations of psychoactive drugs.
- **Gamma-aminobutyric acid (GABA) analog**
    - *Pregabalin*. It was the first drug to be approved by the US FDA in 2007. Pregabalin reduces pain and improves sleep and quality of life, so it can be recommended for the treatment of these symptoms in patients with FM. It must be noted that a recent study comparing the efficacy of Duloxetine and Pregabalin concludes a higher efficacy of duloxetine for the treatment of pain in patients with FM [61].
- **Other pharmacotherapies**, like opioids (e.g., tramadol), dopamine agonist (e.g., ropinirole, pramipexole, or rotigotine), cannabinoids (e.g., Nabilone), or sodium oxybate, do not seem to support its use for treating FM [62–65].

5.2 Nonpharmacological options

- **Exercise**. Exercise is known to be beneficial for overall health. Incorporation of some physical exercise with strengthening and stretching program as a part of FM treatment shows significant effects in reducing pain and related FM symptoms. Recent evidence suggests that exercise may regulate the immune- and stress-related responses [66–68].
- **Transcranial stimulation**. Two types of noninvasive brain stimulation methods have been used to treat the cognitive and affective disorders [69]:

transcranial magnetic stimulation (TMS) and transcranial direct current stimulation (tDCS). TMS sends a brief electrical current from an electromagnetic coil that is placed against the patient's scalp, creating a regional magnetic field that affects neural activity. tDCS sends a weak electrical current through a pair of electrodes placed on the scalp in the region of interest. The current is considered to help modulate the neural activity, possibly in a polarity specific way [70, 71]. It appears that both TMS and tDCS may modulate mood, but the effects on pain may be marginal.

- **Psychological and behavioral modalities**

  - **Psychological treatment**

There is great evidence of the effectiveness of cognitive behavioral therapy on pain control, physical discomfort, and mood in patients with FM [72]. Similarly, behavioral therapy has shown efficacy in reducing the number of medical visits.

Other treatments, such as relaxation techniques, used in isolation for the sole purpose of controlling pain, have not proven effective. On the other hand, despite some positive results, there is no scientific evidence to recommend hypnosis and other forms of therapy.

In any case, it seems that the best option is the use of "multicomponent therapies," specifically those based on the combination of physical exercise, cognitive behavioral intervention strategies, and drugs. They have proven effective in managing pain and improving the quality of life and physical capacity of patients.

- **Alternative therapies**

Today there is no scientific evidence on the effectiveness of certain treatments, at least for being recommended: acupuncture, homeopathy, ozone therapy, dietary supplements, Qi-Gong, Reiki, or Taichi [73].

Finally, the beneficial effect of chiropractic treatment and massage in the treatment of FM has not been sufficiently demonstrated, and therefore, its use is not recommended.

Appendix 1

And who is Mya?
"El entusiasta"
www.elentusiasta.es

The H.G. Wells Museum
Second day of the fatigue, Sunday. In the twenty-first century

News: and where's Mya?

Yesterday, the *Sculpture* of Pain was stolen, a fifteenth-century masterpiece, highly valued by the *Experts of Life*. It belongs to the stage of the Spanish flamboyant gothic. It's an alabaster sculpture made by Sebastián de la Esperanza. It symbol-izes medieval culture; the accompanying book personifies Wisdom.

It was transferred in March 1999, from the Cathedral of Sigüenza to the recently opened H.G. Wells Museum.

The *Commissioner of Righteousness* has asked to cooperate with the country's officials to investigate the clues in depth.

This morning, the main authorities of the emotions, have established the action plan and the resources they will provide to clarify the events that occurred.

At the moment, the museum officials have not made authorized statements. At 7:30 pm, the director called a press conference at the headquarters of the feelings (25 Transcendence St.), to make the first manifestations of what happened.

A reward is offered to all those who care about visibility.

Myalgia

Mya reads the news and decides to go to the museum. She cannot accept another day of tiredness and fatigue.

The H.G. Wells Museum is a building without defined forms. A weird-speaking drone with fraudulent voice announces: "free admission." There is a large uneven corridor where three rooms are placed on the right side and one more on the left.

What do they hide?

Mya enters into the first of the rooms in the right: "*The Room of the White Coats.*" Although *Painting One* greets her kindly, it can only spend 5 minutes because there are too many visitors. It examines her quickly and recommends talking to *Painting Two*. Then, the latter gives her some futuristic capsules and asks her to come back at another time. Finally, a whisper leads her to *Painting three*, which tells her that it has something for pain. It scares her because she hadn't explained anything.

She comes out very confused, and stays absorbed in the middle of "*The Family Room,*" right next to the caution tape that the *Art Police* had put to cordon off the scene. She hears peaceful voices. Being suspended in the air, the *legless chairs* tell her that they are almost no longer visited or accompanied. At the beginning of the opening of the museum, it was the most frequented room, but now they are not important to them or simply do not know how to look at them. On the ceiling of this lugubrious room there is a *Deco Lamp* that looks at the walls with the complicity of the years. From a distance it seems to say: "I already knew that sooner or later it would happen." The always silent *Deco Lamp* addresses the intrigued **Mya** sharing its thoughts: "They have never watched us, they don't care, people come and go, they look at us but they don't see us. They extract what we have inside but they give us nothing back. The one who hung us performed his function. The one who repairs us, from time to time, also believes that he has fulfilled his duty. But now, that doesn't care." And the *Sculpture of Pain* was she left to her fate by a wrong way or did she abandon her privileged place in the museum because of misunderstanding and loneliness?

Curiosity leads her to the "*Just in Time Room,*" where the *Mosaics* are in continuous synchronized motion and almost silent. They ignore her. They prefer not to have eye contact with her. They have lost the habit. They do not recognize visitors because they are missing too much. Their complaints and regrets bore them. They don't feel they are part of the team.

Once she visited the rooms on the right of the corridor, she went to the left side, to the "*Not Near Room.*" Those who were next to the stolen sculpture. And since their disappearance they have not even asked again. *Sculptures with no eyes* look her up and down, without any empathy. She prefers to think they have not seen her. She listens to a secure voice, which comes from the *Spokesman of the Council of Emotions*, who starts the meeting. It is necessary to face the fact of theft and start making decisions. Find out who has been the guilty before it is judged by the *Court of Righteousness*.

After 5 hours, the members of the council were still trying to assess what could have happened with the sculpture. The clues confused them. The *Query Painting* had not manifested yet. Its strokes made a slight movement. Everyone else looked paying more attention than on other occasions, but they didn't understand why the picture wasn't able to talk.

Mya, as she did not know anything about it, felt a greater curiosity for the painting. She waited just to see what it was doing. Its images were as clocks with distorted shapes and its light was different from the rest. Would it know who was the guilty of the disappearance? What were the reasons of its differences? Would it be able to reach others with harmony? What a different museum! All its elements express those they feel and hear! She exclaimed.

Suddenly, several coordinated voices arise:

- *Painting Two*: "We were drawn to remember the decay of those who live depending on something or someone."
- *Sculpture Eight*: "We were built to remember that principles exist."
- *Mosaic Fifteen*: "We were just to remember that the senses exist."
- *Frame Ten*: "We were to remember the transcendence."

Everyone directed their forms to *Painting Seven*, which looked at the ground for a few seconds and shouted with no-voice: "Please, let's change something about our past!"

From this moment on, they understood why the *Pain* with their *Sculpture* had decided to leave.

Author details

José Vicente Martínez-Quiñones[1*], Mar Martínez Gamarra[2]
and Ignacio Jáuregui-Lobera[3]

1 Department of Neurosurgery, Mutua de Accidentes de Zaragoza, Zaragoza, Spain

2 Storytelling Spanish Association (ASEST), Zaragoza, Spain

3 Department of Molecular Biology and Biochemical Engineering, University of Pablo de Olavide of Seville, Seville, Spain

*Address all correspondence to: jvmartinez@maz.es

References

[1] Kuner R, Flor H. Neural circuits of chronic pain. Neuroscience. 2018;**387**:1-3

[2] Sancassiani F, Machado S, Ruggiero V, Cacace E, Carmassi C, Gesi C, et al. The management of fibromyalgia from a psychosomatic perspective: An overview. International Review of Psychiatry. 2017;**29**(5):473-488

[3] Branco JC, Bannwarth B, Failde I, Abello Carbonell J, Blotman F, Spaeth M, et al. Prevalence of fibromyalgia: A survey in five European countries. Seminars in Arthritis and Rheumatism. 2010;**39**(6):448-453

[4] Sumpton J, Moulin D. Fibromyalgia. In: Biller J, Ferro JM, editors. Handbook of Clinical Neurology, Vol. 119 (3rd series). Neurologic Aspects of Systemic Disease; Part I. Elsevier BV; 2014. pp. 513-524

[5] Bennett R, Friend R, Marcus D, Bernstein C, Han BK, Yachoui R, et al. Criteria for the diagnosis of fibromyalgia: validation of the modified 2010 preliminary ACR criteria and the development of alternative criteria. Arthritis Care and Research. 2014;**66** (9):1364-1373

[6] Burton AR. Neurasthenia. Journal of the National Medical Association. 1925; **17**(1):16-18

[7] Gowers WR. A lecture on lumbago: its lessons and analogues. BMJ. 1904;**1**: 117-121

[8] Fletcher E. Fibrositis. Postgraduate Medical Journal. 1937;**13**(143):324-329

[9] Smythe HA, Moldofsky H. Two contributions to understanding of the fibrositis syndrome. Bulletin on the Rheumatic Diseases. 1977;**28**:928-931

[10] Wolfe F, Cathey MA. The epidemiology of tenders points: A prospective study of 1520 patients. The Journal of Rheumatology. 1985;**12**: 1164-1168

[11] Bested AC, Marshall LM. Review of Myalgic Encephalomyelitis/Chronic Fatigue Syndrome: an evidence-based approach to diagnosis and management by clinicians. Reviews on Environmental Health. 2015;**30**(4):223-249

[12] Kissling W, Mendel R, Förstl H. The burn-out syndrome: prevalence, symptoms, differential diagnosis and treatment. Deutsche Medizinische Wochenschrift. 2014;**139**(50):2587-2596

[13] Benjamin S, Morris S, McBeth J, Macfarlane GJ, Silman AJ. The association between chronic widespread pain and mental disorder: A population-based study. Arthritis and Rheumatism. 2000;**43**:561-567

[14] McBeth J, Macfarlane GJ, Hunt IM, Silman AJ. Risk factors for persistent chronic widespread pain: a community-based study. Rheumatology (Oxford). 2001;**40**:95-101

[15] Wolfe F, Walitt B. Culture, science and the changing nature of fibromyalgia. Nature Reviews Rheumatology. 2013;**9**(12):751-755

[16] Nicholas M, Vlaeyen JW, Rief W, Barke A, Aziz Q, Benoliel R, et al. The IASP classification of chronic pain for ICD-11: Chronic primary pain. Pain. 2019;**160**:28-37

[17] Treede R-D, Rief W, Barke A, Aziz Q, Bennett MI, Benoliel R, et al. Chronic pain as a symptom or a disease: The IASP Classification of Chronic Pain for the International Classification of Diseases (ICD-11). Pain. 2019;**160**:19-27

[18] Kool MB, Geenen R. Loneliness in patients with rheumatic diseases: The significance of invalidation and lack of

social support. The Journal of Psychology. 2012;**146**:229-241

[19] Adams LM, Turk DC. Psychosocial factors and central sensitivity syndromes. Current Rheumatology Reviews. 2015;**11**:96-108

[20] Wolfe F, Smythe HA, Yunus MB, Bennett RM, Bombardier C, Goldenberg DL, et al. The American College of Rheumatology 1990 Criteria for the Classification of Fibromyalgia. Report of the Multicenter Criteria Committee. Arthritis and Rheumatism. 1990;**33**(2): 160-172

[21] Wolfe F, Clauw DJ, Fitzcharles MA, Goldenberg DL, Katz RS, Mease P, et al. The American College of Rheumatology preliminary diagnostic criteria for fibromyalgia and measurement of symptom severity. Arthritis Care & Research (Hoboken). 2010;**62**(5): 600-610

[22] Wolfe F, Clauw DJ, Fitzcharles MA, Goldenberg DL, Häuser W, Katz RS, et al. Fibromyalgia criteria and severity scales for clinical and epidemiological studies: A modification of the ACR Preliminary Diagnostic Criteria for Fibromyalgia. The Journal of Rheumatology. 2011;**38**(6):1113-1122

[23] Crawford BK, Piault EC, Lai C, Bennett RM. Assessing fibromyalgia-related fatigue: content validity and psychometric performance of the Fatigue Visual Analog Scale in adult patients with fibromyalgia. Clinical and Experimental Rheumatology. 2011;**29**(6 Suppl 69):S34-S43

[24] Bennett RM. Clinical manifestations and diagnosis of fibromyalgia. Rheumatic Diseases Clinics of North America. 2009;**35**(2):215-232

[25] Bennett RM, Jones J, Turk DC, Russell IJ, Matallana L. An internet survey of 2,596 people with fibromyalgia. BMC Musculoskeletal Disorders. 2007;**8**:27

[26] Turk DC, Adams LM. Using a biopsychosocial perspective in the treatment of fibromyalgia patients. Pain Management. 2016;**6**(4):357-369

[27] Wilson HD, Robinson JP, Turk DC. Toward the identification of symptom patterns in people with fibromyalgia. Arthritis and Rheumatism. 2009;**61**(4): 527-534

[28] Wolfe F, Brähler E, Häuser W. Fibromyalgia prevalence, somatic symptom reporting, and the dimensionality of polisymptomatic distress: Results from a survey of the general population. Arthritis Care and Research. 2013;**65**(5):777-785

[29] Meeus M, Nijs J. Central sensitization: a biopsychosocial explanation for chronic widespread pain in patients with fibromyalgia and chronic fatigue syndrome. Clinical Rheumatology. 2007;**26**(4):465-473

[30] Brummett CM, Bakshi RR, Goesling J, Leung D, Moser SE, Zollars JW, et al. Preliminary validation of the Michigan Body Map. Pain. 2016;**157**(6):1205-1212

[31] Neblett R, Cohen H, Choi Y, Hartzell MM, Williams M, Mayer TG, et al. The Central Sensitization Inventory (CSI): establishing clinically significant values for identifying central sensitivity syndromes in an outpatient chronic pain sample. The Journal of Pain. 2013;**14**(5):438-445

[32] Kroenke K. Physical symptom disorder: a simpler diagnostic category for somatization-spectrum conditions. Journal of Psychosomatic Research. 2006;**60**:335-339

[33] Rubin JJ. Psychosomatic pain: new insights and management strategies. Southern Medical Journal. 2005;**98**: 1099-1110

[34] Ehrlich GE. Pain is real; fibromyalgia isn't. The Journal of Rheumatology. 2003;**30**:1666-1667

[35] McCarberg BH. Clinical overview of fibromyalgia. American Journal of Therapeutics. 2012;**19**(5):357-368

[36] Fitzcharles MA, Yunus MB. The clinical concept of fibromyalgia as a changing paradigm in the past 20 years. Pain Research and Treatment. 2012; **2012**:184835

[37] Buskila D, Atzeni F, Sarzi-Puttini P. Etiology of fibromyalgia: the possible role of infection and vaccination. Autoimmunity Reviews. 2008;**8**(1):41-43

[38] Arnold LM, Hudson JI, Hess EV, et al. Family study of fibromyalgia. Arthritis and Rheumatism. 2004;**50**(3): 944-952

[39] Holliday KL, McBeth J. Recent advances in the understanding of genetic susceptibility to chronic pain and somatic symptoms. Current Rheumatology Reports. 2011;**13**(6):521-527

[40] Burke NN, Finn DP, McGuire BE, Roche M. Psychological stress in early life as a predisposing factor for the development of chronic pain: Clinical and preclinical evidence and neurobiological mechanisms. Journal of Neuroscience Research. 2017;**95**(6): 1257-1270

[41] Scarinci IC, McDonald-Haile J, Bradley LA, Richter JE. Altered pain perception and psychosocial features among women with gastrointestinal disorders and history of abuse: a preliminary model. The American Journal of Medicine. 1994 Aug;**97**(2): 108-118

[42] Yunus MB. Editorial Review: An update on central sensitivity syndromes and the issues of nosology and psychobiology. Current Rheumatology Reviews. 2015;**11**:70-85

[43] Murgatroyd C, Spengler D. Epigenetics of early child development. Frontiers in Psychiatry. 2011;**2**:16

[44] Ablin J, Neumann L, Buskila D. Pathogenesis of fibromyalgia— a review. Joint, Bone, Spine. 2008;**75**(3): 273-279

[45] Limer KL, Nicholl BI, Thomson W, Mcbeth J. Exploring the genetic susceptibility of chronic widespread pain: The tender points in genetic association studies. Rheumatology. 2008;**47**(5):572-577

[46] Beggs S. Long-term consequences of neonatal injury. Canadian Journal of Psychology. 2015;**60**:176-180

[47] Schwaller F, Fitzgerald M. The consequences of pain in early life: Injury-induced plasticity in developing pain pathways. The European Journal of Neuroscience. 2014;**39**:344-352

[48] Clos-Garcia M, Andrés-Marin N, Fernández-Eulate G, Abecia L, Lavín JL, van Liempd S, et al. Gut microbiome and serum metabolome analyses identify molecular biomarkers and altered glutamate metabolism in fibromyalgia. eBioMedicine. 2019;**46**: 499-511

[49] Wolfe F, Häuser W, Walitt BT, Katz RS, Rasker JJ, Russell AS. Fibromyalgia and physical trauma: The concepts we invent. The Journal of Rheumatology. 2014;**41**(9):1737-1745

[50] Palagini L, Carmassi C, Conversano C, Gesi C, Bazzichi L, Giacomelli C, et al. Transdiagnostic factors across fibromyalgia and mental disorders: Sleep disturbances may play a key role. A clinical review. Clinical and Experimental Rheumatology. 2016;**34**: S140-S144

[51] Plazier M, Ost J, Stassijns G, De RD, Vanneste S. Pain characteristics in fibromyalgia: Understanding the multiple dimensions of pain. Clinical Rheumatology. 2015;**34**:775-783

[52] Chinn S, Cadwell W, Gritsenko K. Fibromyalgia pathogenesis and

treatment options update. Current Pain and Headache Reports. 2016;**20**:25-35

[53] Walker J, Holloway I, Sofaer B. In the system: Patients' experiences of chronic back pain. Pain. 1999;**80**: 621-628

[54] Helgeson VS. Two important distinctions in social support: Kind of support and perceived versus received. Journal of Applied Social Psychology. 1993;**23**:825-845

[55] Belle D. Gender differences in the social moderators of stress. In: Barnett RC, Biener L, Baruch GK, editors. Gender and Stress. Nueva York: Free Press; 1987. pp. 257-277

[56] Weber RP. Basic Content Analysis. Newbury Park, CA: Sage Publications; 1990

[57] Jáuregui-Lobera I. Cuestiones de género. Zaragoza: Libros Certeza; 2007

[58] Jáuregui-Lobera I, Martínez-Gamarra M, Montes-Martínez M, Martínez-Quiñones JV. Storytelling as instrument of communication in health contexts. Journal of Negative and No Positive Results. 2020;**5**

[59] Okifuji A, Gao J, Bokat C, Hare BD. Management of fibromyalgia syndrome in 2016. Pain Management. 2016;**6**(4): 383-400

[60] Government of Spain. Fibromyalgia. Madrid (Spain): Ministry of Health, Social Policy and Equality; 2011

[61] Bidari A, Moazen-Zadeh E, Ghavidel-Parsa B, Rahmani S, Hosseini S, Hassankhani A. Comparing duloxetine and pregabalin for treatment of pain and depression in women with fibromyalgia: an open-label randomized clinical trial. DARU. 2019;**27**:149-158

[62] Bennett RM, Kamin M, Karim R, Rosenthal N. Tramadol and acetaminophen combination tablets in the treatment of fibromyalgia pain: A double blind, randomized, placebo-controlled study. The American Journal of Medicine. 2003;**114**(7):537-545

[63] Holman AJ, Myers RR. A randomized, double-blind, placebo-controlled trial of pramipexole, a dopamine agonist, in patients with fibromyalgia receiving concomitant medications. Arthritis and Rheumatism. 2005;**52**(8):2495-2505

[64] Skrabek RQ, Galimova L, Ethans K, Perry D. Nabilone for the treatment of pain in fibromyalgia. The Journal of Pain. 2008;**9**(2):164-173

[65] Scharf MB, Baumann M, Berkowitz DV. The effects of sodium oxybate on clinical symptoms and sleep patterns in patients with fibromyalgia. The Journal of Rheumatology. 2003;**30**(5): 1070-1074

[66] Kelley GA, Kelley KS, Jones DL. Efficacy and effectiveness of exercise on tender points in adults with fibromyalgia: A meta-analysis of randomized controlled trials. Art. 2011; **2011**:125485

[67] Busch AJ, Webber SC, Brachaniec M, et al. Exercise therapy for fibromyalgia. Current Pain and Headache Reports. 2011;**15**(5):358-367

[68] Mist SD, Firestone KA, Jones KD. Complementary and alternative exercise for fibromyalgia: A meta-analysis. Journal of Pain Research. 2013;**6**: 247-260

[69] Jáuregui Lobera I, Martínez Quiñones JV. Neuromodulation in eating disorders and obesity: A promising way of treatment? Neuropsychiatric Disease and Treatment. 2018;**14**:2817-2835

[70] Galhardoni R, Correia GS, Araujo H, et al. Repetitive transcranial magnetic stimulation in chronic pain: A review of the literature. Archives of Physical Medicine and Rehabilitation. 2015;**96**(4 suppl):S156-S172

[71] Boyer L, Dousset A, Roussel P, et al. rTMS in fibromyalgia: A randomized trial evaluating QoL and its brain metabolic substrate. Neurology. 2014;**82** (14):1231-1238

[72] Bernardy K, Klose P, Welsch P, Häuser W. Efficacy, acceptability and safety of Internet-delivered psychological therapies for fibromyalgia syndrome: A systematic review and meta-analysis of randomized controlled trials. European Journal of Pain. 2019;**23** (1):3-14

[73] Lauche R, Cramer H, Häuser W, Dobos G, Langhorst J. A Systematic overview of reviews for complementary and alternative therapies in the treatment of the fibromyalgia syndrome. Evidence-based Complementary and Alternative Medicine. 2015;**2015**:610615

5

Psychological and Societal Implications of Projecting the Shadow on the Feminine in Tibetan Buddhist Contexts

Anne Iris Miriam Anders

Abstract

Idealizing and medicalizing of methods ascribed to Buddhism has led to individualizing their structural and societal challenges. Although the long-undervalued need for introspection may get addressed, people are now caught under the cloak of spirituality hoping for quick enlightenment or a panacea solving mental diseases. Thus, at this point, the impact of decontextualizing concepts, unreflectively copying feudal structures into Tibetan Buddhist seminar- and meditation-centers, as well as of lacking knowledge required for the gradual application-oriented learning processes taught in traditional Buddhist philosophy have become clear. This shows in recent testimony of economical, psychological, and physical abuse in international Tibetan Buddhist organizations. The violence against individuals and man-made trauma in such contexts need to get analyzed before the background of neologisms, that is concepts allowing for arbitrariness and violence in the name of spirituality, as well as of the sophisticated systems of rationalizing damage and silencing trauma and victims. Furthermore, though those in the '*inner circles*' run the risk of traumatization and of being held accountable, it is women who are at higher risk, particularly those who engage in secret relationships. Thus, in terms of treatment, the collectively projecting the shadow on the feminine, leading to an attitude of exploitation and control against women, requires consideration.

Keywords: trauma, silencing of trauma, depression, psychosis, Buddhism, inner circle, secret consort, manipulation, exploitation, abuse, guru yoga, double bind, indoctrination in Buddhist groups, Vajrayāna, rationalization, decontextualization of concepts, cults, crazy wisdom, karma purification, pure view, Buddhist meditation, Buddhist seminar centers, Buddhist philosophy, mindfulness, mental diseases, rlung disease, unconscious, dakini

1. Introduction

In international Tibetan Buddhist seminar-, meditation-, and retreat-centers, patterns of violence and exploitation have developed over the past decades. Recently, economical, psychological, and physical abuse [1–12] was reported. It has evolved against the background of structures that systematically devalue and control the

feminine. Such structures effect on the individuals of the respective groups and engrave into their bodies and minds. Thus, in a cultural-insensitive, unreflected transfer of knowledge of Buddhist philosophy and respective training techniques, the culturally ingrained ways in dealing with the feminine and its unconscious attitudes were absorbed. A visualization concept of females merely forming the passive counterparts to male characters, their devaluation in comments and acquired behavior patterns as well as misunderstood visualization techniques leading to narcissistic self-aggrandizing patterns contribute to confusion. This disorientation in turn not only forms the basis for developing self-devaluation and uncertainty regard-ing the individuals social positions in the groups, but also causes a *double bind*-based inability to act. Thus, one option seems to be the proximity to the spiritual master, the identifying of women with the male master, which somehow is supposed to define their position and seemingly would enhance their spiritual progress towards enlightenment as well. The undefined social positions of women in such groups, which encourage projecting undesirable aspects onto them, and sexualized aspects, such as the role of a secret lover, pose a cultural challenge for them. However, besides uncertainties due to a lack of cultural socialization, and the opportunities for honest communication on this issue, usually prevented by vows of secrecy, damage to group members is incurred by those regarding themselves as Vajrayāna practitioners,
even preaching Vajrayāna, for whom gender equality ought to be standard in their training. Thus, in neglecting individual and institutional betrayal trauma [13], the implicit traumatization of people, despite being undeniable injuries, has been successfully silenced for decades. And control of the feminine has also been achieved by projecting the shadow, one's own unwanted aspects, at the women.

Moreover, the narrative of Buddhism being a panacea for mental health not only misinterprets its spiritual methods to be psychological or medical ones. Damage is also caused by seducing and misleading sick individuals and by misinterpreting any trauma of those severely injured by the leadership or group members. Thus, the shadows behind the devaluation of females and seducing some of them into neglected social positions reveal a blind spot in Tibetan Buddhism and its seminar-, meditation-, and retreat-centers in the West, where it has continued to grow over decades. In rationalizing misconduct of the leadership and their helpers to be '*crazy wisdom*' [1, 2, 5, 8] or even so-called '*karma purification*' [1, 2], it was possible to even cover the injury to individuals and structural defects.

Due to the ongoing efforts to whitewash, denigrate those concerned, and silence the required discourse on leadership responsibility and accountability in the respec-tive international contexts and head organizations, it is now crucial to broaden the perspective and consider the societal impact of such offences which, even as Buddhism and spirituality, have already been injuring and traumatizing many people. In the following subchapter, the descriptions of eleven probands are presented.

2. Narratives of members of Buddhist groups

2.1 Methods

Qualitative data of the research project *TransTibMed* from eleven participants in different international Tibetan Buddhist groups are presented covering the following eleven questions: *Which kind of abuse or violence have you experienced in Buddhist groups; how did you react to abuse or violence; how have your experiences in Buddhist groups had an impact on you; which kind of indoctrination, abuse, or violence against others have you witnessed; how have you reacted in the face of this indoctrination, violence, or abuse towards others; how did the experiences in Buddhist groups change you;*

how did the experiences in Buddhist groups change your relationships and your ways of relating to others; *how did your experiences in Buddhist groups change the way you work*; and *have you parted with one or more Buddhist groups or teachers? If so, why?*

The questions *when you think of abuse in Buddhist groups - the abuse of people who have been manipulated and of minors, including sexual abuse - how do you think and feel about it? How do you evaluate the responsibility in the group? Who is responsible for what* and *why do we allow male Buddhist teachers to not only denigrate but also exploit women for their own (mostly hidden) agendas in the name of spirituality* were replied to by others and one person who also replied to the above.

Probands were recruited through information at university, the *German Buddhist Union (DBU)*, and indirectly through (former) group members informing others at social networks.

2.2 Recent testimony

All probands presented wrote about their experiences in international Tibetan Buddhist organizations. Some of them were in several groups. All together, these statements refer to eleven different international Buddhist organizations. In order to protect the individuals, the names of the respective organizations are not provided here.

The following results are structured as follows: All answers of one person are presented in one subchapter. The first nine questions were replied to by #1, #2, #3, #4, and #8 and the last two questions were replied to by #3, #5, #6, #7, #9, #10, and #11. The first six persons (#1–#6) are female and #7–#11 are male.

Questions are written in italics and the replies in straight letters. All answers of probands in German were translated by the author.

2.2.1 #1

Which kind of abuse or violence have you experienced in Buddhist groups?: "Psychological abuse - gaslighting (stating everything is simply in my mind), manipulation to accept abuse by the abuser himself stating that he was my teacher, that everything 'is empty' therefore he couldn't be an abuser. Psychological abuse through an email attack to my workplace claiming I am having a nervous breakdown" (#1).

How did you react to abuse or violence: "At the time of the individual abuse within [...] I felt inadequate, I did not acknowledge that the perpetrator should be able to take some responsibility for their behaviors. I felt abandoned and inadequate because of the way the group reacted to the abuse - they did not acknowledge it had happened and when I disclosed it they did not view it as abuse. I was minimized by the 'spiritual director' when I disclosed it to her - she said that my 'practice was enduring suffering'. At the time this made me feel more inadequate. Later I understood this as a minimizing activity, and I became very angry about six months later after reading testimonies of other former members. Following my workplace receiving an email from [...] management using a fake identity I experienced rage, could not concentrate, my boundaries were poor, I turned to alcohol to cope, I experienced suicidality. I felt paranoid, I did not understand how much danger I might be in or not. I did not know who could help, I felt abandoned by people who did not understand and could not help me. I had digestion problems due to the anxiety and shame for several months. I had little energy and could not exercise, experienced stiffness and rigidity in my face, I had slow speech and slow processing speed. I dissociated frequently e.g. not remembering where I had put things, where I had parked my car. I had nightmares about being murdered by the leadership" (#1).

How have your experiences in Buddhist groups had an impact on you: "Severe post traumatic stress, anxiety, shame, and post traumatic growth. I am now connected to people who I find kind and who listen to me and appreciate my perspective on the groups. I therefore feel heard and understood, and no longer gaslighted" (#1).

Which kind of indoctrination, abuse, or violence against others have you witnessed: "I witnessed long term members so highly indoctrinated that they repeated teach-ings verbatim all the time, they did not have vocabulary from outside the group anymore. I saw people force the teachings on each other to invalidate the other per-sons feelings and dismiss their needs. I have read testimonies and seen evidence of threats against former members - threats to ruin peoples reputations and livelihoods. I heard people with mental health problems be spoke about disrespectfully" (#1).

How have you reacted in the face of this indoctrination, violence, or abuse towards others: "At the time I believed what was said about former members - that they had 'lost patience in their spiritual path' or had 'developed an angry mind and were blaming the centre'. When I came to realize that this was gaslighting of whistle-blowers (after leaving) I became very distressed that the centre could avoid taking responsibility for people's wellbeing by blaming their 'mind' for everything. When I saw the threats and character assassination of former members I went into shock, and then experienced righteous anger" (#1).

How did the experiences in Buddhist groups change you: "I now understand spiritual abuse and am very sensitive to coercion. I am suspicious of all spiritual teachers. I only trust survivors of abuse and a few friends and family. I have more highly developed critical thinking skills and enjoy being disobedient. I now struggle to follow rules I believe are unnecessary, I trust my intuition more" (#1).

How did the experiences in Buddhist groups change your relationships and your ways of relating to others: "I recognise my needs and when someone is not good for me, I do not automatically put other people first. I do not practice accepting everything, I feel more in touch with righteous anger. I try to communicate my emotions more. I trust few people, especially religious people" (#1).

How did your experiences in Buddhist groups change the way you work: "I am suspi-cious of meditation and mindfulness, I read all about the under reported adverse effects. I understand abusive systems of power and abusive group dynamics. I don't trust cognitive therapies so much anymore, I only trust interventions that are also systemic" (#1).

Have you parted with one or more Buddhist groups or teachers? If so, why: "Yes both [...] after reading testimonies of abuse and reading cultic studies literature, I under-stand that they are personality cults and that they do not understand trauma. They claim to help you with stress and teach you mindfulness when they actually believe you should be practising dissociation from your emotions. They have obscured and whitewashed serious abuse, appointed only internal safeguarding officers who are invested in the continuation of the movements, and who are interested in saving their reputations" (#1).

2.2.2 #2

Which kind of abuse or violence have you experienced in Buddhist groups: "Sexual assaults, however without violence, we were servile, so there was no need for it. Men were instrumentalized, delegated by relocation, assigned as secretaries of centers, to work for the Lama was an honour, sometimes for little or no payment, many did not longer pursue their own lives, partnerships were interrupted, separations and uniting were arranged" (#2).

How did you react to abuse or violence: "I did not perceive it as such. It was only when my best friend revealed herself to me that I could see it as abuse on her and then on me as well" (#2).

The questions *how have your experiences in Buddhist groups had an impact on you* and *which kind of indoctrination, abuse, or violence against others have you witnessed* were not answered by #2.

How have you reacted in the face of this indoctrination, violence, or abuse towards others: "later I also learned about sexual assaults against very young women" (#2).

How did the experiences in Buddhist groups change you: "have become more suspi-cious, but also more adult and autonomous" (#2).

How did the experiences in Buddhist groups change your relationships and your ways of relating to others: "Sometimes one gets arrogant, considering oneself as something better, but one also becomes more compassionate. That we are all essentially the same and can simply be on equal level with each other has reached me and I have internalized it to this day. In a therapeutic context it has helped to make encounters on equal level, but also endangered for much closeness and confluence" (#2).

The questions *how did your experiences in Buddhist groups change the way you work* and *have you parted with one or more Buddhist groups or teachers? If so, why* were not answered by #2.

2.2.3 #3

Which kind of abuse or violence have you experienced in Buddhist groups?: "spiri-tual, psychological, emotional" (#3).

How did you react to abuse or violence: "Anger, helplessness, eventually some deference to my teacher for survival and to maintain my position in the group. Basically you have to tell him he is right and you are wrong to preserve your standing as a student" (#3).

The question *how have your experiences in Buddhist groups had an impact on you* was not answered by #3.

Which kind of indoctrination, abuse, or violence against others have you witnessed: "Gaslighting, shaming, slander, emotional manipulation, violation of confidential-ity, outright lies, telling the Executive Director to fire someone because 'she was too neurotic', psychologizing every single student, punishment sending people away from group retreats into solitary or banning people from retreats" (#3).

How have you reacted in the face of this indoctrination, violence, or abuse towards others: "I was often not aware or stood by quietly and watched" (#3).

How did the experiences in Buddhist groups change you: "Sustained attention, strength to do multi day ritual, I am not afraid to be alone in the woods, I accept pain and negative experiences as just part of life. I feel a tremendous union with the divine available in my body. I regularly experience space that feels between life and death, no self, and primordial. I will also never ever become a student of a male spiritual teacher again. I will never give my power away to any human teacher ever again. I have learned a lot about this and still feel very hurt" (#3).

The questions *how did the experiences in Buddhist groups change your relationships and your ways of relating to others*, *how did your experiences in Buddhist groups change the way you work* and *have you parted with one or more Buddhist groups or teachers? If so, why* were not answered by #3.

When you think of abuse in Buddhist groups—the abuse of people who have been manipulated and of minors, including sexual abuse—how do you think and feel about it? How do you evaluate the responsibility in the group? Who is responsible for what: "Angry. Sad. Helpless. The teachers are responsible for the abuse, the board of directors is responsible for not intervening and for allowing a spiritual director who is also paid employee to have veto power over the board (absolute control of the whole organization, which is legally questionable and the board knew it)" (#3).

Why do we allow male Buddhist teachers to not only denigrate but also exploit women for their own (mostly hidden) agendas in the name of spirituality: "We all participate in patriarchy. Tibetan Buddhism encourages mind control, submissiveness, and patriarchal hierarchy. I believe that we allow it because we are so disconnected from our own power that we are willing to let some guy and some exotic tradition tell us what to do. We are eager to hand the reigns over, and Tibetan Buddhism in its sleek ways explains why we should. I believe that men have been suing the tradi-tion for their own agendas for so many centuries that perhaps it has only become a vehicle for patriarchal abuse and I seriously question if the Vajrayana is of benefit in the world now" (#3).

2.2.4 #4

#4 did not answer the question: *which kind of abuse or violence have you experienced in Buddhist groups?*

How did you react to abuse or violence: "I got super angry with myself, blaming myself very badly for not being good enough" (#4).

How have your experiences in Buddhist groups had an impact on you: "Lack of trust, no direction in life, I cannot see my future, I'm afraid of making decisions, I feel helpless and good for nothing" (#4).

Which kind of indoctrination, abuse, or violence against others have you witnessed: "Later on I heard for a community member that the senior teacher had sexual abuse on different women. Even one of the women contacted me and [was] telling me her story. Also I saw people leaving abruptly and getting very confused. Some left with anger. And I heard in the community that there was a woman who got crazy and left. Whatever that means. I guess mentally ill" (#4).

How have you reacted in the face of this indoctrination, violence, or abuse towards others?: "I was blaming myself and asking help from others. I saw everyone else right and I thought they are the best people on Earth, I wanted to get back to the community. I was scared of my family. The community members were immaculate and wise. They even sent me pictures, messages, poems I couldn't understand because I so much wanted to figure out the messages behind" (#4).

How did the experiences in Buddhist groups change you: "I doubt myself, I had better periods but I keep falling back. I lost trust in life, I lost trust in myself and others, I have a lot of tension and fear in me. I cannot imagine to be capable of anything. Study or move away from my parents" (#4).

How did the experiences in Buddhist groups change your relationships and your ways of relating to others: "I can be still opened but deep down I have fear, doubt and it is not easy to trust people in a deeper level. I feel alone" (#4).

How did your experiences in Buddhist groups change the way you work: "I cannot imagine myself to have a job with responsibility. I don't work much a week and sometimes I just sleep for the whole day" (#4).

Have you parted with one or more Buddhist groups or teachers? If so, why: "Yes, two groups, because I had psychosis and got sick" (#4).

2.2.5 #5

When you think of abuse in Buddhist groups—the abuse of people who have been manipulated and of minors, including sexual abuse—how do you think and feel about it? How do you evaluate the responsibility in the group? Who is responsible for what: "I think leaders of Buddhist groups are individuals and it is unavoidable to find some 'black sheep' among them. Certainly I regret such incidents and would feel a serious betrayal of trust if I were to experience this from someone at the centre where I frequently visit. Once someone in the group hears about such, I believe it is their responsibility to communicate to stop it" (#5).

Why do we allow male Buddhist teachers to not only denigrate but also exploit women for their own (mostly hidden) agendas in the name of spirituality: "I would not allow this, but have not had any experience with it, usually I would take action or at least distance myself in case this would not be possible" (#5).

2.2.6 #6

When you think of abuse in Buddhist groups—the abuse of people who have been manipulated and of minors, including sexual abuse—how do you think and feel about it? How do you evaluate the responsibility in the group? Who is responsible for what: "Abuse is unethical and illegal and we always have an obligation to stop it. I don't think most groups are capable of policing themselves. They are too insular and secretive and outside law enforcement should be contacted. I tried to contact the Dalai Lama and other leaders repeatedly, but they never respond" (#6).

Why do we allow male Buddhist teachers to not only denigrate but also exploit women for their own (mostly hidden) agendas in the name of spirituality: "Because some people actually believe these men have special rights and powers and don't have the balls to stand up for people being exploited. People are blinded by robes and spiritual authority and it's dangerous" (#6).

2.2.7 #7

When you think of abuse in Buddhist groups—the abuse of people who have been manipulated and of minors, including sexual abuse—how do you think and feel about it? How do you evaluate the responsibility in the group? Who is responsible for what: "This should not happen at all and ought to lead to an immediate criminal report. The person abusing is responsible, however, depending on the circumstances, also the group involved and the structures prevailing within it. The veneration of the teacher in Tibetan Buddhism unfortunately also creates conditions for abuse, be it physical or authoritative, even if the teachings clearly do not provide for that. In my opinion, Tibetan Buddhism needs some effort towards adjustment to at least make abuse more difficult" (#7).

Why do we allow male Buddhist teachers to not only denigrate but also exploit women for their own (mostly hidden) agendas in the name of spirituality: "Teachers are often held sacrosanct, and criticism of them is mostly unwanted. Sometimes a strong relationship of superiority/subordination can be seen, which facilitates abuse" (#7).

2.2.8 #8

Which kind of abuse or violence have you experienced in Buddhist groups: "Humiliation, exposure, psychological violence, repression, deprivation of healthy self-esteem, intrigues, defamation campaigns, systematic manipulation and lies. Theft: do not take what is not given = misuse of tied donations" (#1) [cited in 2].

How did you react to abuse or violence: "denial, reality negation, rationalization, first insights, perception, evaluation, attempts to communicate, departure" (#8).

How have your experiences in Buddhist groups had an impact on you: "I no longer conform to any group consensus I consider inappropriate. I insist on discussing openly without individual participants manipulating others first. I advocate transparency and truthfulness, even if this is not popular, including financial issues, and try to convey democratic values. My position is that ethics could make a difference, before talking about philosophy and religion" (#8).

Which kind of indoctrination, abuse, or violence against others have you witnessed: "Anyone at [...] should have seen quite a lot. For me, these subtle constant manipulations have been the worst, and that behind the scenes the violence was brutal" (#8).

How have you reacted in the face of this indoctrination, violence, or abuse towards others: "First I rationalized. I found many 'old students' so unpleasant that I considered more drastic measures to possibly be an option. Today I look at it differently. I do not count the eight letter writers among the 'old students', nor all students of [...]. After realizing that all of this at [...] is a dead end, and being frustrated to find out my fellow sanghaists lacked understanding, I left. They were in a 'tunnel'. Particularly the many people afraid of losing their 'dzogchen', whatever that might mean to the individual" (#8).

How did the experiences in Buddhist groups change you: "Now I look at the world more openly, in its entirety, with all of its problems and opportunities" (#8).

How did the experiences in Buddhist groups change your relationships and your ways of relating to others: "I live quite isolated, beyond my professional and family life. I keep considerable distance from Buddhists" (#8).

How did your experiences in Buddhist groups change the way you work: "I take care of myself and my environment as much as I can. People who want to preach to me, I send away" (#8).

Have you parted with one or more Buddhist groups or teachers? If so, why: "Of all of them. My disgust with Buddhist groups is an impulse way too strong to be ignored. It either will subside or it doesn't. I am a Buddhist who pretends he is not" (#8).

2.2.9 #9

When you think of abuse in Buddhist groups—the abuse of people who have been manipulated and of minors, including sexual abuse—how do you think and feel about it? How do you evaluate the responsibility in the group? Who is responsible for what: "I feel angry and a huge sense of injustice about it, because it totally goes against the spirit of Buddhism, which is compassion, kindness, and bringing people to enlightenment. The teacher and the Buddhist institution the teacher is affiliated with is responsible" (#9).

Why do we allow male Buddhist teachers to not only denigrate but also exploit women for their own (mostly hidden) agendas in the name of spirituality: "It is an issue to do with the dominant patriarchal society we are part of today, where men are in positions of authority. This, unfortunately has extended to religion" (#9).

2.2.10 #10

When you think of abuse in Buddhist groups—the abuse of people who have been manipulated and of minors, including sexual abuse—how do you think and feel about it? How do you evaluate the responsibility in the group? Who is responsible for what: "Every single person has his share of responsibility, even if he acted in blind trust. These are mitigating circumstances, of a sort. In [...]: The higher the position, the greater is the degree of blindness. And the fish is always stinking from its head. Those at the top of an authoritarian structure, and who, due to their position as lama per se are endowed with particular abilities, ought to take responsibility for the consequences of their actions. Responsibility in groups is usually given to older students, who might have been accordingly indoctrinated and bring the relevant skills. Sociological studies might show 80% of leadership in Western Buddhist groups are female, except for the top positions. A psychologist and Buddhist, who I know well, even claims that women are more susceptible to manipulating behaviors in these positions" (#10).

Why do we allow male Buddhist teachers to not only denigrate but also exploit women for their own (mostly hidden) agendas in the name of spirituality: "Ignorance, lack of awareness, lack of ethical conscience. This is true for all genders, although it is mainly women who are currently victims of male offenders. Mostly all is well, as long as one isn't victimized oneself" (#10).

2.2.11 #11

When you think of abuse in Buddhist groups—the abuse of people who have been manipulated and of minors, including sexual abuse—how do you think and feel about it? How do you evaluate the responsibility in the group? Who is responsible for what: "Disgusted and annoyed. Everyone is responsible in particular the people who know directly about it and keep silent. However I know some people did try to bring abuse to light in the group I knew many years ago. Everything was ignored. They kept files they later gave to an investigation. Yet the group or the lama has still not admitted abuse" (#11).

Why do we allow male Buddhist teachers to not only denigrate but also exploit women for their own (mostly hidden) agendas in the name of spirituality: "Because it happens behind closed doors and unless the women themselves speak out it is difficult to prove. Also Tibetan Buddhism like most religions use fear of hell and damnation to silence. Also women are told they are dakini and as such special with special merit when they die" (#11).

2.3 Interpretation

The current issues in so-called Buddhist centers unfold against the background of oversimplifications of terms and concepts of Buddhist philosophy as well as of damaging neologisms. In particular, however, traditional application-oriented learning processes crucial for understanding and teaching are missing. The individual effects of these substantial and structural deficiencies are evident as health dam-age, specifically mental health, and traumatization of group members. Unreflected decontextualized use of Buddhist terminology and concepts and the neologisms in these contexts thus negatively impact on group dynamics and the health of a group and its members. Since the indoctrination described by the testimonies and the traumatization is still attempted to be denied by the mainstream within these organi-zations as well as the victims silenced [2], the latter are not compensated in any ways by precisely these organizations which have often previously enriched themselves on them. Furthermore, by propagating Buddhism a panacea for mental diseases, even persons with mental disorders are misled in highly irresponsible ways. Although oaths of secrecy associated with seemingly Buddhist concepts render it difficult for those affected to talk, testimonies regarding indoctrination and systematic abuse causing trauma and mental illness are available now. However, a high number of unrecorded cases of those, who for various reasons are unable to communicate, ought to be assumed.

The kind of abuse described by the probands covers psychological abuse (#2, #3), especially those aspects of the students' submission, which serve as a basis for sexual assault (#2), the indoctrinative interpretations that are suggesting the abuse itself would take place in the mind of the student (#1) only, as well as psychological violence (#8). This questioning of one's own autonomous understanding of situations and even one's perception leads to a continuous state of disorientation, which initially may contribute to psychological damage and is particularly important to consider in later processes of treatment. By means of neologisms such as '*karma purification*' and '*crazy wisdom*', which serve to rationalize any misconduct of group leaders and entourage towards the goal of the students' enlightenment, a form of dependence is constructed, in which they even bind themselves to the insulting leadership. In such ways their identification processes [14] are enhanced and self-reliance and autonomy reduced.

Emotional abuse (#3) was presented as humiliation (#8), exposure (#8), and repression (#8), which explains the very reduction in self-esteem (#8) of students in such groups. However, by using misunderstood visualizations of the Vajrayāna, also narcissistic tendencies get encouraged, resulting in severe arrogance, particularly among those seeking to establish themselves in positions of authority in such contexts, and in such ways forming a kind of spiritual narcissism. This, in turn, may explain their lack of empathy and compassion towards the victims, even whilst still proclaiming Buddhist compassion.

The abuse of authority for slandering any current or former students was reported as interfering with lies even at the workplace, outside the so-called Buddhist organization (#1). The lies (#8), intrigues (#8), and defamation campaigns (#8) mentioned have a huge impact on the individuals, particularly when used to irritate or destroy their reputation, social networks, and income. Since one has grown accustomed to such situations in these contexts, it seems necessary to emphasize that such is far from the basic ethical values taught within traditional Tibetan Buddhism.

The indoctrination saying the abuser would be allowed for the abuse, because of being a spiritual teacher (#1) already indicates an utterly inappropriate way of defining spiritual authority. Groups propagating such dangerous concepts concern-ing their spiritual teacher, devoid of ethics and adherence to national legislation, together with any authorities imposing their authoritative rules at will, endanger group members as well as visitors.

Any manipulation of students, interpreting the work for a lama, who is regarded a spiritual authority in the group, being an honor (#2), which in turn meant sexual abuse of servile (female) students (#2) and the instrumentalization of men for all kinds of little or unpaid services (#2), as well as systematic manipulation (#8), were also described as abuse (#2). Interpreting work for a spiritual authority as honor already indicates narcissistic group dynamics, where autonomous authentic training of Buddhist ethics and meditation has been replaced by rivalry over physical proximity to the leadership, which in turn has been redefined and also implies power over the group through identification processes. Thus, such concepts shape not only the group's structures and behavior patterns but also its economic handling, that is expecting donations for certain group members. Furthermore, manipulation is not only for complying with financial and other service expectations, but often people are played off against each other and exchanged after their exploitation at will. Over the years of affiliation, however, these kinds of interactions, which are accompanied by psychological and financial dependencies as well as mental identification processes, can cause serious damage. Theft in the sense of misuse of tied donations (#8) was also mentioned to be abuse. And the manipulation with the conceptual distortion of the Buddhist concept of emptiness used to explain away abuse and abuser (#1) severely devaluates Buddhist philosophy and undermines sound and informed terminological and conceptual discourse.

The testimony of indoctrination, abuse, or violence against others was described as follows: subtle constant manipulations (#8), highly indoctrinated long-term members lacking vocabulary from outside the group (#1), and repeating verbatim all the time (#1). For so-called Buddhist seminar- and retreat-participants the follow-ing methods were described: psychologizing every single student (#3), emotional manipulation (#3), violation of confidentiality (#3), gaslighting (#3), shaming (#3), slander (#3), and outright lies (#3). Someone also testified disrespectful speech about people with mental health problems (#1). Furthermore, blackmailing of the management was described, such as telling the executive director to fire some-one because of being diagnosed neurotic (#3) by nonprofessionals. Furthermore, there is testimony on punishment in the form of sending people away from group into solitary retreats or banning people from retreats (#3) and brutal violence behind the scenes (#8). Someone interpreted dismissing people's needs by invalidating their feelings (#1) through forcing what was called 'teachings' on them. There is also testimony on threats to ruin people's reputations and livelihoods (#1) and on sexual abuse of different women by a senior teacher (#4). Whereas sexual abuse of minors is a clearly defined a criminal offense, currently also severely manipulated and indoctrinated adults, who have mostly initially made their way up to the '*inner circle*' [2, 5] and have then moved on to physical proximity or agreed to the position of secret lovers, claim the same for themselves. Thus, the overloaded phrase of 'sexual abuse' in current contextual discourses ought to be further differentiated, taking into account unequal balance of power, indoctrination, seduction, untrue promises, coercive control, self-responsibility of adults, as well as victimizing collaborators and witnesses. Moreover, the dynamics of controlling the feminine, which have been adopted unreflectively from Tibetan Buddhism, manifest in seemingly impersonal attitudes towards the women concerned, which thus results in a high number of victims.

Three successive states of individual reaction to indoctrination, abuse or violence in the respective Buddhist group showed: continuous close affiliation, critical reflec-tion, and departure. For the period of close affiliation to a group helplessness (#3), denial (#8), feeling of inadequacy (#1), not acknowledging that the perpetrator should be able to take some responsibility for their behaviors (#1), feeling aban-doned and inadequate because of the reactions of the leadership and group to the abuse (who did not view it as abuse) (#1), oneself not perceiving abuse and violence as such, but only understanding it when seeing it on someone else first (#2) and anger (#3) were reported. One person severely turned against herself and reported getting seriously angry at herself (#4) with putting herself down (#4). Another person in high position in her group and dependent on financial terms told she has taken over the opinion of the teacher to preserve her own standing and maintain her position in the group (#3). Thus, these replies also may show some implications and limitations of holding positions in such groups. In phase two, the period of reflection and doubts, there were communication attempts before departure (#8). In phase three, after departure from the group, there were feelings to be abandoned by those who did not understand and could not help (#1), anxiety and shame for several months causing digestion problems (#1), frequent dissociation (#1), which might have been accompanied by stiffness and rigidity in the face (#1), little energy (#1), and slow speech and slow processing speed (#1). Furthermore, doubts regard-ing the dangers (#1) with nightmares about being murdered by the leadership (#1), lack of concentration (#1), poor boundaries (#1), turning to alcohol to cope (#1), and suicidality (#1) were reported. Reading testimonies of former members (#1) was reported having caused anger. And the workplace receiving an email from the so-called Buddhist organization's management, who was even using a fake identity (#1), caused rage (#1).

The above three successive states of individual reaction were reported to be accompanied by two inner processes when observing indoctrination, abuse, or violence of others: the identifying and indoctrinating phase and the reflection phase. These observations show concepts and behavior far from the attitude of traditional Buddhist practice of having the individual's autonomy, awareness and self-reflection as its basis. At the period of being indoctrinated, identifying and merging with the leadership, management or group expectations reactions such as lack of one's own awareness of it (#3), standing quietly (#3) and watching (#3), which could be interpreted as a kind of freezing in shock about what was seen, as well as rationalizing (#8) and even believing what was said about former members (#1) were reported. Someone did not respond to the question directly, but stated sexual assaults against very young women (#2). Yet another person told she was even blaming herself (#4) for the above behavior of other group members while regarding everyone else right. At the period of reflection, when interpreting the issues leading to decisions, someone described realizing all of it a dead end (#8) and his frustration about his fellows narrowing their understanding like in a 'tunnel' (#8) before he left. Others responded to the manipulation and indoctrination tactics in the group with shock and later righteous anger (#1), because of the threats and character assassination of former members (#1) as well as with high distress about the center avoiding to take responsibility by blaming people's 'mind' for anything (#1).

The question on how the person was changed him- or herself by their experiences in these groups was replied to with some positive aspects such as sustained attention (#3), strength to do multi-day ritual (#3), being not afraid to be alone in the woods (#3), and the feeling of union with the divine (#3). However, the positively connotated aspect of accepting pain and negative experiences as just a part of life (#3) may already endanger this individual in highly manipulative contexts. Aspects with negative connotations, such as doubting oneself (#4), not being able to imagine to be capable of anything (#4), having a lot of tension and fear (#4), as well as having lost trust in oneself and others (#4) and in life (#4), were reported as well. People also described having become more suspicious (#2), particularly of all spiritual teachers (#1), being sensitive to coercion (#1) and understanding spiritual abuse (#1), the latter of which may not only protect the individual but also enable them to protect others from unreasonable nonsense and misuse. The phrase spiri-tual abuse might be interpreted as people being seduced into giving up their own strength as if dependent on a master providing them access to their own spirituality. Furthermore, with reporting greater autonomy (#2) and trusting one's own intuition more (#1), an individual process of change was addressed, which is also found in phrases such as becoming more adult (#2), having developed critical thinking skills (#1), and probably even in enjoying being disobedient (#1) after experienc-ing abuse in highly authoritative structures to some extent. Also, the result of a process, such as looking at the world more openly (#8), was referred to, and deci-sions were shared such as never becoming a student of a male spiritual teacher again (#3) and never ever giving one's power away to any human teacher (#3).

The scope of the personal impact of these experiences in Buddhist groups was described with adverse effects such as severe self-devaluation (#4), posttrau-matic stress (#1), and feelings of helpless (#4), shame (#1), and anxiety (#1). Furthermore, lack of trust (#4) was described at the interpersonal level, which might impact considerably on future relationships and work decisions. Although the fear of making decisions (#4) and loss of direction in life (#4) may come up in an early period of leaving an abusive group, they sometimes continue for even years. The refusal to conform to any group consensus considered inappropriate (#8) is often part of the separating process and might stay as a lesson learned. Furthermore, there are positive connotations for a time period after having left the group and making new personal and working relationships, which were called new connections to kind people (#1) and posttraumatic growth (#1). Also, the values of the person were described to be discussing openly without individual participants manipulating others first (#8) and advocating transparency and truthfulness (#8), even if this is not popular, including financial issues (#8), as well as trying to convey democratic values (#8) and ethics (#8). The reflection of absorbed values and integration of one's own value system are aspects of the process of separation, which often occur long after the physical separation. Sometimes this also encompasses referring to traditional basic Buddhist ethics. In therapeutic processes, it takes place in the phase of dealing with introjects and in the phase of integration. The impact on relationships and ways of relating to others was described as getting arrogant sometimes (#2) for the period in the group, which is regarding oneself higher or more spiritually advanced than others. Negative impact of fear and doubt with feeling lonely and difficulties to trust people (#4) was described as well. Furthermore, it was said recognizing one's own needs (#1), which seems to be a key issue to reconnect to oneself, not practicing accepting everything (#1) and not automatically putting other people first (#1), trusting few people (#1), as well as trying to communicate emotions more (#1), which may show as becoming more compassionate (#2) or feeling in touch with righteous anger (#1). The making of encounters on equal level at a therapeutic context with dangers for too much conflu-ence (#2) was an impact for a professional therapist. Someone also shared keeping a considerable distance from Buddhists (#8) and living quite isolated beyond profes-sional and family life (#8).

The impact on one's work was described as taking care to the best of one's abilities of oneself and surrounding (8), understanding abusive systems of power and abusive group dynamics (#1) and also as suspiciousness of meditation and mindfulness (#1). A young person shared a highly negative impact for her life saying she could not imagine herself at a job with responsibility (#4), she would not work much (#4) and sometimes sleep for the whole day (#4).

The following two questions refer to open letters and ongoing investigations widely discussed in the context. They were asked to understand not only the persons' opinion but also their position in the group and their behavior. Not everyone replied to the questions: *when you think of abuse in Buddhist groups—the abuse of people who have been manipulated and of minors, including sexual abuse—how do you think and feel about it? How do you evaluate the responsibility in the group? Who is responsible for what?* Whereas someone told abuse to be unethical and illegal (#6) and in this way referred to basic values, another person simply stripped the leadership of its exaggerated superiority saying the leaders of Buddhist groups were individuals and it would be unavoidable to find some 'black sheep' among them (#5). #7 judged that it should not happen at all and ought to lead to an immediate criminal report. Someone replied the veneration of the teacher in Tibetan Buddhism unfortunately would also create conditions for abuse (#7). Reports on one's own feelings range from helpless (#3), sadness (#3), and anger (#3) to disgust and annoyance (#11). Furthermore, someone told to regret such incidents (#5) and feel a serious betrayal of trust (#5). Someone reported feeling anger and a huge sense of injustice about it (#9) and gave reasons for such behavior going against the spirit of Buddhism, which would be defined as compassion, kindness, and bringing people to enlightenment (#9). Regarding the assignment of responsibilities, one woman said people always have an obligation to stop abuse (#6), and similarly another person told it would be the responsibility of anyone hearing about abuse to communicate to stop it (#5). A man told the person abusing is responsible (#7), however, depending on the circumstances, also the group involved, and the structures prevailing within (#7). Another man told that the teacher and the Buddhist institution the teacher is affiliated with were responsible (#9) and someone else that every single person had his share of responsibility, even if they acted in blind trust (#10), and that the latter would be mitigating circumstances (#10). Furthermore, one woman regarded the leadership and its teachers to be responsible for the abuse (#3) and the board of directors for not intervening (#3) and she analyzed challenging power structures allowing for abuse (#3). #6 assumed most of these so-called Buddhist groups would not be capable of policing themselves (#6) arguing them to be too insular (#6) and secretive (#6) and outside law enforcement (#6). This woman also reported having tried to contact the Dalai Lama and other leaders repeatedly without ever having received any response (#6). Someone else told that Tibetan Buddhism would need some effort towards adjustment to at least make abuse more difficult (#7), and #10 analyzed the degree of higher position in the group to positively correlate with the degree of blindness (#10). He continued to elaborate that responsibility in groups were usually given to older students, who might have been be accordingly indoctri-nated and bring the relevant skills (#10). He argued they ought to take responsibil-ity for the consequences of their actions (#10). Yet another person replied that everyone would be responsible, in particular those people who knew but kept silent (#11). This person then reported to know some people who were first ignored when they tried to bring abuse to light in the group (#11) and that neither the lama nor his group would have admitted abuse (#11), even after they later have given the files to an investigation (#11). Despite singularizing individuals with shifting the issues on them, the persons in the groups acting in such ways are "agents in violent betrayal" [15].

The question *why do we allow male Buddhist teachers to not only denigrate but also exploit women for their own (mostly hidden) agendas in the name of spirituality* was replied to as follows: Someone telling to have no experience with it assumes she would not allow this (#5) by taking action (#5) or at least distancing herself (#5). A man called it ignorance, lack of awareness, and lack of ethical conscience (#10) and elaborated this to be true for all genders, although currently mainly women were victims of male offenders (#10) and that as long as one is not victimized oneself (#10) people would perceive everything to be fine (#10). Another man ana-lyzed the secrecy behind closed doors (#11) telling unless the women themselves speak out, it would be difficult to prove (#11). He described the fear of hell used in Tibetan Buddhism for silencing (#11) and the seduction with calling the women a dakini promising them special merit at the time of their death (#11). Another man analyzed it as an issue to do with the dominant patriarchal society (#9), where men are in positions of authority having extended to religion (#9). A man analyzed that teachers would be often held sacrosanct (#7), telling criticism of them were mostly unwanted (#7). Furthermore, he argued the strong relationship of superiority facilitating abuse (#7). One women responded with participation in patriarchy (#3) accused what she thinks is Tibetan Buddhism encouraging mind control, submissiveness, and patriarchal hierarchy (#3) and interprets people disconnected from their own power (#3) being willing to let someone tell them what to do (#3). She accused men suing the tradition for their own agendas for many centuries (#3) and regards what she has learned to be so-called Vajrayana even a vehicle for patriarchal abuse (#3). Another woman argued with attributing special rights and powers to certain men (#6), saying people were blinded by robes and spiritual authority, judging this to be dangerous (#6). She also attributes lack of courage to protect those exploited (#6).

Thus, the opening of any closed elitist circles to the wider societal discourse, the democratization processes required within the strictly hierarchical struc-tures of Tibetan Buddhist centers and a supervised training of group members in traditional interpretations of Buddhist terms, concepts and ethics as well as the urgently needed cultural discourses are a vital condition for differenti-ated, linguistically and scientifically sound processes of knowledge transfer and exchange. However, whereas these concerns contribute to overcoming structural and conceptual inadequacies, the view of and behavior towards women remains a key issue. Particularly, the tacit transfer of projecting the shadow onto the female and the implicit mechanisms of their control ought to be reflected and addressed. In this context, the role and function of a teacher's secret lover and unreflective copying culturally shaped structures and behavior with regards to her are crucial. Given the lack of reference within their own cultural context, this raises questions about the psychological effects of such kind of social isolation of these women as well as about their secret position of power, which is even defined highly desirable in some circles. This issue raises further questions about leadership responsibility with regard to the group dynamics induced by it and the effects on the women concerned and their self-responsibility. The societal challenge of correcting individual damages that have been recurring throughout generations, which nega-tively impact on the knowledge of Buddhism itself, however, is directly opposed to the current mainstream of secrecy and individualizing these issues as so-called *'bad karma'* [1, 2] in such contexts. But although those who still draw their indi-vidual profits from these structures try to influence their followers with refusing to listen to the victims and authoritative and confusing definitions, such as trauma being even the aggression of the victim, and in such ways continue to manipulate seminar participants and publicly ridicule and slander victims, now the wider social surrounding has started to counteract the strategy of individualizing issues.

3. Conclusion

Lacking intercultural exchange of scientific knowledge and its integration into the education in Buddhist philosophy and Tibetan medicine resulted in oversimplification and misguided practice.

Furthermore, the collective projection of the shadow onto the feminine reveals through the current individual and structural challenges in these contexts. This pattern being passed down through generations and unreflectively transferred to Western centers has contributed to forming a subculture spreading internationally under Buddhist cover, with its own secrecy rules, use of language in rationalizing neologisms for the silencing of trauma and the traumatized [2] and trauma dynamics. Ignoring the unconscious in teacher-student relationships and group dynamics has led to the superelevation of persons, even loosing ethics, which form the basis of every Buddhist tradition. Thus, based on the demands for identification with the spiritual master and his entourage, mental diseases were induced.

For individuals coming from Buddhist contexts, it is therefore important to replace the convenient ways of handing over responsibility, which are leading to patterns of dependency and serving exploitation, with freedom to autonomy along with self-responsibility regarding their own training and ethics. The autonomy in one's own spirituality can never be substituted by an intermediary who is regarded as the sole access to one's own resource. And the role of the lineage holder in Vajrayāna is not meant for such.

Society, which provides care for the shamelessly exploited, diseased, and traumatized people, now faces several challenges. Apart from prevention through dismantling common idealizations and providing information about the circumstances, terminology involved in indoctrination and the dangers in hypnotising techniques or dissociation sold for so-called Buddhist meditation, it is crucial to develop treatment concepts for those with complex diseases to provide therapeutic care. Furthermore, broadening of the perspective is needed to enable improve-ment of these closed systems with their seminar-, meditation-, and retreat-centers, particularly concerning education as well as conveying human rights and national legislation to those group members who assume their spiritual masters and entourage are above legislation. For preserving the knowledge of Buddhist philosophy and practice, curing the transgenerational patterns of traumatization of individuals, compensating victims and deciding on how to deal with perpetrators, accomplices and collaborators are crucial.

Acknowledgements

This research was funded by the German Federal Ministry of Education and Research, grant reference number 01UL1823X.

Author details

Anne Iris Miriam Anders
Institute of Social and Cultural Anthropology, Ludwig Maximilians University
Munich, Germany

*Address all correspondence to: miriam.anders@campus.lmu.de

References

[1] Anders AIM. Psychische Auswirkungen von Machtmissbrauch in buddhistischen Gruppierungen und essenzielle Aspekte bei psychotherapeutischen Interventionen für Betroffene. SFU Forschungsbulletin. 2019;7(1):32-49. DOI: 10.15135/2019.7.1.32-49. Available in English from: https://www.en.transtibmed.ethnologie.uni-muenchen.de/publications/index.html

[2] Anders AIM. Silencing and oblivion of psychological trauma, its unconscious aspects, and their impact on the inflation of Vajrayāna. An analysis of cross-group dynamics and recent developments in Buddhist groups based on qualitative data. Religion. 2019;**622**:1-23. DOI: 10.3390/rel10110622

[3] An Olive Branch. Shambhala Final Project Report [Internet]. 2019. Available from: https://www.dropbox.com/s/eloezy0vc0nhgro/AOB_FinalReport_March2019_final.pdf?dl=0 [Accessed: 20 March 2019]

[4] An Olive Branch. Report on the Shambhala Listening Post [Internet]. 2019. Available from: https://www.dropbox.com/s/111arue9y4gtk73/AOB_ListeningPostReport_March2019_final.pdf?dl=0 [Accessed: 20 March 2019]

[5] Baxter K. Report to the boards of trustees of: Rigpa fellowship UK, and Rigpa fellowship US. Outcome of an investigation into allegations made against Sogyal Lakar (also known as Sogyal Rinpoche) in a letter dated 14 July 2017 [Internet]. 2018. Available from: https://static1.squarespace.com/static/580dbe87e6f2e16700cb79fe/t/5b8f7c1e1ae6cfb38491e668/1536130081917/Lewis+Silkin+report.pdf [Accessed: 15 May 2020]

[6] Ex-OKC born-kids. 40 Years of Abuse in the name of Dharma [Internet]. 2020. Available from: https://okcinfo.news/en/timeline/ [Accessed: 01 June 2020]

[7] Morman C, Leslie L, Fitch L, Ellerton D, Canepa A. An Open Letter to the Shambhala Community from Long-Serving Kusung [Internet]. 2019. Available from: https://drive. google.com/file/d/1W3fN12nEY-l0U2yejz3O4vcqaCMfusIa/view?fbclid=IwAR0Qo3zbWkJ3E5wjPUhLoVwOJnKwZee_AAzA79kvgj9K6DcOfh5uU7p5pM0 [Accessed: 16 February 2019]

[8] Standlee M, Sangye D, Pistono M, Standlee J, Price G, et al. Open letter to Sogyal Lakar [Internet]. 2017. Available from: https://www.lionsroar. com/wp-content/uploads/2017/07/Letter-to-Sogyal-Lakar-14-06-2017-.pdf [Accessed: 15 May 2020]

[9] The Charity Commission. New Charity Inquiry: Rigpa Fellowship. Charity Commission investigates Rigpa Fellowship [Internet]. 2018. Available from: https://www.gov.uk/government/news/new-charity-inquiry-rigpa-fellowship [Accessed: 15 May 2020]

[10] Winn AM. Project Sunshine: Final Report A Firebird Year Initiative to Bring Light and Healing to Sexualized Violence Embedded Within the Shambhala Community [Internet]. 2018. Available from: www. andreamwinn.com/pdfs/Project_ Sunshine_Final_Report.pdf [Accessed: 01 June 2020]

[11] Winn AM, Merchasin C. Buddhist Project Sunshine Phase 3 Final Report The Nail: Bringing Things to a Clear Point A 2-Month Initiative to Bring Activating Healing Light to Sexualized Violence at the Core of the Shambhala Buddhist Community [Internet]. 2018. Available from: andreamwinn.com/project_sunshine/Buddhist_Project_Sunshine_Phase_3_Final_Report.pdf [Accessed: 01 June 2020]

[12] Winn AM, Edelman R, Merchasin C, Monson E, Women Survivors. Buddhist Project Sunshine Phase 2 Final Report. A 3-month Initiative to Bring Healing Light to Sexualized Violence at the Core of the Shambhala Buddhist Community [Internet]. 2018. Available from: andreamwinn.com/project_sunshine/Buddhist_Project_Sunshine_Phase_2_Final_Report.pdf [Accessed: 01 June 2020]

[13] Dockler L, Mueller J. Introduction to the special issue on institutional and betrayal trauma. Journal of Aggression, Maltreatment and Trauma. 2017;**26, 1**: 1-2. DOI:10.1080/10926771.2016.1263707

[14] Jung CG. Die Beziehungen zwischen dem Ich und dem Unbewußten. 2nd ed. Dt. Taschenbuch-Verlag: München; 2014

[15] Gentile K. Assembling justice: Reviving nonhuman subjectivities to examine institutional betrayal around sexual misconduct. Journal of the American Psychoanalytic Association. 2018;**66**(4):647-678. DOI: 10.1177/0003065118797138

6

Post-Traumatic Stress Disorder in Children and Adolescents: Some Recent Research Findings

Yuanyuan Li, Ya Zhou, Xiaoyan Chen, Fang Fan, George Musa and Christina Hoven

Abstract

Childhood trauma can have a profound effect on development, with a lifelong impact on physical growth, psychological development, and mental health. This chapter provides a framework for adolescent health professionals to understand the impacts of traumatic stress on children and adolescents. This chapter mainly takes the Wenchuan Earthquake studies in China as an example, and reviews recent research findings on epidemiological characteristics of PTSD and related mental disorders, as well as on possible influencing factors and mechanisms for post-traumatic adaptation in children and adolescents. Important intervention strategies for PTSD in children and adolescents are introduced. Prospects for future research are also discussed.

Keywords: PTSD, comorbidity, post-traumatic adaptation, protective and risk factors, treatments, children, adolescents

1. Introduction

Exposure to potentially traumatic events such as hostilities of school shootings, terrorist attacks, threats of war, destruction of public property, suicide bombings, and natural disasters is highly frequent among young people across the world. Many children appear to be confronted with one or more potentially traumatic events while growing up. As children and adolescents have limited coping strategies and are less capable of effectively protecting themselves, they are more vulnerable to traumatic disaster than adults. It was reported that, in the immediate aftermath of such events, a high percentage of children will experience symptoms of Post-traumatic Stress Disorder (PTSD) with approximately 20–30% going on to develop the full disorder in the first 6 months [1]. However, due to the special stage of their physical and mental development, unique features of pediatric PTSD have less been studied. Fortunately, there is growing recognition of the fact that traumatic events can have severe and lasting impacts on children, and clinicians are becoming increasingly sensitive to the psychological needs of young survivors of traumatic events.

Depending upon the developmental stage and level of cognitive and emotional maturity, the symptomatology of PTSD in children are expected to be different from that in adults [2]. Prevalence and symptomatology of PTSD also vary greatly among children and adolescents depending upon the traumatic event itself, the severity and duration of exposure, and the child's demographic variables such as gender, age, and ethnicity. For example, rates of PTSD diagnosis are higher among girls, middle school children, and Hispanics [3–5]. Interpersonal traumas, such as sexual and physical assaults, are more likely to result in PTSD than exposure to natural or technological disasters [2, 6]. In addition, numerous psychological, family, and social factors such as parental mental status and, prolonged life disruption could also affect children and adolescents' post-trauma adaptation and recovery [7, 8]. Currently, PTSD is increasingly viewed as a potentially serious disorder in children and adolescents, because of not only the intense suffering it wreaks on young people, but also its adverse effects on biological, psychological, and social development [9]. Left untreated, PTSD can persist for years, increase the children's risk of developing other disorders, and impair their psychosocial functioning in future life [10].

In this chapter, we will take the Wenchuan Earthquake studies in China as an example to introduce current research results of PTSD and related mental disorders, their influencing factors and mechanisms, and intervention strategies in adolescents. The Wenchuan Earthquake is an 8.0-magnitude earthquake that struck Wenchuan County in China's south-western Sichuan Province on May 12, 2008. This massive disaster left 69,197 people dead, 374,176 injured, 18,222 listed as missing, and at least 4.8 million people were rendered homeless in the earthquake affected areas. Moreover, a number of subsequent earthquakes have ravaged south-western China during the years after the Wenchuan Earthquake. Since this earthquake, researchers in China have conducted a series of studies to examine the impacts of earthquake exposure on mental health development among Chinese children and adolescents. For example, Fan and his colleagues established the Wenchuan Earthquake Adolescents Health Cohort (WEAHC) [11], which is a 6-wave longitudinal study across 10 years in a cohort of 2250 adolescents exposed to this disaster. The WEAHC project examined longitudinal epidemiological characteristics of various disaster-related mental health disorders (i.e., PTSD, depression, anxiety, sleep disturbances, etc.), and collected psychological, familial, and genetic data with the aim of exploring potential etiologies of these disorders. In addition to the WEAHC project, other research teams have also conducted longitudinal investigations of child and adolescent earthquake survivors in China since 2008. All these studies have offered novel insights into the epidemiology, symptomology, related risk and proactive factors, and preventive and intervening measures for PTSD and comorbid disorders in Chinese children and adolescents. In this chapter, we will introduce important findings from the WEAHC study as well as these other studies.

Specific issues of this chapter are as follows: (1) assessment of post-traumatic stress disorder in children and adolescents; (2) epidemiological characteristics of PTSD among children and adolescents; (3) possible mechanisms for PTSD in children and adolescents; (4) post-traumatic growth; (5) psychological and pharmacological treatments for children and adolescents with PTSD.

2. Assessment of post-traumatic stress disorder in children and adolescents

There is consensus that core symptoms for the diagnosis of PTSD in children over the age of 7 years are almost similar to those used for adults. However, below this age (particularly below the age of 5 years), there is less agreement on the criteria for diagnosis. Nevertheless, trauma-affected symptoms in younger children are gradually being identified, such as regression to immature behaviors (becoming more anxious and clingy, and having difficulty settling to sleep), aggression (becoming irritable, having temper tantrums, or displaying destructive behavior), repetitive reenactment in play or drawings, and nightmares may occur less frequently [12]. We also need to be able to identify children and adolescents symptomatology as it relates to their functioning in different contexts.

Children may not report their psychological reactions to the trauma unless they are specifically asked about aspects of trauma [13]. Due to cognitive immaturity, children may not be given the opportunities to talk about the event. Even having the opportunity, limited cognitive and expressive language skills of children may make it difficult to infer their thoughts and feelings smoothly. However, since parents and teachers have often been shown to be poor reporters of symptoms in children [2], directly asking the children about their symptoms is almost always required.

To date, more evaluation tools have been developed to evaluate the reactions and symptoms of children and adolescents exposed to traumatic events. The evaluation tools can be roughly divided into two categories: subjective instruments and (semi-) structured interview tools.

2.1 Subjective instruments

Self-rating or other-rating (usually reported by parents or caregivers) scales are considered as effective tools for screening PTSD in children and adolescents, which can reflect the current stress response of the patient to a certain extent, and are convenient for large-scale use in the trauma-exposed population.

2.1.1 Impact of Event Scale-Revised, IES-R

The Impact of Event Scale-Revised (IES-R) is a self-report measure of current subjective distress in response to a specific traumatic event [14]. Although originally developed for adults, this scale is useful to monitor post-traumatic stress symptoms as well as to track progress with interventions among individuals over the age of 7 years [15].

IES-R is a revised version of the Impact of Event Scale [16], which consists of 22-item, with 3 core symptom clusters of PTSD: intrusion (8 items related to intrusive thoughts, nightmares, intrusive feelings, and imagery associated with the traumatic event), avoidance (8 items related to avoidance of feelings, situations, and ideas), and hyperarousal (6 items related to difficulty concentrating, anger and irritability, psychophysiological arousal upon exposure to reminders and hypervigilance). IES-R requests subjects to report on the degree of distress rather than the frequency of the symptoms and takes approximately 10 min to complete and score with no special training required to administer the questionnaire. It also showed good reliability, validity, and sensitivity to change.

2.1.2 The Children's Revised Impact of Event Scale, CRIES-13

The Children's Revised Impact of Event Scale (CRIES-13) with good reliability and validity as well as a stable factors structure, is a brief child-friendly measure designed to screen children at risk for PTSD. It has been used to screen a large number of at-risk-children following multiple types of traumatic events [17]. According to the DSM criteria with 17 PTSD symptoms across three symptom clusters, CRIES revealed a three-factor solution corresponding to the intrusion (4 items), avoid-ance (4 items), and arousal (5 items) subscales. Higher scores reflect children's higher risk with PTSD. According to Smith et al. [18], the scores were related to the children's level of traumatic exposure, anxiety, and depression, as well as distress reported from mothers and teachers.

2.1.3 Child PTSD Symptom Scale, CPSS

The Child PTSD Symptom Scale [19] is a self-report measure of PTSD severity among 8–18 years old children, which is in accordance with the diagnostic criteria in the Diagnostic and Statistical Manual of Mental Disorders (DSM–IV 4th ed. [20]). It seems well understood by children and is relatively quick for them to administer. The CPSS indexes the frequency of the 17 PTSD symptoms (DSM–IV), with each item rated on a 4-point Likert-type scale (0 = not at all, 1 = once a week or less, 2 = 2–4 times a week, 3 = 5 or more times per week). The impact of symptoms on daily function is also measured with seven dichotomously scored items that include aspects such as schoolwork and relationship with one's family [21].

The CPSS can be used as a continuous measure of symptom severity (ranging from 0 to 51), and a cutoff of 11 or above was found to have sensitivity of 95% and specificity of 96% [21]. Foa et al. [19] also reported that the 17 symptom items could be scored dichotomously to generate a DSM–IV consistent diagnosis of PTSD.

2.1.4 The UCLA PTSD Reaction Index for DSM-IV, revision 1 (UCLA CPTSD-RI)

In 1985, the UCLA PTSD Reaction Index, a screening questionnaire based on DSM diagnostic criteria to assess post-traumatic stress reactions among children and adolescents was developed by UCLA Trauma Psychiatry Program.

The UCLA PTSD-RI is a self-report instrument showing satisfactory reliability and validity [22–24], which has been used widely around the world for the measurement of childhood PTSD [25]. The 33-item scale contains two parts: (1) a section with 13 questions (scored dichotomously) that aligned with DSM-IV criterion A (the objective and subjective experiences and memories of the traumatic event); (2) a section with 20 questions map directly onto the DSM-IV criterion B (intrusion), criterion C (sense of "numbness" and avoidance), and criterion D (arousal) for PTSD, with each item scored from 0 (never or rarely) to 4 (most or all of the time).

2.2 Structured and semi-structured diagnostic interview schedules

These interview tools have strict implementation procedures, and must be used by professionals or strictly trained surveyors to objectively evaluate the subject's symptoms. Because these tools provide greater diagnostic reliability, they have become major assets in assessing treatment efficacy, epidemiological patterns of psychopathology, and the continuity and validity of psychiatric syndromes appearing in children and adolescents [26]. The contents of most of these interview schedules are generally symptom-based, but differ in format.

2.2.1 The schedule for affective disorders and schizophrenia for school-age children-present and lifetime version, K-SADS-PL

K-SADS-PL is a semi-structured diagnostic interview schedule used by a child and adolescent psychiatry specialists to ascertain both lifetime and current status of mental illness in children and adolescents, which is DSM-IV compatible. It is formatted to interview both parents and children. Score sheet margin notations are required if the worst current episode symptoms have resolved. This later information is needed to determine whether diagnostic criteria are still met for the disorder. Therefore, symptoms rated in the current episode may not be those that the child is experiencing at the time of the interview [26].

2.2.2 Mini international neuropsychiatric interview for children and adolescents, MINI-KID

MINI-KID is a structured clinical diagnostic interview designed to assess the presence of psychiatric disorders according to ICD-10 and DSM-IV criteria in children and adolescents aged 6–17 years without mental retardation. It is a brief but valid and reliable diagnostic instrument that can be used in clinical settings in psychiatry [27]. MINI-KID can be easily conducted by a trained surveyor, which allows it easy to be used in large-scale epidemiological investigations. MINI has been translated into over 40 different languages and validity and reliability have been reported over 7 different languages [27].

When selecting the appropriate evaluation tool and formulating an evaluation plan, the surveyors need to consider factors based on their own knowledge background, the familiarity of the tools and the objective conditions. The surveyors should first consider the purpose and object of the assessment. For example, a simple and reliable self-report questionnaire is more appropriate to use in large-scale epidemiological surveys, while a more comprehensive and diagnose assessment method seems more suitable for individual assessment. In the selection and planning of assessment tools, the following factors should be considered: the type and severity of trauma, the evaluation of risk and protective factors, the evaluation of children's social functions, the characteristics of children and adolescents' psychological development in different ages, assessments of parents' mental health. In addition, it should be noted that cultural differences may weaken their original effects.

3. Epidemiological characteristics of PTSD among children and adolescents

Due to the lack of relatively mature investigative tools and ethical reasons, the epidemiological characteristics of PTSD in children and adolescents are less studied than that in adults, and research has been mostly focused on children or adolescents at an advanced age. Findings from earlier studies indicate that the prevalence of PTSD in children and adolescents is lower than in adults. But with the development of various survey tools and methods, more and more studies show that the prevalence of PTSD in children and adolescents is not lower than that in adults. In 2002, La Greca et al. [28] reviewed the prevalence of PTSD of children exposed to natural or man-made disasters, and found that 5–10% of the children meet the diagnostic criteria for PTSD. In other traumatic contexts, such as fires, sexual assaults and wars, surveys show that the prevalence of PTSD in children ranges from 25 to 75%.

After the 2008 Wenchuan Earthquake, a large number of studies have been done among child and adolescent earthquake survivors. As stated above, a representative research project is the WEAHC established by Fan et al. [11] in Dujiangyan City, one of the 10 worst affected areas by the Wenchuan Earthquake. A large sample of 2250 adolescents was enrolled in the initial survey conducted at 6 months post-earthquake. Among them, 1573 were followed-up subsequently at 12, 18, 24, and 30 months post-earthquake. Data were collected on adolescents' mental health problems (i.e.,

PTSD, depression, anxiety, and sleep disturbances), earthquake-related stressors (i.e., earthquake exposure and negative life events post-earthquake), psychosocial and familial factors (e.g., trait resilience, coping styles, social support, and parenting styles), and behavioral/social functioning (e.g., prosocial behaviors and academic performance). Five years and a half after the earthquake (October and November 2013), another screening survey on mental health problems were conducted among 3501 adolescents (some were from the original cohort). Based on survey results, 512 adolescents were enrolled for individual clinical interviews and provided their oral mucosal samples for genetic analysis. Data from the WEAHC study provided great opportunity to investigate longitudinal epidemiological characteristics of mental disorders among Chinese adolescent earthquake survivors, as well as to explore the psychosocial and genetic mechanisms underlying these disorders. Aside from the WEAHC, longitudinal investigations of child and adolescent earthquake survivors have also been conducted by other research teams in China after 2008. Yet, many of them were limited by small sample sizes, few survey waves, or short follow-up duration. Regarding epidemiological characteristics of PTSD among child and adolescent earthquake survivors, some major findings from the WEAHC study and other studies are as follows.

First, the WEAHC study showed that prevalence estimates of probable PTSD were 21.0, 23.3, 13.5, and 14.7% at 6, 12, 18, and 24 months after the earthquake [11]. The rates tended to be higher at 12 and 24 months, suggesting an "anniversary reaction" in adolescents' post-earthquake mental adaptation process. This highlights the importance of providing adolescents with more intensive mental health support around the anniversary dates. In addition, the effects of trauma exposure in childhood can continue into adulthood. For example, data from Wenchuan Earthquake samples found that the prevalence of PTSD among the young adults 8.5 years later after they experienced the 2008 Wenchuan Earthquake was still as high as 4.75% [29].

Second, there are individual differences in the long-term change of PTSD symptoms among adolescent earthquake survivors. The WEAHC study observed five different patterns of the PTSD trajectories [30]: resistance (minimal or no symptoms over time, 65.3% of the sample), recovery (initially moderate/severe symptoms followed by a gradual return to pre-trauma functioning, 20.0%), relapsing/remitting (symptoms displaying a cyclical course, 3.3%), delayed dysfunction (initially minimal/no symptoms followed by elevated symptoms, 4.2%), and chronic dysfunction (moderate or severe symptoms over time, 7.2%). Different types of trajectories have their own characteristics, and those who show the latter three patterns are at high risk for PTSD. Post-disaster psychological intervention should focus on prevention, and it is necessary to identify high-risk populations to enhance the pertinence and effectiveness of the intervention.

Third, clinical presentations are exceedingly complex and children with PTSD are at increased risk of having comorbid psychiatric diagnoses. Depression and anxiety disorder have been reported to be common comorbid disorders associated with PTSD [31]. Consistent with previous studies based in western countries, research on the post-traumatic psychological consequences of adolescents after the Wenchuan Earthquake have also proved the prevalence of the comorbidity of PTSD and other mental disorders [32, 33]. One publication from the WEAHC study [34] examined the associations of adolescent survivors' PTSD symptoms, depression, generalized anxiety disorder (GAD), separation anxiety disorder (SAD), panic disorder, social phobia, conduct disorder, and attention deficit hyperactivity disorder (ADHD) at 1 and 1.5 years post-earthquake. Results showed that 91.9 and 94.0% of the adolescents with PTSD symptoms had at least one comorbid psychiatric disorder at 1 and 1.5 years post-earthquake, respectively. 54.3 and 50.4% of those without PTSD symptoms had at least one other psychiatric disorder. Compare to behavior problems, PTSD symptoms were more likely to co-occur with subtypes of anxiety or depression symptoms. Adolescents who were identified as having PTSD comorbid with depression or SAD at half year were more likely to have PTSD symptoms over time. Longitudinal analyses showed that depression, GAD, and SAD symptoms at 1 year post-earthquake predicted higher levels of PTSD symptoms at 1.5 years post-earthquake. In turn, increased PTSD symptoms predicted increases in GAD and panic disorder symptoms. The reason of the high prevalence of PTSD and comorbid depression/anxiety may be due to the shared variance resulting from the overlapping symptoms between PTSD and other mental disorders [35]. These findings suggest that specific multi-modal assessments and treatments targeting both PTSD and its comorbid disorders are warranted.

Forth, different environmental and psychological factors have different impacts on post-traumatic adaptations among adolescents with different characteristics. For example, positive coping styles and social support resources have positive effect on post-traumatic adaptation [36], and adolescents with different characteristics (i.e., different ages) need to be trained with different coping skills to guide them in seeking and take good use of various social support resources. In addition, the predictive effects of environmental factors such as negative life events on the post-traumatic psychopathology of certain groups (such as those with high resilience) diminished over time. The design of post-traumatic mental disorder intervention strategies and mental health education efforts should consider the characteristics of different individuals, focus on individuals at high risk for continuing, relapsing or delayed mental symptoms, and fully consider various environmental/ psychological factors in implementing targeted intervention.

Finally, the occurrence of post-traumatic mental disorder shows familial aggregation, and the interaction between susceptible genes and family environmental factors have impact on adolescents' post-traumatic mental disorder. HPA axis-related genes and serotonin transporter genes have been evidenced to have a role in various stress-related physical and mental illnesses [37]. The WEAHC study examined the relationship between glucocorticoid receptor gene (NR3C1), one of the key genes involved in the HPA axis regulation, and anxiety disorders in adolescent earthquake survivors. NR3C1 polymorphisms rs6191 GG genotype, rs6196 AA genotype, and rs41423247 GG genotype were found associated with decreased risk of anxiety disorders. There was also a significant interaction between rs41423247 genotypes and maternal warmth in predicting adolescent anxiety disorders; that is, rs41423247 GG genotype was linked with reduced risk of anxiety disorders only when maternal warmth was high. In another case-control study conducted 3 years following the Wenchuan Earthquake, 183 adolescents with the average age of 15 years (64 adolescents diagnosed with PTSD and 119 controls) were investigated. The results showed that serotonin transporter gene polymorphisms (i.e., 5-HTTLPR and 5-HTTVNTR) and earthquake exposure had a significant interaction effects on PTSD of the adolescents. Specifically, when a teenager who carrying an S allele exposed to high level of earthquake exposure, he/she would have a fourfold increased risk in developing PTSD [38]. These findings highlight the importance of considering family and genetic variables in developing interventions. Exposure to traumatic events in early life may influence individuals' gene expression through epigenetic modification, which would have long-term and even lifetime effects on their physical and mental function in the future. Future research on the epigenetic mechanisms underlying the relationship between genetic etiologies, family factors and adolescent PTSD is warranted, to further explore the disease etiology.

4. Possible mechanisms for PTSD in children and adolescents

4.1 Biological factors

4.1.1 Genetic factors

Studies have shown that the occurrence of PTSD may be associated with genetic susceptibility. Xian et al. [39] assessed 3304 monozygotic and dizy-gotic male-male twin pair members with PTSD and found that genetic factors have an impact on all PTSD symptoms. On one hand, stress can induce the abnormal expression of cognition and neuroendocrine related genes, which eventually leads to the occurrence of PTSD. For example, abnormal expres-sion of Corticosterone-related genes may cause PTSD. On the other hand, the development of PTSD may be related to gene polymorphism. At present, most candidate genes for PTSD are located in dopamine system and serotonin system. For example, a meta-analysis showed that 5-hydroxytryptaminentransporter (5-HTT) gene polymorphism is closely related to post-stress affective disorder. In addition, glucocorticoid receptor genes, GABA-A receptors, BDNF genes et al. have been reported to be related to PTSD. It is worth noting that the pathogenic genes of neuropsychiatric diseases are pleiotropic, that is, one genotype can be susceptible to several different mental diseases. Pleiotropy is clearly mani-fested in PTSD. For example, the incidence of anxiety and affective disorders in patients with PTSD is much higher than that in the general population. Finally, PTSD is often comorbid with many mental illnesses, such as depression and suicidal tendencies, which made its clinical features complex and diverse. As a result, the homogeneity of the research sample decreases, which further increases the difficulty of genetic research.

4.1.2 Neuroendocrine changes

The role of HPA axis dysfunction in the pathogenesis of PTSD in adults has been extensively researched and explained. Previous studies have found that cortisol levels decreased in adult patients with PTSD, which could also predict the patients' PTSD level after 6 months [40]. Low cortisol levels may strengthen the memory of traumatic events and increase individuals' subjective distressing experience. This kind of distressing experience can change individual's psychological functioning, delay their recovery and increase their adverse reactions, which may affect the ability of the victim to cope with traumatic experience, and in turn, lead to the occurrence of PTSD. However, Lipschitz et al. [41] found that the suppression of salivary cortisol following low-dose dexamethasone in adolescent PTSD patients showed no difference from those who experienced traumatic events without PTSD and healthy non-traumatized controls, while PTSD subjects with co-occurring depression showed higher salivary cortisol level before and after this experiment compared to controls.

4.1.3 Neuroimaging findings

Brain is a human organ that processes emotions and thoughts. Evidence has identified the changes in brain imaging among adults with PTSD. However, due to immature neurodevelopment, it is thought that the brain changes of children and adolescents with PTSD may be different from those in adults. We reviewed the current neuroimaging findings in children and adolescents and summarize the main findings below:

I. Prefrontal cortex and cognitive impairment: A study conducted by Carrion in 2010 found that in children with PTSD, the decrease in the volume of the left prefrontal cortex was related to their plasma cortisol levels before bed, suggesting that this area may be related to cortisol imbalance in children. In the study of functional magnetic resonance imaging (fMRI), it was found that the key areas of the prefrontal cortex of children with PTSD could not reach the activation level of children of normal age when performing cognitive functions. The above studies suggest that changes in the structure and function of the prefrontal cortex may be related to children's susceptibility to PTSD and cognitive impairment caused by PTSD.

II. Hippocampus and memory, behavioral abnormalities: A series of studies in children and adolescents with PTSD and PTSS have reported inconsistent findings within the hippocampal volumetric and memory as well as behavioral abnormalities. For example, a longitudinal study found that the severity of PTSS and corticosteroid levels can serve as independent predictors of children's hippocampal volume reductions 1 year later [42]. However, De Bellis [43] found that the hippocampal volume of children with PTSD was significantly larger compared to normal controls. In addition, this study also found that hippocampal volume was positively correlated with age at onset of PTSD. Therefore, the researchers hypothesized that the increase in hippocampal volume may be related to behavioral abnormalities such as attention impairment in children with PTSD [43]. Another fMRI study reported the relationship between hippocampus and memory among young PTSD subjects. This study found that during a verbal memory task, the activation of the right hippocampus of the children decreased; while children's avoidance and numbing symptoms was related to reduced activation of the left hippocampus [44]. It's worth noting that, most of these studies were cross-sectional design, future longitudinal study studies with neuropsychological measures as well as trauma control subjects are needed to clarify the role of hippocampal functioning in the development of PTSD in children and adolescents.

4.2 Sociopsychological factors

4.2.1 Trauma type and traumatic exposure level

Mass disasters such as natural disasters, large-scale human-induced accidents, spree shootings, war and terrorism, all have been shown to exert deleterious impacts on children and adolescents. The level of exposure also has consistently been associated with later post-traumatic stress reactions following various types of trauma [45]. These distinctions are likely to result in different effects. For example, many studies conducted after Wenchuan Earthquake all reported that different levels of earthquake exposure level could positively predict adolescents' PTSD at different time points post-earthquake [32, 46].

In addition, the severity of disaster exposure includes objective exposure level (e.g., direct exposure such as death, disappearance and/or injury of family members, house damage, property loss and direct witness of traumatic events) and the severity of subjective fear. Studies examining the impact of trauma exposure on PTSD have found that PTSD is more directly affected by objective exposure, and social support plays a moderating role in the relationship between objective exposure and PTSD [47].

4.2.2 Personality characteristics

Studies have shown that children and adolescents' negative personality characteristics are associated with their PTSD symptoms. For example, it was reported that neuroticism was significantly related to PTSD, and emotion-oriented coping partly mediated the effect of neuroticism on PTSD symptoms [48]. Extraversion was reported to have significant indirect effects on both PTSD and post-traumatic growth through social support [49]. Further, An et al. [50] longitudinally investigated the contribution of personality in the development of PTSD and found that neuroticism was an independent and significant predictor of subsequent PTSD. In addition, gratitude was reported to be a protective factor of relieving PTSD symptoms [51].

4.2.3 Cognitive models

PTSD is thought to be maintained by a range of cognitive and behavioral strategies that the individual uses to control the current threat [52]. At an early stage of a traumatic event, children and adolescents' cognitive reconstruction of the disaster and the reorganization of post-traumatic broken memory all influence the occurrence of PTSD [53]. Their problematic appraisals of the trauma and/or its aftermath are also considered to increase the risk of developing PTSD. Dunmore et al. [54] found that cognitive processing style during assault (mental defeat, mental confusion, detachment); appraisal of assault sequelae (appraisal of symptoms, perceived negative responses of others, permanent change); negative beliefs about self and world; and maladaptive control strategies (avoidance/safety seeking) could significantly predict PTSD in the 9 months follow-up. Thus, misunderstanding of traumatic events can lead to secondary trauma.

4.2.4 Social support

Social support is a robust protective factor for post-traumatic mental health [55]. Supportive social environment can not only provide individuals with necessary coping resources, but also provide them with a safe environment, reduce their experience of subsequent negative life events, and encourage them to think positively about traumatic events, thereby helping to reduce the negative impact of traumatic events on individuals and promote positive changes after trauma. Much literature on adolescent exposure to Wenchuan Earthquake also suggested the positive protective effect of social support on alleviating PTSD. For example, Zhao et al. [56] found that social support (both subjective support and support availability) improved the quality of life of the earthquake survivors with PTSD symptoms. Moreover, Wu et al. reported that among all the social support resources, the support of parents and teachers is the most important [47].

4.2.5 Age and gender

There are gender differences in children and adolescent's defense and coping styles, as well as the effects of social support, which have important influence on their post-traumatic reactions. Many studies have found that girls are more likely to have PTSD symptoms than boys following disasters [30, 33, 57]. Generally, female more often use strategies such as repression and fantasy to deal with traumatic events [58]. Second, there are also gender differences in the neuroendocrine reaction caused by trauma. Girls have more adverse physical and psychological reactions after trauma, which may further aggravate girls' PTSD symptoms [59].

Children's experience of danger, their perception and understanding of trauma, susceptibility to parental distress, own coping styles and skills, and memory of trauma may vary with ages. Most studies suggest a positive relation-ship between PTSD and children's age after the earthquake [30]. However, another study reported that at 1 month after the earthquake, the incidence of PTSD in survivors under 15 years of age was significantly higher than that in survivors over 15 years [60]. Age differences are also shown in children's experience of specific post-traumatic symptoms and previous studies results are mixed. For preschool children, they may display more overt aggression and destructiveness as well as behavioral re-enactments of the traumatic event. While, the reactions of children over the age of 8–10 years, are more similar to those manifested by adults [61]. Inconsistent research conclusions may be related to differences in stressors, study criteria, measurement and distance from stressors. For example, a study of earthquake reported that there was an interaction between age and distance from the epicenter, younger children in areas closer to the epicenter showed severer PTSD symptoms while older children in areas far away from the epicenter showed severer PTSD symptoms [62]. The reason may be that in areas far away from the epicenter, older children are more likely to follow media coverage of the earth-quake and experience alternative trauma; younger children are more susceptible to direct trauma exposure. All these current explanations are tentative and should be interpreted cautiously, also, future studies are suggested to further illustrate these possible explanations and explain with caution due to the complex nature of PTSD.

4.2.6 Family factors

Family environmental factors (e.g., poor parent-child relationship and family adversity) are risk factors that accelerate PTSD. In addition, as family members sometimes encounter a disaster simultaneously, children's and parents' post-disaster symptoms can be highly interactive [63, 64]. Parents' response after the trauma event affects children's judgment of the event, and their coping styles are imitated by children. In addition, given mothers are primary caregivers of children, maternal poor psychological states, continued focus on the disaster event, or changes in family support could be a risk factor for children's post-traumatic symptoms. Moreover, some studies also suggest that the incidence of PTSD is substantially related to genetic factors. Xian et al. [39] investigated 3304 monozygotic and dizygotic male–male twin pair subjects to examine whether and to what degree genetic and environmental contributed to PTSD. The results showed that genetic and family environmental factors have influence on all PTSD symptoms, the liability for PTSD being 20.0% due to genetic contribution specific to PTSD.

5. Post-traumatic growth among children and adolescents exposed to Wenchuan Earthquake

PTSD is a prevalent psychiatric disorder in adolescents after traumatic events. However, researchers found personal growth in the aftermath of traumatic events [65, 66]. Tedeschi and Calhoun [67] used the term post-traumatic growth (PTG) to describe these positive outcomes after struggling with a traumatic experience. Dimensions of PTG encompass recognition and elaboration of personal strengths, enhanced interpersonal relationships, and positive changes in life priorities [68]. Prior studies revealed that survivors may develop PTG in spite of different types of traumatic events [69, 70]. For example, Jin et al. [71] found that the PTG prevalence among adolescents after the earthquake was even up to 51.1%.

Take the trends of PTG in Chinese adolescent sample as example. One study found that the average PTG was 2.96 (ranging from 0 to 5) among adolescents 1 year after the Wenchuan Earthquake, suggesting the relative high level of PTG among adolescent survivors. Further analysis found that PTG in this time showed significant difference in gender (female was higher than that of male) and, insignificant difference was found in grades. However, a decreased tendency of PTG (average mean = 2.77) after 2.5 years was observed in Wenchuan Earthquake [72].

After 3.5 years of Wenchuan Earthquake, the average of PTG was 2.78, and there were significant differences in gender and grades. Specifically, female had higher PTG than male, and junior students was lower than that of senior students [73]. This research group followed the development of PTG among this adolescent sample, and found the average of PTG was 2.68 after 4.5 years earthquake. Further analysis of the results at 8.5 years after the earthquake were similar to 3.5 years after the earthquake, with average mean was 2.80, a higher female and ethnic minorities level of PTG than that of male and Chinese Han population (the majority ethnic of the Chinese population), and lower levels of PTG among junior students than that among senior students [29].

The relationship between PTSD and PTG has been one of the interested areas among researchers. A review of 77 papers showed that the relationship was ambiguous [74]. The particular reason that accounts for this unclear relationship is that most studies employed cross-sectional rather than longitudinal designs, making it impossible for us to establish a definitive causal relationship. Some study of Wenchuan Earthquake examined the longitudinal relationships between PTSD and PTG among adolescents. A three-wave, cross-lagged study found that PTSD reported at 3.5 and 4.5 years after the earthquake both could predicted PTG 4.5 and 5.5 years after the earthquake, respectively, while PTG did not predict PTSD during the 3 years follow-up. This study suggests that, after exposure to traumatic events, PTSD and PTG can coexist in individuals, and the relieved PTSD symptoms do not indicate the improvement of PTG [75]. This relationship between PTSD and PTG may be because that cognitive pathways to PTSD and PTG is different. For example, deliberate rumination leads to PTG whereas intrusive rumination elicits PTSD in a long time after trauma [76].

From previous mentioned studies, the PTG level of adolescents was highest at 1 year after the earthquake, and although it has declined slightly since then, it has remained at a high level for a long time. That phenomenon could be explained that traumatic events like the earthquake might bring psychological stresses, and it is this stresses that may encourage adolescent survivors to use positive coping ways to overcome the negative outcomes because of traumatic events. During this coping process, having a new interpretation and understanding of traumatic events may help adolescents achieve personal growth. As the negative effects of traumatic events on individuals decreased when time passes, therefore, this decreased situation not only eases the stresses of traumatic events, but also reduces the incentive for individuals to implement PTG. Meanwhile, female may be better than male to develop PTG and senior survivors may be more likely to develop PTG than junior students. Moreover, the racial disparities in PTG level suggest that cultural factors may need to be consider in PTG research. Together, all these suggest that the relationships between gender and PTG is stable over time, the same result was observed when grade differences were considered.

6. Treatments for children and adolescents with post-traumatic stress disorder

6.1 Psychological treatments

Young people with PTSD may suffer from major depression, aggression, and conduct disorder [77, 78]. They may also be more likely to have suicidal ideation and attempts [79]. Left untreated, PTSD can lead to negative effects on sufferers' adulthood, such as college drop-out [80] and lower quality of life [81]. The National Child Traumatic Stress Network (NCTSN) suggests that trauma treatments should not only help children receive timely and appropriate treatments to recover from traumatic events but also build their resilience to cope with future stress more successfully. Hence, the identification of high-risk children and adolescents and providing them with appropriate and timely treatments are essential and imperative.

Currently, the number of treatment models for PTSD has proliferated. The first-line treatments encompass trauma-focused CBT (i.e., TF-CBT) [82, 83] and Prolonged Exposure for Adolescents (i.e, PE-A) [84]. Traditionally, components of treatments include: psychoeducation about PTSD, affective modulation and cognitive processing, behavioral activation, relaxation skills, trauma narrative, in vivo mastery of trauma reminders, conjoint parent-child sessions, and future safety and development [85, 86]. Furthermore, cognitive behavioral interventions for trauma in schools (CBITS) [87, 88] and trauma and grief component therapy for adolescents (TGCT) [89] are also welcomed as efficient ways to treat traumatized youths mainly due to available resources of schools. Eye Movement Desensitization and Reprocessing (EMDR), using dual-stimulation exercises to lower emotional arousal of the traumatic triggers [90], is evidenced as a promising method for youths with PTSD [91, 92]. Given the various and effective aspects of intervention, different treatments can be employed as a combination to gain a superior result. For example, TF-CBT combined with supportive therapy and a psychodynamic form (.i.e., play therapy) showed a better result [93]. Though it is true that forms of treatments have made progress, they are subject to some drawbacks such as high drop-out rates [94–96]. It is mainly because the nature of trauma symptoms (especially avoidance) leads participants to be unwilling to address the traumatic event directly and reprocess the details of their suffering [97]. It is therefore difficult to see the long-term efficacy and benefits of treatments if participants have poor adherence.

Unlike traditional CBT interventions, mindfulness-based interventions (MBIs), as "third-wave" cognitive behavioral treatments, were proposed to solve this high drop-out problem. Mindfulness is characterized by paying attention to one's experience in the present moment in a non-judgmental manner [98]. There are some theoretical reasons to explain the potential mechanisms why mindfulness may reduce PTSD. Mindfulness interventions can help the sufferers to improve the ability to distinguish the past and present, so as to lower the re-experiencing symptoms [99] of post-traumatic stress disorder. In addition, increasing sufferers' capability to tolerate distressing memories, thoughts, and feelings when employing mindfulness interventions may be more likely to reduce avoidance of distressing memories [100]. Furthermore, hyperarousal of PTSD could decrease because of the training in stress reduction and relaxation [101]. Within MBIs, Mindfulness-based stress reduction (MBSR) and Mindfulness-based cognitive therapy (MBCT) were widely cited in the background of MBIs. Compared with trauma-focused therapies, MBIs showed equally efficacious and significantly lower drop-out rate [102], and were well-accepted for PTSD treatments of youths [103]. Despite the prior research showed positive effects of MBIs in youth with PTSD, the mean effect size among youths is still lower than adults. Hence, some adaptive programs should be developed to gain satisfying results among youths [104] by shortening the session length, for example, from 90 to 30–45 min. Second, different exercises are suggested to provide specific needs for youths, such as more body scans and drawings. Third, children are more dependent on caregivers; inviting caregivers to treatment sessions should also be concerned.

In addition, art therapy is another promising intervention programmer, which promotes expression and healing. It is acknowledged that traumatic memories are sometimes overwhelming, and difficult to express in words alone [105]. Art therapy as an alternative approach can help sufferers to access the traumatic memory safely [106]. More importantly, young children are often unable to provide coherent descriptions about the traumatic event mainly due to their limited language capacity [107], making it difficult for clinicians to offer suitable interventions in helping these young children. Some previous empirical studies have provided preliminary evidence that art therapy could ameliorate PTSD symptoms in children [108, 109]. For example, Lyshak-Stelzer et al. [110] recruited 29 valid participants (14 took a trauma-focused expressive art therapy protocol (TF-ART); 15 completed a treatment-as-usual (TAU) control condition; the average age was 15.07). Results showed that patients in TF-ART had greater reduction in PTSD symptom severity than youth in the TAU condition. To support future research and practice of employing art therapy for PTSD treatment, Spiegel et al. [105] concluded some characteristics that differ from other approaches of treating PTSD: relaxation, non-verbal expression, containment of traumatic material within an object or image, symbolic expression, externalization of traumatic memories and emotions, and enjoying the pleasure that arose from creation. Again, prior studies reported promising results for art therapy in relieving PTSD among youths; however, future studies need to develop more effective and age-appropriate treatments under art therapy structure.

In conclusion, both traditional approaches like TF-CBT and the "third-wave" treatments like mindfulness-based interventions provide positive preliminary evidence in PTSD treatments among youths. Although the various interventions provide necessary helps in mitigating PTSD, it is still far way to go in developing PTSD treatments among youths. Future studies should expand the sample size, use randomized controlled trials and offer long follow-up assessments after treatments to make more definitive conclusions about the efficacy of PTSD treatments among youths. Also, researchers and practitioners need to continue to contribute to developing adaptive interventions in youths.

6.2 Pharmacological treatments

To date, experiences with efficacious pharmacological interventions used for children and adolescents with PTSD are relatively lack. A common consensus is that adopting some targeted pharmacological treatments for young patients, especially for hyperarousal symptoms, sleep problems and psychiatric comorbidity, may improve their life quality and social functions [111, 112].

There was evidence supporting the using of pharmacological treatments such as serotonin-selective reuptake inhibitors (SSRIs), divalproex sodium (DVP), atypical antipsychotics and beta-receptor antagonism in reducing PTSD symptoms among children and adolescents. SSRIs have been proved their effects in treating youths with depression and anxiety disorders [113]. Overall, SSRIs are safe and well-tolerated, but it is important to note that they may increase the risk of suicide in children and adolescents in addition to the common anticholine side effects [114, 115]. DVP was reported to be effective for treating core PTSD symptoms in a randomized controlled clinical trial (high dose of DVP conditions: 500–1500 mg/day compared with dose conditions: <250 mg/day) [116]. Atypical antipsychotics agents (i.e., risperidone, quetiapine, clozapine) and anti-adrenergic agents (i.e., clonidine) are often used in treating children with PTSD, schizophrenia, bipolar disorder, or psychotic symptoms in children. A study provided preliminary evidence that patients presented rapid and sustained improvement across all symptom clusters of acute stress disorders with minimal to no adverse effects after using moderate dosages of risperidone [117]. Other studies reported that beta-receptor antagonism (propranolol) [118, 119] and clonidine had significant effects on alleviating PTSD symptoms in children [120]. Further, pharmacological treatments are highly suggested to combine with TF-CBT or other trauma-centered therapy [121, 122]. Given methodological limitations, e.g., small sample sizes and few well-designed clinical trials, these findings should be interpreted cautiously.

Some important points when using pharmacological treatments in children and adolescence with PTSD should be noticed. First, are they and their parents willing to take part in pharmacological interventions. Second, those who comorbid with depression or other serious mental illnesses should be highly concerned. Moreover, specific developmental characteristics should be considered when adopting pharmacological treatments. The response effects of pharmacological treatments may vary with age, weight, gender, mental health as well as absorption, distribution, metabolism, and excretion of medication. Taken together, future studies should ideally take into account these developmental factors when applying pharmacological approaches.

7. Summary

Taking the Wenchuan Earthquake studies in China as an example, this chapter introduces some current research results about the epidemiological characteristics of PTSD and related mental disorders in children and adolescents, as well as their influencing factors and mechanisms. Important intervention strategies for PTSD in children and adolescents have also discussed. There are some issues that need further research.

First, apart from mental health effects of disasters on children and adolescents, future research should pay more attention to other aspects of their well-being and functioning, such as academic performance and relationship quality. This can provide an important reference for our in-depth understanding of post-traumatic psychological reactions and behavior changes, and also help to develop integrative interventions beneficial for the overall psychological and behavioral improvement of trauma-exposed children and adolescents. Second, considering the possible coexistence of PTSD and PTG, it is necessary to study the relationship between PTSD and PTG within longitudinal data with the aim of clarifying the relationship between these two variables, it is necessary to study the relationship between PTSD and PTG within longitudinal data. As mentioned, previous studies have mainly analyzed the mechanism of PTSD or PTG from a single perspective, ignoring the coexistence characteristics of them, making it difficult to effectively compare the differences between the two mechanisms. Therefore, future research can incorporate PTSD and PTG into a model at the same time, so as to determine the similarities and differences between the two mechanisms. Third, clinical intervention research from the perspective of integrating the remission of PTSD and promotion of PTG is needed. In the past, traumatic research mainly focused on the remission of individual PTSD, and developed related intervention methods, and also tested its effects through empirical studies. However, overall clinical empirical research on the promotion of PTG in the treatment for PTSD is still very rare. Therefore, research on psychological intervention for PTSD from the integration perspective of PTSD remission and PTG promotion at the same time is an important issue to be explored in the future. Fourth, future research should explore effective genetic, neuroendocrine, and neuroimaging related biomarkers, which may be of utility in developing new treatments and evaluating treatment outcomes.

Author details

Yuanyuan Li[1], Ya Zhou[2], Xiaoyan Chen[1], Fang Fan[1*], George Musa[3] and Christina Hoven[3]

1 School of Psychology, Center for Studies of Psychological Application, and Key Laboratory of Mental Health and Cognitive Science of Guangdong Province, South China Normal University, Guangdong, China

2 Department of Psychology, Lund University, Lund, Sweden

3 Department of Child and Adolescent Psychiatry, New York State Psychiatric Institute, Columbia University, New York, USA

*Address all correspondence to: fangfan@scnu.edu.cn

References

[1] Schnurr PP, Friedman MJ, Bernardy NC. Research on posttraumatic stress disorder: Epidemiology, pathophysiology, and assessment. Journal of Clinical Psychology. 2002;**58**(8):877-889

[2] Kar N. Psychological impact of disasters on children: Review of assessment and interventions. World Journal of Pediatrics. 2009;**5**(1):5-11

[3] DiGrande L, Perrin MA, Thorpe LE, Thalji L, Murphy J, Wu D, et al. Posttraumatic stress symptoms, PTSD, and risk factors among lower Manhattan residents 2 ~ 3 years after the September 11, 2001 terrorist attacks. Journal of Traumatic Stress. 2008;**21**(3):264-273

[4] Galea S, Ahern J, Resnick H, Kilpatrick D, Bu cuvalas M, Gold J, et al. Psychological sequelae of the September 11 terrorist attacks in New York City. New England Journal of Medicine. 2002;**346**(13):982-987

[5] Schlenger WE, Caddell JM, Ebert L, Jordan BK, Rourke KM, Wilson D, et al. Psychological reactions to terrorist attacks. Journal of the American Medical Association. 2002;**288**(5):58I-588I

[6] Shaw JA. Children, adolescents and trauma. Psychiatric Quarterly. 2000;**71**(3):227-243

[7] Comer JS, Fan B, Duarte CS, Wu P, Musa GJ, Mandell DJ, et al. Attack-related life disruption and child psychopathology in New York city public schoolchildren 6-months post-9/11. Journal of Clinical Child & Adolescent Psychology. 2010;**39**(4):460-469

[8] Shi X, Zhou Y, Geng F, Li Y, Fan F. Posttraumatic stress disorder symptoms in parents and adolescents after the Wenchuan Earthquake: A longitudinal actor-partner interdependence model. Journal of Affective Disorders. 2017;**226**:301

[9] Kirsch V, Wilhelm FH, Goldbeck L. Psychophysiological characteristics of ptsd in children and adolescents: A review of the literature. Journal of Traumatic Stress. 2011;**24**(3):370-372

[10] Bolton D, O'Ryan D, Udwin O, Boyle S, Yule W. The longterm effects of a disaster experienced in adolescence: II: General psychopathology. Journal of Child Psychology and Psychiatry. 2000;**41**(4):513-523

[11] Fan F, Zhou Y, Mo L, Zhang W, Xie J, Liu X, et al. Cohort profile: The Wenchuan Earthquake adolescent health cohort study. International Journal of Epidemiology. 2017; **46**(1):27-28

[12] Tareen A, Garralda ME, Hodes M. Post-traumatic stress disorder in childhood. Archives of Disease in Childhood-Education and Practice. 2007;**92**(1):ep1-ep6

[13] Wolfe DA, Sas L, Wekerle C. Factors associated with the development of post traumatic stress disorder among child victims of sexual abuse. Child Abuse & Neglect. 1994;**18**:37-50

[14] Creamer M, Bell R, Failla S. Psychometric properties of the impact of event scale—Revised. Behaviour Research and Therapy. 2003;**41**(12):1489-1496

[15] Motlagh H. Impact of event scale-revised. Journal of Physiotherapy. 2010;**56**(3):203

[16] Horowitz M, Wilner N, Alvarez W. Impact of event scale: A measure of subjective stress. Psychosomatic Medicine. 1979;**41**(3):209-218

[17] Perrin S, Meiser-Stedman R, Smith P. The Children's Revised Impact of Event Scale (CRIES): Validity as a screening instrument for PTSD. Behavioural and Cognitive Psychotherapy. 2005;**33**(4):487-498

[18] Smith P, Perrin S, Yule W, Rabe-Hesketh S. War exposure and maternal reactions in the psychological adjustment of children from Bosnia-Hercegovina. The Journal of Child Psychology and Psychiatry. 2001;**42**(3):395-404

[19] Foa EB, Johnson KM, Feeny NC, Treadwell KR. The Child PTSD Symptom Scale: A preliminary examination of its psycho-metric properties. Journal of Clinical Child Psychology. 2001;**30**:376-384. DOI: 10.1207/S15374424JCCP3003_9

[20] American Psychiatric Association. Diagnostic and Statistical Manual of Mental Disorders. 4th ed. Washington; 1994

[21] Nixon RD, Meiser-Stedman R, Dalgleish T, Yule W, Clark DM, Perrin S, et al. The Child PTSD Symptom Scale: An update and replication of its psychometric properties. Psychological Assessment. 2013;**25**(3):1025

[22] Lonigan CJ, Shannon MP, Taylor CM, Finch AJ Jr, Sallee FR. Children exposed to disaster: II. Risk factors for the development of post-traumatic symptomatology. Journal of the American Academy of Child & Adolescent Psychiatry. 1994;**33**(1):94-105

[23] Frederick C. Psychic trauma in victims of crime and terrorism. In: Vanden Bos GR, Bryant BK, editors. Cataclysm, Crisis and Catastrophes: Psychology in Action Master Lecture Series. Washington, DC: American Psychiatric Press; 1987. pp. 55-108

[24] La Greca AM, Siiverman WK, Vemberg EM, et al. Symptoms of posttraumatic stress in children following hurricane Andrew. Journal of Consulting and Clinical Psychology. 1996;**64**:712-723

[25] Steinberg AM, Brymer MJ, Decker KB, Pynoos RS. The University of California at Los Angeles post-traumatic stress disorder reaction index. Current Psychiatry Reports. 2004;**6**(2):96-100

[26] Ambrosini PJ. Historical development and present status of the schedule for affective disorders and schizophrenia for school-age children (K-SADS). Journal of the American Academy of Child & Adolescent Psychiatry. 2000;**39**(1):49-58

[27] Adamowska S, Adamowski T, Frydecka D, Kiejna A. Diagnostic validity polish language version of the questionnaire MINI-KID (Mini international neuropsychiatry interview for children and adolescent). Comprehensive Psychiatry. 2014;**55**(7):1744-1750

[28] La Greca AM. Traumatic stress disorders in children and adolescents. In: Traumatic Stress Disorders in Children & Adolescents Oxford Handbooks. 2012

[29] Wu X, Wang W, Zhou X, Chen Q, Lin C. Investigation on mental health state of adolescents after 8.5 years of Wenchuan Earthquake. Xinli Fazhan Yu Jiaoyu. 2018;**34**:80-89

[30] Fan F, Long K, Zhou Y, Zheng Y, Liu X. Longitudinal trajectories of post-traumatic stress disorder symptoms among adolescents after the Wenchuan Earthquake in China. Psychological Medicine. 2015;**45**(13):2885-2896

[31] Brady KT, Killeen TK, Brewerton T, Lucerini S. Comorbidity of psychiatric disorders and posttraumatic stress disorder. The Journal of Clinical Psychiatry. 2000;**61**(Suppl 7):22-32

[32] Wang L, Long D, Li Z, Armour C. Posttraumatic stress disorder symptom structure in Chinese adolescents exposed to a deadly earthquake. Journal of Abnormal Child Psychology. 2011;**39**(5):749

[33] Fan F, Zhang Y, Yang Y, Mo L, Liu X. Symptoms of posttraumatic stress disorder, depression, and anxiety among adolescents following the 2008 Wenchuan Earthquake in China. Journal of Traumatic Stress. 2011;**24**(1):44-53

[34] Geng F, Zhou Y, Liang Y, Zheng X, Li Y, Chen X, et al. Posttraumatic stress disorder and psychiatric comorbidity among adolescent earthquake survivors: A longitudinal cohort study. Journal of Abnormal Child Psychology. 2019;**47**(4):671-681

[35] Salcioglu E, Basoglu M, Livanou M. Post-traumatic stress disorder and comorbid depression among survivors of the 1999 earthquake in Turkey. Disasters. 2007;**31**(2):115-129

[36] Zheng Y, Fan F, Liu X, Mo L. Life events, coping, and posttraumatic stress symptoms among Chinese adolescents exposed to 2008 Wenchuan Earthquake, China. PLoS One. 2012;**7**(1)

[37] Oberlander TF, Weinberg J, Papsdorf M, Grunau R, Misri S, Devlin AM. Prenatal exposure to maternal depression, neonatal methylation of human glucocorticoid receptor gene (NR3C1) and infant cortisol stress responses. Epigenetics. 2008;**3**:97-106

[38] Tian Y, Liu H, Guse L, Wong TK, Li J, Bai Y, et al. Association of genetic factors and gene- environment interactions with risk of developing posttraumatic stress disorder in a case-control study. Biological Research for Nursing. 2015;**17**(4):364-372. DOI: 10.1177/1099800415588362

[39] Xian H, Chantarujikapong SI, Scherrer JF, Eisen SA, Lyons MJ, Goldberg J, et al. Genetic and environmental influences on posttraumatic stress disorder, alcohol and drug dependence in twin pairs. Drug and Alcohol Dependence. 2000;**61**(1):95-102

[40] Meewisse ML, Reitsma JB, De Vries GJ, Gersons BP, Olff M. Cortisol and post-traumatic stress disorder in adults: Systematic review and meta-analysis. The British Journal of Psychiatry. 2007;**191**(5):387-392

[41] Lipschitz DS, Rasmusson AM, Yehuda R, Wang S, Anyan W, Gueoguieva R, et al. Salivary cortisol responses to dexamethasone in adolescents with posttraumatic stress disorder. Journal of the American Academy of Child & Adolescent Psychiatry. 2003;**42**(11):1310-1317

[42] Carrion VG, Weems CF, Reiss AL. Stress predicts brain changes in children: A pilot longitudinal study on youth stress, posttraumatic stress disorder, and the hippocampus. Pediatrics. 2007;**119**(3):509-516

[43] Tupler LA, Bellis MDD. Segmented hippocampal volume in children and adolescents with posttraumatic stress disorder. Biological Psychiatry. 2006;**59**(6):523-529

[44] Carrion VG, Haas BW, Garrett A, Song S, Reiss AL. Reduced hippocampal activity in youth with posttraumatic stress symptoms: An FMRI study. Journal of Pediatric Psychology. 2010;**35**(5):559-569

[45] Pine DS, Cohen JA. Trauma in children and adolescents: Risk and treatment of psychiatric sequelae. Society of Biological Psychiatry. 2002;**51**:519-531

[46] Ma X, Liu X, Hu X, Qiu C, Wang Y, Huang Y, et al. Risk indicators for post-traumatic stress disorder in adolescents exposed to the 5.12 W enchuan earthquake in China. Psychiatry Research. 2011;**189**(3):385-391

[47] Wu X, Zhang Y, Lin C, Zang W. The effect of disaster exposure on PTSD of primary and secondary students: Mediating and moderating effects. Psychological Development and Education. 2013;**29**:641-648

[48] Wang L, Chen W, Zhang XL, Shi JN. Coping as a mediator of the relationship between personality and PTSD symptoms among surviving adolescents of the Wenchuan Earthquake. Chinese Journal of Clinical Psychology. 2011;**19**:89-91

[49] Jia X, Ying L, Zhou X, Wu X, Lin C. The effects of extraversion, social support on the posttraumatic stress disorder and posttraumatic growth of adolescent survivors of the Wenchuan Earthquake. PLoS One. 2015;**10**(3):e0121480

[50] An Y, Fu F, Wu X, Lin C, Zhang Y. Longitudinal relationships between neuroticism, avoidant coping, and posttraumatic stress disorder symptoms in adolescents following the 2008 Wenchuan Earthquake in China. Journal of Loss and Trauma. 2013;**18**(6):556-571

[51] Zheng Y-H, Fan F, Ting-chen, CFL. Relationship between gratitude and symptoms of post-traumatic stress disorder among adolescents: Mediation of social support and resilience. Psychological Development and Education. 2011;**5**:12

[52] Ehring T, Ehlers A, Glucksman E. Do cognitive models help in predicting the severity of posttraumatic stress disorder, phobia, and depression after motor vehicle accidents? A prospective longitudinal study. Journal of Consulting and Clinical Psychology. 2008;**76**(2):219

[53] Ehlers A, Clark DM. A cognitive model of posttraumatic stress disorder. Behaviour Research and Therapy. 2000;**38**:319-345

[54] Dunmore E, Clark DM, Ehlers A. A prospective investigation of the role of cognitive factors in persistent posttraumatic stress disorder (PTSD) after physical or sexual assault. Behaviour Research and Therapy. 2001;**39**(9):1063-1084

[55] Shallcross SL, Arbisi PA, Polusny MA, Kramer MD, Erbes CR. Social causation versus social erosion: Comparisons of causal models for relations between support and PTSD symptoms. Journal of Traumatic Stress. 2016;**29**(2):167-175

[56] Zhao C, Wu Z, Xu J. The association between post-traumatic stress disorder symptoms and the quality of life among Wenchuan Earthquake survivors: The role of social support as a moderator. Quality of Life Research. 2013;**22**(4):733-743

[57] Wang W, Fu W, Wu J, Ma X, Sun X, Huang Y, et al. Prevalence of PTSD and depres—Sion among junior middle school students in a rural town far from the epicenter of the Wenchuan Earthquake in China. PLoS One. 2012;**7**(7):e41665

[58] Tolin DF, Foa EB. Sex differences in trauma and posttraumatic stress disorder: A quantitative review of 25 years of research. Psychological Bulletin. 2006;**132**(6):959-992

[59] Olff M, Langeland W, Draijer N, Oersons B. Gender differences in posttraumatic stress disorder. Psychological Bulletin. 2007;**133**(2):183-204

[60] Lau JTF, Yu X, Zhang J, et al. Psychological distress among adolescents in Chengdu, Sichuan at 1 month after the 2008 Sichuan earthquake. Journal of Urban Health Bulletin of the New York Academy of Medicine. 2010;**87**(3):504-523

[61] Dyregrov A, Yule W. A review of PTSD in children. Child and Adolescent Mental Health. 2006;**11**(4):176-184

[62] Groome D, Soureti A. Post-traumatic stress disorder and anxiety symptoms in children exposed to the 1999 Greek earthquake. British Journal of Psychology. 2004;**95**(3):387-397

[63] Lambert JE, Holzer J, Hasbun A. Association between parents' PTSD severity and children's psychological distress: A meta analysis. Journal of Traumatic Stress. 2014;**27**(1):9-17

[64] Shi X, Zhou Y, Geng F, Li Y, Zhou J, Lei B, et al. Posttraumatic stress disorder symptoms in parents and adolescents after the Wenchuan Earthquake: A longitudinal actor-partner interdependence model. Journal of Affective Disorders. 2018;**226**:301-306

[65] Cryder CH, Kilmer RP, Tedeschi RG, Calhoun LG. An exploratory study of posttraumatic growth in children following a natural disaster. American Journal of Orthopsychiatry. 2006;**76**:65-69

[66] Linley PA, Joseph S. Positive change following trauma and adversity: A review. Journal of Traumatic Stress. 2004;**17**:11-21

[67] Tedeschi RG, Calhoun LG. Trauma & Transformation: Growing in the Aftermath of Suffering. Thousand Oaks, CA: SAGE Publications; 1995

[68] Tedeschi RG, Calhoun LG. The posttraumatic growth inventory: Measuring the positive legacy of trauma. Journal of Traumatic Stress. 1996;**9**:455-471

[69] Cho D, Park CL. Growth following trauma: Overview and current status. Terapia Psicológica. 2013;**31**:69-79

[70] Kira IA, Aboumediene S, Ashby JS, Odenat L, Mohanesh J, Alamia H. The dynamics of posttraumatic growth across different trauma types in a Palestinian sample. Journal of Loss and Trauma. 2013;**18**:120-139

[71] Jin YC, Xu JP, Liu DY. The relationship between post traumatic stress disorder and post traumatic growth: Gender differences in PTG and PTSD subgroups. Social Psychiatry and Psychiatric Epidemiology. 2014;**49**:1903-1910

[72] Ying LH, Lin CD, Wu XC, Chen CS, Greenberger E, An YY. Trauma severity and control beliefs as predictors of posttraumatic growth among adolescent survivors of the Wenchuan Earthquake. Psychological Trauma: Theory, Research, Practice, and Policy. 2014;**6**:192-198

[73] Zhou X, Wu X, An Y, Chen H, Long C. Social support mediate the associations between gratitude and post-traumatic growth in middle school students at three years after Wenchuan Earthquake. Psychological Development and Education. 2014;**30**:68-74

[74] Helgeson VS, Reynolds KA, Tomich PL. A meta-analytic review of benefit finding and growth. Journal of Consulting and Clinical Psychology. 2006;**74**(5):797-816

[75] Zhou X, Wu X, Chen J. Longitudinal linkages between posttraumatic stress disorder and posttraumatic growth in adolescent survivors following the Wenchuan Earthquake in China: A three-wave, cross-lagged study. Psychiatry Research. 2015;**228**(1):107-111

[76] Zhou X, Wu X. The relationship between rumination, posttraumatic stress disorder, and posttraumatic growth among Chinese adolescents after earthquake: A longitudinal study. Journal of Affective Disorders. 2016;**193**:242-248

[77] Allwood MA, Dyl J, Hunt JI, Spirito A. Comorbidity and service utilization among psychiatrically hospitalized adolescents with posttraumatic stress disorder. Journal of Psychological Trauma. 2008;**7**(2):104- 121. DOI: 10.1080/19322880802231791

[78] Yang P, Yen CF, Tang TC, Chen CS, Yang RC, Huang MS, et al. Posttraumatic stress disorder in adolescents after Typhoon Morakot-associated mudslides. Journal of Anxiety Disorder. 2011;**25**(3):362-368. DOI: 10.1016/j.janxdis.2010.10.010

[79] Chemtob CM, Madan A, Berger P, Abramovitz R. Adolescent exposure to the world trade center attacks, PTSD symptomatology, and suicidal ideation. Journal of Trauma Stress. 2011;**24**(5):526-529. DOI: 10.1002/jts.20670

[80] Duncan RD. Childhood maltreatment and college drop-out rates: Implications for child abuse researchers. Journal of Interpersonal Violence. 2000;**15**(9):987-995. DOI: 10.1177/088626000015009005

[81] Goenjian AK, Roussos A, Steinberg AM, Sotiropoulou C, Walling D, Kakaki M, et al. Longitudinal study of PTSD, depression, and quality of life among adolescents after the Parnitha earthquake. Journal of Affective Disorders. 2011;**133**(3):509-515. DOI: 10.1016/j.jad.2011.04.053

[82] Cohen JA, Deblinger E, Mannarino AP, Steer RA. A multisite, randomized controlled trial for children with sexual abuse–related PTSD symptoms. Journal of the American Academy of Child & Adolescent Psychiatry. 2004;**43**(4):393-402. DOI: 10.1097/01.chi.0000111364.94169.f9

[83] Silverman WK, Ortiz CD, Viswesvaran C, Burns BJ, Kolko DJ, Putnam FW, et al. Evidence-based psychosocial treatments for children and adolescents exposed to traumatic events. Journal of Clinical Child & Adolescent Psychology. 2008;**37**(1):156- 183. DOI: 10.1080/15374410701818293

[84] Foa EB, McLean CP, Capaldi S, Rosenfield D. Prolonged exposure vs supportive counseling for sexual abuse-related PTSD in adolescent girls: A randomized clinical trial. Journal of the American Medical Association. 2013;**310**(24):2650-2657. DOI: 10.1001/jama.2013.282829

[85] Keeshin BR, Strawn JR. Psychological and pharmacologic treatment of youth with posttraumatic stress disorder: An evidence-based review. Child and Adolescent Psychiatric Clinics of North America. 2014;**23**(2):399-411x. DOI: 10.1016/j.chc.2013.12.002

[86] Smith P, Dalgleish T, Meiser-Stedman R. Practitioner review: Posttraumatic stress disorder and its treatment in children and adolescents. Jouranl of Child Psychology Psychiatry. 2019;**60**(5):500-515. DOI: 10.1111/jcpp.12983

[87] Allison AC, Ferreira RJ. Implementing cognitive behavioral intervention for trauma in schools (CBITS) with Latino Youth. Child and Adolescent Social Work Journal. 2017;**34**(2):181-189. DOI: 10.1007/s10560-016-0486-9

[88] Morsette A, Swaney G, Stolle D, Schuldberg D, van den Pol R, Young M. Cognitive Behavioral intervention for trauma in schools (CBITS): School-based treatment on a rural American Indian reservation. Journal of Behavior Therapy and Experimental Psychiatry. 2009;**40**(1):169-178. DOI: 10.1016/j.jbtep.2008.07.006

[89] Layne CM, Saltzman WR, Poppleton L, Burlingame GM, Pasalic A,

Durakovic E, et al. Effectiveness of a school-based group psychotherapy program for war-exposed adolescents: A randomized controlled trial. Journal of American Academy of Child and Adolescent Psychiatry. 2008;**47**(9):1048-1062. DOI: 10.1097/CHI.0b013e31817eecae

[90] van den Hout MA, Engelhard IM. How does EMDR work? Journal of Experimental Psychopathology. 2012;**3**(5):724-738. DOI: 10.5127/jep.028212

[91] De Roos C, van der Oord S, Zijlstra B, Lucassen S, Perrin S, Emmelkamp P, et al. Comparison of eye movement desensitization and reprocessing therapy, cognitive behavioral writing therapy, and wait-list in pediatric posttraumatic stress disorder following single-incident trauma: A multicenter randomized clinical trial. Journal of Child Psychology and Psychiatry. 2017;**58**(11):1219-1228

[92] Diehle J, Opmeer BC, Boer F, Mannarino AP, Lindauer RJ. Trauma-focused cognitive behavioral therapy or eye movement desensitization and reprocessing: What works in children with posttraumatic stress symptoms? A randomized controlled trial. European Child & Adolescent Psychiatry. 2015;**24**(2):227-236. DOI: 10.1007/s00787-014-0572-5

[93] Sánchez-Meca J, Rosa-Alcázar AI, López-Soler C. The psychological treatment of sexual abuse in children and adolescents: A meta-analysis. International Journal of Clinical and Health Psychology. 2011;**11**(1):67-93

[94] Cohen JA, Mannarino AP, Knudsen K. Treating sexually abused children: 1 year follow-up of a randomized controlled trial. Child Abuse & Neglect. 2005;**29**(2):135-145. DOI: 10.1016/j.chiabu.2004.12.005

[95] Schottenbauer MA, Glass CR, Arnkoff DB, Tendick V, Gray SH. Nonresponse and dropout rates in outcome studies on PTSD: Review and methodological considerations. Psychiatry. 2008;**71**(2):134-168. DOI: 10.1521/psyc.2008.71.2.134

[96] Stallard P. Psychological interventions for post-traumatic reactions in children and young people: A review of randomised controlled trials. Clinical Psychology Review. 2006;**26**(7):895-911. DOI: 10.1016/j.cpr.2005.09.005

[97] Schneider SJ, Grilli SF, Schneider JR. Evidence-based treatments for traumatized children and adolescents. Current Psychiatry Reports. 2013;**15**(1):332. DOI: 10.1007/s11920-012-0332-5

[98] Cullen M. Mindfulness-based interventions: An emerging phenomenon. Mindfulness. 2011;**2**(3):186-193. DOI: 10.1007/s12671-011-0058-1

[99] Muller-Engelmann M, Wunsch S, Volk M, Steil R. Mindfulness-based stress reduction (MBSR) as a standalone intervention for posttraumatic stress disorder after mixed traumatic events: A mixed-methods feasibility study. Frontiers in Psychology. 2017;**8**:1407. DOI: 10.3389/fpsyg.2017.01407

[100] Follette V, Palm KM, Pearson AN. Mindfulness and trauma: Implications for treatment. Journal of Rational-Emotive & Cognitive-Behavior Therapy. 2006;**24**(1):45-61. DOI: 10.1007/s10942-006-0025-2

[101] Wahbeh H, Goodrich E, Goy E, Oken BS. Mechanistic pathways of mindfulness meditation in combat veterans with posttraumatic stress disorder. Jouranal of Clinical Psychology. 2016;**72**(4):365-383. DOI: 10.1002/jclp.22255

[102] Frost ND, Laska KM, Wampold BE. The evidence for present-centered therapy as a treatment for posttraumatic stress disorder. Journal of Trauma Stress. 2014;**27**(1):1-8. DOI: 10.1002/jts.21881

[103] Zoogman S, Goldberg SB, Hoyt WT, Miller L. Mindfulness interventions with youth: A meta-analysis. Mindfulness. 2014;**6**(2):290-302. DOI: 10.1007/s12671-013-0260-4

[104] Borquist-Conlon DS, Maynard BR, Brendel KE, Farina ASJ. Mindfulness-based interventions for youth with anxiety: A systematic review and meta-analysis. Research on Social Work Practice. 2019;**29**(2):195-205. DOI: 10.1177/1049731516684961

[105] Spiegel D, Malchiodi C, Backos A, Collie K. Art therapy for combat-related PTSD: Recommendations for research and practice. Art Therapy. 2006;**23**(4):157-164. DOI: 10.1080/07421656.2006.10129335

[106] Talwar S. Accessing traumatic memory through art making: An art therapy trauma protocol (ATTP). The Arts in Psychotherapy. 2007;**34**(1):22-35. DOI: 10.1016/j.aip.2006.09.001

[107] Feldman R, Vengrober A. Posttraumatic stress disorder in infants and young children exposed to war-related trauma. Journal of the American Academy of Child & Adolescent Psychiatry. 2011;**50**(7):645-658. DOI: 10.1016/j.jaac.2011.03.001

[108] Berger R, Pat-Horenczyk R, Gelkopf M. School-based intervention for prevention and treatment of elementary-students' terror-related distress in Israel: A quasi-randomized controlled trial. Journal of Trauma Stress. 2007;**20**(4):541-551. DOI: 10.1002/jts.20225

[109] Ugurlu N, Akca L, Acarturk C. An art therapy intervention for symptoms of post-traumatic stress, depression and anxiety among Syrian refugee children. Vulnerable Children and Youth Studies. 2016;**11**(2):89-102. DOI: 10.1080/17450128.2016.1181288

[110] Lyshak-Stelzer F, Singer P, Patricia SJ, Chemtob CM. Art therapy for adolescents with posttraumatic stress disorder symptoms: A pilot study. Art Therapy. 2007;**24**(4):163-169. DOI: 10.1080/07421656.2007.10129474

[111] Cohen JA et al. AACAP work group on quality issues. Practice parameter for the assessment and treatment of children and adolescents with posttraumatic stress disorder. Journal of the American Academy of Child & Adolescent Psychiatry. 2010;**49**(4):414-430

[112] Davis LL, Frazier EC, Williford RB, Newell JM. Long-term pharmacotherapy for post-traumatic stress disorder. CNS Drugs. 2006;**20**(6):465-476

[113] Cohen JA, Mannarino AP, Perel JM, Staron V. A pilot randomized controlled trial of combined trauma-focused CBT and sertraline for childhood PTSD symptoms. Journal of the American Academy of Child & Adolescent Psychiatry. 2007;**46**(7):811-819

[114] Bridge JA, Iyengar S, Salary CB, Barbe RP, Birmaher B, Pincus HA, et al. Clinical response and risk for reported suicidal ideation and suicide attempts in pediatric antidepressant treatment: A meta-analysis of randomized controlled trials. Journal of the American Medical Association. 2007;**297**(15):1683-1696

[115] Seedat S, Stein DJ, Ziervogel C, Middleton T, Kaminer D, Emsley RA, et al. Comparison of response to a selective serotonin reuptake inhibitor in children, adolescents, and adults with posttraumatic stress disorder. Journal of Child and Adolescent Psychopharmacology. 2002;**12**(1): 37-46

[116] Steiner H, Saxena KS, Carrion V, Khanzode LA, Silverman M, Chang K. Divalproex sodium for the treatment of PTSD and conduct disordered youth: A pilot randomized controlled clinical trial. Child Psychiatry and Human Development. 2007;**38**(3):183-193

[117] Meighen KG, Hines LA, Lagges AM. Risperidone treatment of preschool children with thermal burns and acute stress disorder. Journal of Child and Adolescent Psychopharmacology. 2007;**17**(2):223-232

[118] Alarcón RD, Glover S, Boyer W, Balon R. Proposing an algorithm for the pharmacological management of posttraumatic stress disorder. Annals of Clinical Psychiatry. 2000;**12**(4):239-246

[119] Famularo R, Kinscherff R, Fenton T. Propranolol treatment for childhood posttraumatic stress disorder, acute type: A pilot study. American Journal of Diseases of Children. 1988;**142**(11):1244-1247

[120] Harmon RJ, Riggs PD. Clonidine for posttraumatic stress disorder in preschool children. Journal of the American Academy of Child & Adolescent Psychiatry. 1996;**35**(9):1247-1249

[121] March JS. Combining medication and psychosocial treatments: An evidence-based medicine approach. International Review of Psychiatry. 2002;**14**(2):155-163

[122] Strawn JR, Keeshin BR, DelBello MP, Geracioti TD Jr, Putnam FW. Psychopharmacologic treatment of posttraumatic stress disorder in children and adolescents: A review. Journal of Clinical Psychiatry. 2010;**71**(7):932

7

Use of Falun Gong to Address Traumatic Stress among Marginalized Clients

Margaret Trey and Cirecie West-Olatunji

Abstract

Although mental health service providers have focused on the effects of trauma and related interventions for decades, little is known about pervasive and historic trauma, particularly for socially marginalized individuals. Thus, clinical issues associated with sociopolitical oppression have been under-investigated. Coupled with the lack of sufficient cultural competence when working with diverse clients, mainstream clinicians frequently lack adequate case conceptualization skills and culturally sensitive interventions to assist clients from diverse backgrounds. Using traumatic stress as a framework for exploring evidence-based interventions to address long-term, pervasive marginalization and its psychological effects, the authors propose that mindfulness techniques are particularly beneficial to this client population. The authors reviewed culture-centered interventions to address traumatic stress for marginalized client populations, focusing on the mindfulness practice of Falun Gong. Recommendations for practice include the inclusion of traumatic stress theory and techniques in pre-service training, professional development training for practitioners focusing on mindfulness techniques with clients assessed with historical trauma, and Web-based training for clinical faculty to enhance their knowledge about traumatic stress, historical trauma, and associated interventions for clients from marginalized communities. The authors offer recom-mendations for future research that focuses on studies exploring the usefulness of Falun Gong in working with clients with traumatic stress.

Keywords: Falun Gong, Falun Dafa, meditation, mindfulness, traumatic stress

1. Introduction

Scholars have most recently begun to investigate the impact of pervasive micro aggressions and other forms of systemic oppression on individuals from culturally and socially marginalized groups. Researchers have suggested that trauma affected clients report emotional and psychological impairment, such as depression and anxiety [1]. Other investigators have found that problems interpersonal conflicts and substance abuse problems are evident. Educational researchers have also explored traumatic stress and academic achievement and assert that severe persistent stress due to environmental factors, such as racism, can negatively impact children's academic performance [2, 3]. The authors use traumatic stress theory as a framework for exploring effective interventions to decrease symptomology due to systemic oppression.

The purpose of this paper is to outline the benefits of Falun Gong, an ancient Chinese mind-body and spiritual discipline, as a mindfulness intervention when working with culturally marginalized clients. The authors provide an overview of the clinical issues associated with historical trauma and then present Falun Gong as an alternative solution for ameliorating the effects of social marginalization. The authors suggest that Falun Gong is beneficial in addressing the psychological, physical, academic, and financial needs of these particular types of clients. Recommendations for practice include expanded training on Falun Gong as a clinical intervention and an enhancement of the curriculum in various mental health-training programs to include more emphasis on mindfulness and, more particularly, Falun Gong. Suggestions for future research focus on developing a national study exploring the impact of Falun Gong practices on traumatic stress symptoms for culturally marginalized clients.

2. The effects of historical trauma on marginalized populations

How individuals cope with trauma is dependent upon their social positioning prior to the onset of traumatic experiences. Some groups of people, such as poor people, the elderly, culturally diverse, and mentally/physically impaired, are dispro-portionately affected by traumatic events and experiences based upon institutional-ized and historical biases in society. Lack of access to institutional resources and lack of power to control those institutions creates a cycle of socio-cultural abuse that threatens the psyche of culturally diverse individuals.

Yet, mental health professionals have been slow to acknowledge clinical issues related to pervasive trauma & chronic stress due to cultural hegemony [4]. For culturally diverse clients, for example, this has meant diagnoses based upon models of normalcy for middle-class Whites. Research has shown that systemic oppression has deleterious physical and mental health effects. Traumatic stress and psychological distress have been shown to be evident in several studies. Some of the outcomes of systemic oppression are noted in physical/psychological health [1–3] and education disparities [2, 5].

2.1 Cultural and clinical competence

For the most part, traditional perspectives in the behavioral sciences have focused on the client as a poorly functioning individual. An ecological approach con-siders the possibility of a malfunctioning system and its impact on the client [6]. In analyzing some hypotheses to explain why clinicians have been slow to incorporate systemic interventions into their roles and responsibilities, one study suggests that clinicians may "underestimate the power of resources other than their values, skills, and personalities" ([7], p. 33).

An eco-systemic perspective in examining trauma aids in understanding and conceptualizing the needs of culturally diverse communities. Concentrating on the African American experience, researchers have begun investigating the cor-relates between historical trauma and oppression [1, 8–10]. Additional work in this area by Seaton [11] revealed that, in particular, due to racism, African Americans experience more stressful events than European Americans. In summarizing the Differential Exposure Hypothesis (DEH), Seaton suggested that racism, bias, and discrimination are detrimental to African Americans because they are disproportionately placed at higher risk for psychological disorders. Eco-systemic interventions incorporate an understanding of those external influences that impact an individual's functioning [6].

Over the past two decades, mental health practitioners across all disciplines have become increasingly aware of the need for clinicians to involve themselves in the role of advocate for their clients [12–14]. Clinicians need to consider their clients within the context of their families and communities, as well as their social, cultural, and religious systems [15]. Additionally, assessment and treatment models are needed to intervene with clients who have been impacted by systemic oppression. Clinicians can explore relevant themes to address the context of systemic oppression and the related traumatic experiences. Intervening for trauma due to systemic oppression is necessary for recovery. Through their expanded awareness of sociocultural oppression, clinicians can become healers as well as advocates for their clients [14].

2.2 Traumatic stress theory

Chronic stress/pervasive trauma, related to systemic oppression, is transgenerational in nature: this is contextualized by historical and systemic oppression resulting in discriminatory legislation and racism in the U.S. Current effects of systemic oppression and trauma may be additive to the historical trauma experienced by previous generations [3]. Many of the problems reported by individual trauma survivors also are reported by their partners, including individual stress symptoms, isolation, poor relationship quality, and reduced intimacy. The available literature suggests that trauma and trauma symptoms affect not only the individual but also the people with whom traumatized persons have a significant relationship (e.g., spouses, partners, and children). However, this literature on the systemic effects of trauma is predominantly clinical in nature [16].

Trauma is experienced intergenerationally despite the absence of direct exposure to a traditional traumatic stimulus as evidenced from the study of Jewish Holocaust survivor's children [17]. This study was also extended to the family members of veterans from World War II and the Vietnam War, indigenous peoples, individuals and groups living under repressive regimes, those experiencing domes-tic violence and crime, and those living with infection and life-threatening diseases. Symptoms may include depression, anxiety, suicidal ideation and behavior, sub-stance abuse, and violence.

Effective interventions with culturally diverse clients: (a) build on existing knowledge within the client's worldviews, (b) maintain client empowerment and agency, (c) demonstrate reciprocity in the transformation process, and (d) honor the historical and contextual forms of healing within the client's familial and community networks. Some examples of these types of interventions include the use of story circle and other forms of narrative storytelling. More recently, clini-cal research has explored the benefits of meditation and mindfulness is assisting trauma-affected clients. Both of these types of interventions can be useful in working with culturally diverse clients.

2.3 Story circle

Story circle is a tool to build equal partnerships that foster better understanding and communication among participants with like interests, thereby creating a stronger sense of community [18]. The story circle is oral and affective in nature. Stories tell individuals about their whole selves. Clients have the opportunity to share their feelings, thoughts and emotions with other people. They free their spirit in a way that is incomprehensible to outsiders. The term outsiders, refers to either observers of the story circle, or other cultures that may not be familiar with storytelling traditions in their society. The story circle tends to create a comfortable environment that encompasses warmth and trust. The facilitator's job is to make sure each person connects the themes and patterns that the stories have created. All stories should connect in some way or another. It is also appropriate for members of the story circle to challenge one another after the storytelling has taken place. When it is time to process, members should discuss where they felt connected and focus on feelings and thought processes. The facilitator should also let everyone share responsibility for keeping track of time because it can last a while. Also, a follow-up activity should be conducted for the group as well.

2.4 Mindfulness/meditation and emergent practices

There is plentiful evidence to show that Eastern meditation and mindfulness techniques have beneficial effects on our personal and work life [19–22]. One study showed that participants reported significant reduction in anxiety, depression, and stress levels after a 10-week mindfulness meditation program [20]. Other studies indicated that meditation could alter brain function and even change the physical structure of the human brain, impacting the concept of lifelong neuroplasticity [23–26]. Weaver [22] noted some of these studies showed that even novice or inexperienced meditators can rewire their brains and reap the benefits of meditative practices. These modified Eastern meditative and mindfulness techniques have shown to be beneficial effects.

As more people are seeking peace, inner balance, and wellbeing through medita-tion and mindfulness practices, there is a mushrooming of interest from those in the helping profession to integrate these ancient practices into their work [27–32]. A survey by the *Psychotherapy Networker* revealed 41.4% of about 2600 therapists reported integrating certain mindfulness techniques into their professional prac-tice [29]. An online survey by *Counseling Today,* a publication of the American Counseling Association (ACA), indicated that 87% of counselors reported adopt-ing an integrated practice with mindfulness approaches into their professional work with clients [28]. Writers, like Meyers [28], regard meditation as a form of mindfulness based technique.

Today, Falun Gong is one of the fastest emergent Chinese spiritual and medita-tive movement practices that is spreading throughout the world [31–33]. Large scale studies conducted in mainland China showed the tremendous health and wellness effects of Falun Gong [32, 34–36]. Likewise, various studies outside of mainland China and around the world indicated Falun Gong's beneficial effects [33, 37–39]. There were two studies outside of China that stood out. The first was the Australian survey completed by the first author under the auspices of The University of South Australia for partial fulfillment of the Doctor of counseling degree examined the health and wellness effects of Falun Gong from the self-reports of Falun Gong practitioners [38]. It was the first empirical study with a diverse sample outside of mainland China [33, 38]. The second one, completed for the partial fulfillment of the Doctor of Philosophy in Psychology at the University of California, Los Angeles, demonstrated that practicing Falun Gong has a beneficial effect and that long-term practice may lead to hemispheric changes in the brain [40, 41].

Falun Gong has not been a subject for much research. Besides these two studies conducted under the auspices of an Australian and a US university respectively, a team of medical doctors and researchers in the United States had undertaken a pilot study to examine the effects of Falun Gong on gene expression and the role of neutrophils in Falun Gong practitioners [42]. Findings from their pilot study revealed superior gene expression, enhanced immunity, and longer lifespan of neutrophils in Falun Gong respondents [42]. The researchers' endeavor provided the first evidence to suggest that practicing Falun Gong could influence immunity, metabolic rate, and cell regeneration. Then there were several publications documented many individuals experiencing health and wellness healing effects after they started practicing Falun Gong [43–45].

3. What is Falun Gong?

Also known as Falun Dafa, Falun Gong is a high-level Chinese self-cultivation practice for overall mind, body, and spiritual improvement [33, 46, 47]. It originated from Northeast China. Over the past two decades since its teacher and founder, Master Li Hongzhi first introduced Falun Gong to the public in 1992, there are numerous terms used to describe Falun Gong [33, 38]. Most non-Falun Gong writers concurred that Falun Gong is a form of qigong [46, 48–51] or a Buddhist qigong system [52]. Other expressions used to describe Falun include traditional Chinese religious practice, or revival of traditional Chinese spiritual practice [49, 53–56], or as a new religious movement [57–60]. Gale and Gorman-Yao [61] described Falun Gong as a cultural movement, while Ackerman [62] referred to the practice as a New Age spiritual movement.

Despite the myriad of descriptive terms and expressions, there is a mutual understanding that Falun Gong is a form of qigong, a comprehensive spiritual meditation discipline, a quasi-religious practice, or a new Chinese religious movement. Human Rights Watch Senior Advisor Spiegel [51] offered a comprehensive definition, describing Falun Gong as a synthesis of qualities:

> *"A form of qigong, an ancient Chinese deep-breathing exercise system sometimes combined with meditation that enthusiasts claim promotes physical, mental, and spiritual well-being by enhancing the flow of vital energy through a person's body. It also includes elements of popular Buddhism and Daoism" (Spiegel, 2002, p. 8).*

Among practitioners, Falun Gong, an ancient Chinese spiritual discipline, is better known as Falun Dafa. The Chinese word "Fa" ([63], p. 390) refers to law or principles in the Buddha School teachings but this is not the same as the Buddhism taught by Buddha Shakyamuni or Siddhārtha Gautama. Penny states in his book, *The Religion of Falun Gong,* that the "falun" in the name Falun Gong "has a different meaning from that in Buddhism" ([64], p. 5). He describes Falun Gong as "the practice of the Wheel of the Law" (p. 5), and that Falun Dafa refers to "the Great Method of the Wheel of the Law" ([64], p. 5).

In *Zhuan Falun*, the complete teachings of Falun Gong, "Dafa," which is pronounced as "Dah-fah" simply means the "Great Law" or the "Great Way" ([63], p. 2). While Falun Dafa is more befitting and widely used in Falun Gong literature, for the purpose of this article that comprises the White Paper, many writers have consistently alluded to this Chinese spiritual discipline as Falun Gong. This is partly because Falun Gong has remained more popular and widely used across different media, popular search engines, and literature by non-Falun Gong people [33, 38].

3.1 Advanced practice with ancient roots

Most Falun Gong literature describes the practice as an ancient Chinese spiritual discipline in the Buddha tradition [31, 33, 38, 47, 65, 66]. Falun Gong, pronounced "Fah-loon Gong," is a high-level, mind-body spiritual system with its roots in both ancient Buddhist and Taoist traditions [63, 67]. The *gong* in Falun Gong and qigong connotes exercise or practice but Falun Gong is not one at the same as practicing qigong. The *gong* in Falun Gong actually pertains to a "high-energy substance that manifests in the form of light, and its particles are fine and its density is high" ([63], p. 5). In Falun Gong, it is the cultivation of this *gong* that facilitates genuine healing, mind-body, and spiritual transformation [63] that many individuals experience. Simply put, Falun Gong, with its moral teachings and fivea meditative exercises, is a popular, tranquil cultivation practice for overall mind-body and spiritual improvement.

At the heart of the practice, Falun Gong teaches three universal principles—Truthfulness, Compassion, Forbearance—or *Zhen, Shan, Ren* in Chinese ([63], pp. 13-17). While some people in the West describe Falun Gong as a "Chinese yoga" ([47], p. 40), Falun Gong exercises are a lot simpler than yoga and do not imitate animal movements, like Indian yoga does. Falun Gong has only four standing exer-cises and one sitting meditation [67]. First introduced to the public in mainland China in 1992, the founder of the practice explains that Falun Gong is an advanced spiritual cultivation discipline and hence a high level form of qigong [63]. Within 7 years—from 1992 to 1999—Falun Gong rose from anonymity to become one of the fastest growing spiritual practices. On July 20, 1999, Falun Gong was illegally banned in mainland China and followers of the practice received the most hor-rendous persecution [33]. At the time, about 100 million people in China were practicing Falun Gong, which means that about one out of 13 Chinese people in mainland China was practicing Falun Gong [68], as a result of the practice's heal-ing benefits.

3.2 Cultivating the heart and mind

A unique characteristic of Falun Gong lies in its focus on heart and mind cultivation and on becoming a morally upright person. Falun Gong is based on the ancient tradition of self-cultivation, transcending ordinary existence toward a higher state of being, and liberating one from the illusions of this material world. Thus, cultiva-tion calls for letting go of desires, being virtuous and uprightness, as well as using special practices techniques to refine both the mind and body [33, 63].

Falun Gong comprises two distinctive aspects—cultivation and practice. Cultivation or self-cultivation is an Eastern concept for mind, body, and spiritual improvement [69] that is a crucial and vital aspect of traditional Chinese culture. Falun Gong underlines *xinxing* cultivation, which is, cultivating the heart and mind [63, 67]. Cultivating the heart denotes improving one's moral character—guided by the principles of truthfulness, compassion, and forbearance [63].

It must be noted that improving one's mind and heart, or moral character, requires a strong main consciousness. In Falun Gong cultivation, it is important that "the mind must be right" ([63], p. 245). According to the teachings of Falun Gong, when one's heart and mind or *xinxing* improves, one's body, mind, and spirit will naturally transform [63] and one will thereby reach optimum health and wellness. So, Falun Gong is more than just a meditation practice; it is a spiritual cultivation discipline for overall body, mind, and spiritual advancement. Of the two—cultivation versus practice—it must be noted that cultivation is far more important than the exercise practice. The latter is merely to strengthen the mechanisms in the body [67].

The practice component of Falun Gong involves a sitting meditation and four standing exercises. Each exercise has specific health-related aims and benefits [67]. Simple, yet beneficial is its health-wellness impact on millions of individuals who turn to Falun Gong for solace. From the integrative counseling perspective, Falun

Gong is a mind-body approach embodying the art of self-care as well as serving as an intervention strategy [37]. Hence, there is potential for its integration into the helping profession [32, 33, 37, 70–74], in particular for addressing traumatic stress among marginalized clients.

3.3 Benefits

Practicing Falun Gong has numerous benefits. Many individuals can attest to it that Falun Gong can help to ease anxiety, stress, and traumatic stress; enhance energy and vitality; and improves the mind and body [43, 44]. Falun Gong has offered inner joy, peace, and serenity, leading to spiritual growth and enlightenment for many individuals. At the 2018 International Conference on Spirituality and Psychology, the first author, who was invited to speak about the viability of Falun Gong integration, presented three case examples on how Falun Gong was able to help individuals to overcome anxiety, depression, and post-traumatic stress disorder [71, 72].

Case story examples illustrate the healing benefits of Falun Gong and its integration feasibility with counseling in helping clients toward self-healing and realizing their varied purpose in life. The ancient art of storytelling helps to provide insight into the healing effects of Falun Gong, allowing individuals who have benefitted from the practice to express their inner world and to create meaning by describing in their own words how Falun Gong has impacted and transformed their lives. For example, voice actor and author Rich Crankshaw is one such individual who has benefited tremendously from the practice. His healing from traumatic stress arising from child hood abuse was empowering: "After three days, my anxiety was lower, my stress level was lower, my depression was not as dominant, and all of a sudden, I understood that I just didn't need to smoke weed or drink beer anymore" ([75], p. 197) . Falun Gong "has been a major part of my ongoing healing and recovery" ([75], p. 198), stated Crankshaw who has an English-Mohawk indigenous ancestry.

Academic research exploring the therapeutic effects of Falun Gong is still lacking. The prevailing body of Falun Gong literature exploring its beneficial effects can be classified into two groups. The first wave of enquiry was in mainland China before the persecution of Falun Gong began on July 20, 1999, while the second movement of scholarly enquiry into the beneficial effects of practicing Falun Gong took place outside of China after 1999. This section revisits some of the studies from both categories. Before 1999, a team of researchers in mainland China completed an extensive survey with a sample size of 12,731 participants from five districts in Beijing [34]. Findings from this massive survey indicated Falun Gong's effectiveness was over 99%, with a 59% cure rate. For physical and mental health, the improve-ment rate was over 80 and 97%, respectively [34].

After the onset of the persecution in 1999, some practitioners in Canada and the United States conducted the North American survey [39]. Findings from this survey supported and reinforced the results from the large-scale Beijing surveys [34]. In 2000, a single-case study for partial fulfillment of a master's degree in social science in counseling showed the beneficial use of Falun Gong in relieving burnout and posttraumatic stress [37]. Additionally, there are two reports worth citing. The first is an independent study conducted in Taiwan, which found that people who prac-tice Falun Gong are physically and mentally healthier than the general Taiwanese population [76]. Respondents reported that practicing Falun Gong helped to eliminate unhealthy and addictive lifestyle habits, such as gambling, cigarette smoking, alcohol addiction, and chewing betel nuts that is a common habit in Asian countries [76]. Lio et al.'s study also highlighted Falun Gong's medical cost-saving potential, showing a 50% decrease in the use of medical health insurance for Falun Gong respondents [76, 77]. In another study, a group of researchers in Russia reported a 73% improvement rate in the respondents' health and wellness [78].

Researchers from Switzerland, Taiwan, UK, and the US did a meta-analysis based on the self-reports from Chinese cancer patients between 2000 and 2015 and found that practicing Falun Gong could significantly improve survival rate for cancer patients [79]. About 97 percent (n = 147, 96.7%) indicated full symptom recovery, with 60 cases confirmed by their doctors [79].

4. Discussion

Falun Gong can be a useful alternative to existing interventions for traumatic stress because of its ability to alleviate anxiety and bring about innerpeace [33, 73]. Contemporary research that explores traumatic stress as it relates to racial bias suggests that individuals often report unhealthy and addictive lifestyles as a means of coping with the daily microaggressions. Falun Gong could help these clients to become more congruent in their perspectives on mind body connection. Falun Gong is likely to target the psychological and physical issues associated with traumatic stress and provide clients with less cognitive distress leading toward better decision-making and help clear negative thought patterns. Falun Gong can also provide clients with a cost-effective intervention that makes it accessible to clients across the socio-economic spectrum.

Moreover, Falun Gong is an intervention that can be conducted within systems, such as family, work, and organization, in much the same way mindfulness and meditation have been introduced into various workplace [21, 80–83]. The use of Falun Gong within the family system is likely to impact interpersonal conflicts that may result from ongoing stressors within the social environment. Parent-child, sibling, and couple interactions can be improved when family members engage in Falun Gong practices and activities together. In this manner, families can share in countering the effects of institutional racism and Falun Gong can serve as a coping mechanism for reducing the associated stress.

Using the mindful practice of Falun Gong in the workplace, employees can become much more productive when they are able to reduce the stress related to workloads and any differential treatment that some members from within the working environment may experience. This would allow for opportunities to clearly think through forms of advocacy for themselves and for others who may be victims of microaggressions in the workplace. On the organizational level, Falun Gong can support members in finding harmony, improving collaboration efforts, and think-ing clearly about strategic goals and initiatives for the organization. Rather than becoming riddled with interpersonal conflicts due to competing demands, issues of power and control among various factions, or challenges caused by lack of member engagement or financial concerns, organizational leaders are able to stay focused on how to work toward a unified goal.

Although Falun Gong, as a mindfulness and meditative practice, is still new to the mental health professions, it is promising as an effective intervention, particularly when working with marginalized clients who experience traumatic stress in a diverse and multiple settings. In fact, various studies have shown that practicing mindfulness and meditation may be beneficial for both the therapists and their clients. For instance, in Germany, a team of researchers found that therapists' personal training in meditation could have favorable impact on clients [84]. The randomized double blind controlled study conducted by Grepmair et al. [84] revealed that it did not matter whether or not the clients themselves practice meditation or know that their therapist practices meditation. Their findings revealed that the outcome was still favorable for the clients.

In another study, Schure et al. [85] emphasized the relevance of preparing counseling students with mindfulness techniques as self-care skills and intervention strategies that students could later incorporate into their professional work. In an earlier study, Gale and Gorman-Yao [61] discussed the health-wellness potential and cultural implications of integrating Falun Gong into nursing for a "cultur-ally appropriate and sensitive nursing care to all clients" (p. 124), a concept that counseling educators and professionals could consider and implement in teaching programs.

5. Recommendations for Practice

Suggestions for improving clinical practice include the inclusion of traumatic stress theory and techniques in pre-service training as well as professional development training for practitioners. Additionally, it is recommended that clinical faculty enhance their knowledge about traumatic stress so that it can be integrated into the various curricula in mental health training programs. Pre-service and practitioner training could focus on integrating Falun Gong in to working with clients assessed with historical trauma. For faculty, web-based training would enhance their knowledge about traumatic stress, historical trauma, and associated interventions for clients from marginalized communities, as well as learning about Falun Gong.

The need for proper training in the mindful practice of Falun Gong via counseling programs in tertiary institutions is crucial. It is hoped an integrated approach with Falun Gong will be part of a training program. While other types of mindfulness techniques are widely taught, there are hardly any institutions that currently offer the mindful practice of Falun Gong as part of their curriculum.

6. Conclusion

The authors offer a recommendation for future research to focus on studies that explore and document the use of Falun Gong to work with clients who have been assessed with traumatic stress. There is a dire need for these studies to provide solid evidence of the positive link between practicing Falun Gong and traumatic stress mainstream and minority communities. For Falun Gong's integration viability, there is thus a need for pioneers in the field to shoulder greater responsibilities, emphasize on-going research, evaluations, and implement proper documenta-tion on the health and wellness effects of Falun Gong, its auxiliary and integrative potential for the health and wellbeing of counseling and health professionals, clients, and the community at large.

Acknowledgements

The authors wish to thank counseling students from the Xavier University of Louisiana who participated in the mindfulness practice of Falun Gong training sessions. Special thanks to Dr. Cirecie West-Olatunji, Professor and Director of the Center for Traumatic Stress Research Center for organizing the double training sessions.

Note

1. This paper and its topic were initially presented at the 2019 International Conference on Spirituality and Psychology in Bangkok, Thailand, by the co-authors. The first author has included more information about Falun Gong from the original White Paper that focuses on integration and the use of Falun Gong to address traumatic stress among marginalized clients.

2. For citation purposes in this book chapter, the authors have used the Fair Winds Press publication of *Zhuan Falun*. However, it is recommended that readers refer to the 2014 hardcover edition of *Zhuan Falun* for references: [86].

Author details

Margaret Trey[1*] and Cirecie West-Olatunji[2]

1 Sibubooks; Center for Psychology and Mind Studies (Researcher & Author of two books on the effects of Falun Gong), New York, USA

2 Center for Traumatic Stress Research, Xavier University of Louisiana, New Orleans, United States

*Address all correspondence to: sibubooks@gmail.com

References

[1] Harrell JP, Hall S, Taliaferro J. Physiological responses to racism and discrimination. American Journal of Public Health. 2003;**93**:243-248. DOI: 10.2105/AJPH.93.2.243

[2] Goodman RD, Miller MD, West-Olatunji CA. Traumatic stress, socioeconomic status, and academic achievement among primary school students. Psychological Trauma Theory Research Practice and Policy. 2012;**4**(3):252. DOI: 10.1037/a0024912

[3] Goodman RD, West-Olatunji CA. Educational hegemony, traumatic stress, and African American and Latino American students. Journal of Multicultural Counseling and Development. 2010;**38**(3):176-186

[4] Ibrahim FA, Roysircar-Sodowsky G, Ohimshi H. Worldview: Recent developments and needed directions. In: Ponterotto JG, Casas JM, Suzuki LA, Alexander CM, editors. Handbook of multicultural counseling. 2nd ed. Thousand Oaks, CA: Sage Publications; 2001. pp. 425-456

[5] West-Olatunji C, Sanders T, Barden S, Behar-Horenstein L. Parenting practices among low-income parents/guardians of academically successful fifth grade African American children. Multicultural Perspectives. 2010;**12**(3):138-144. DOI: 10.1080/15210960.2010.504475

[6] Chung WS, Pardeck JT. Treating powerless minorities through an ecosystem approach. Adolescence. 1997;**32**(127):625-634

[7] Eriksen K. Counselor advocacy: A qualitative analysis of leaders' perceptions, organizational activities, and advocacy documents. Journal of Mental Health Counseling. 1999;**21**:33-49

[8] Danoff-Burg S, Prelow HM, Swenson RR. Hope and life satisfaction in Black college students coping with race-related stress. Journal of Black Psychology. 2004;**30**:208-228

[9] Rich JA, Grey CM. Pathways to recurrent trauma among young Black men: Traumatic stress, substance abuse, and the "code of the street". American Journal of Public Health. 2005;**95**:816-824

[10] Scott LD Jr. Cultural orientation and coping with perceived discrimination among African American youth. Journal of Black Psychology. 2003;**29**:235-256

[11] Seaton EK. An examination of the factor structure of the index of race-related stress among a sample of African American adolescents. Journal of Black Psychology. 2003;**29**:292-307

[12] Bryant-Davis T, Ocampo C. The trauma of racism: Implications for counseling, research, and education. The Counseling Psychologist. 2005;**33**:574-578

[13] Constantine MG, Sue DW. Factors contributing to optimal human functioning in people of color in the United States. The Counseling Psychologist. 2006;**34**(2):228-244. DOI: 10.1177/0011000005281318

[14] Griffen B. Promoting professionalism, collaboration, and advocacy. Counselor Education and Supervision. 1993;**33**:2-9

[15] Boydell KM, Volpe T. A qualitative examination of the implementation of a community-academic coalition. Journal of Community Psychology. 2004;**32**:357-374. DOI: 10.1002/jcop.20010

[16] Frazier KN, West-Olatunji C, St Juste S, Goodman R. Transgenerational trauma & CSA: Reconceptualizing cases involving young survivors of child

sexual abuse. Journal of Mental Health Counseling. 2009;**31**:22-33

[17] Danieli Y. Introduction: History and conceptual foundations. In: Danieli Y, editor. International handbook of multigenerational legacies of trauma. New York: Plenum; 1998. pp. 1-20

[18] Clay L, Olatunji C, Cooley S. Keeping the story alive: Narrative in the African-American church and community. Educational Resource Information Clearinghouse, ERIC No: ED462666; 2001. pp. 1-9

[19] McGee M. Meditation and Psychiatry. Psychiatry (Edgmont). 2008;**5**(1):28-41. Retrieved from: https://www.ncbi.nlm.nih.gov/pmc/articles/PMC2719544/pdf/PE_5_01_28. pdf

[20] Schreiner I, Malcolm JP. The benefits of mindfulness meditation: changes in emotional states of depression, anxiety, and stress. Behaviour Change. 2008;**25**(3):156-168. DOI: 10.1375/bech.25.3.156

[21] Schaufenbuel K. Bringing Mindfulness to the Workplace. 2014. University of North Carolina Kenan-Flagler Business School. Retrieved from: http://www.kenan-flagler.unc.edu/~/media/Files/documents/executive-development/unc-white-paper-bringing-mindfulness-to-the-workplace_final.pdf

[22] Weaver. The Mainstreaming of Mindfulness Meditation. The Week. 2014. Retrieved from: http://theweek.com/articles/448250/mainstreaming-mindfulness-meditation

[23] Davidson RJ, Kabat-Zinn J, SchmumacherJ, RosenkranzM, MullerD, Santorelli SF, et al. Alterations in brain and immune function produced by mindfulness meditation. Psychosomatic Medicine. 2003;**65**(4):564-570

[24] Holzel BK, Carmody J, Evans KC, Hoge EA, Dusek JA, Morgan L, et al. Stress reduction correlates with structural changes in the amygdala [electronic version]. Scan. oxfordjournals.org. 2010;**5**:11-17. DOI: 10.1093/scan/nsp034

[25] Holzel BK, Carmody J, Vangela M, Congletona C, Yerramsettia SM, Garda T, et al. Mindfulness practice leads to increases in regional brain gray matter density. Psychiatry Research: Neuroimaging. 2011;**191**:36-43. DOI: 10.1016/j.pscychresns.2010.08.006

[26] McGreevey S. Meditation's Positive Residual Effects: Imaging Finds Different Forms of Meditation May Affect Brain Structure. 2012. Harvard Gazette. Retrieved from: https://news.harvard.edu/gazette/story/2012/11/meditations-positive-residual-effects/s

[27] Brown AP, Marquis A, Guiffrida D. Mindfulness-based interventions in counseling. Journal of Counseling and Development. 2013;**91**(1):96-104. DOI: 10.1002/j.1556-6676.2013.00077.x

[28] Meyers L. Cultivating a Practice of Mindfulness. Counseling Today. 2016. Retrieved from http://ct.counseling.org/2016/12/cultivating-practice-mindfulness/

[29] Siegel R. West Meets East: Creating a New Wisdom Tradition. 2011, September/October. Psychotherapy Networker. Retrieved from: https://www2.psychotherapynetworker.org/magazine/recentissues/2011-septoct/item/1363-west-meets-east/1363-west-meets-east

[30] Shallcross L. Where East Meets West. 2012. Counseling Today. Retrieved from: http://ct.counseling.org/2012/10/where-east-meets-west/

[31] Trey M. The Study of the Health-Wellness Effects of Falun Gong: Applications to Counseling. In

Spirituality and Counseling Issues: Vistas 2016 Article 25. 2016b. Retrieved from: http://www.counseling.org/docs/default-source/vistas/article_25 58c224f16116603abcacff0000bee5e7.pdf?sfvrsn=6

[32] Trey M. Falun Gong and Its Applications to Counseling: Case Examples. In VISTAS 2017, Article 51. 2017a. Retrieved from: http://www.counseling.org/docs/default-source/vistas/falun_gong.pdf?sfvrsn=4

[33] Trey M. The Mindful Practice of Falun Gong: Meditation for Health, Wellness and Beyond. [2nd edition]. Otisville, NY: Sibubooks LLC; 2020 (In press)

[34] Dan L, Pu R, Li F, Li N, Wang Q, Lu Y, et al. Falun Gong Health Effect Survey of Ten Thousand Cases in Beijing. 1998. Retrieved from http://www.clearwisdom.net/eng/science_eng/survey98_1eng.htm

[35] Summary of Health Surveys Conducted in Mainland China to Assess Falun Gong's Effects on Healing Illness and Maintaining Fitness. 2002. Retrieved from: http://www.pureinsight.org/node/841

[36] Wang Q, Li N, Zheng L, Qu E, Tian X, Jing L. The Effect of Falun Gong on Healing Illnesses and Keeping Fit: A Sampling Survey of Practitioners from Beijing Zizhuyuan Assistance Center [electronic version]. 1998. Retrieved from: http://www.clearwisdom.net/eng/science_eng/survey98_2eng.htm

[37] Lau (Trey) M. Exploring counselors' burnout and alternative coping strategies: Falun Dafa as an alternative coping strategy. In: Unpublished case study for the Master of Social Science (Counseling). Australia: The University of South Australia, Adelaide; 2001

[38] Trey M. The Effect of Falun Gong on Health and Wellness, as Perceived by Falun Gong Practitioners. Otisville, NY: Sibubooks LLC; 2020

[39] Summary of Results from the 1999 Health Survey of Falun Gong Practitioners in North America. 2003. Retrieved from: http://www.pureinsight.org/node/1533

[40] Bendig BW. Cognitive and Physiological Effects of Falun Gong Qigong [doctoral dissertation] UCLA; 2013. Retrieved from: https://escholarship.org/uc/item/4899m047

[41] Bendig BW, Shapiro D, Zaidel E. Group differences between practitioners and novices in hemispheric processing of attention and emotion before and after a session of Falun Gong qigong. Brain and Cognition. 2020;**138**:105494

[42] Li Q , Li P, Garcia GE, Johnson RJ, Feng L. Genomic profiling of neutrophil transcripts in Asian qigong practitioners: A pilot study in gene regulation by mind-body interaction. Journal of Alternative and Complementary Medicine. 2005;**11**(1):29-39. DOI: 10.1089/acm.2005.11.29

[43] Clearwisdom, editor. Life and Hope Renewed: The Healing Power of Falun Dafa. Gillette, NJ: Yih Chyun Corporation; 2005

[44] Clearwisdom, editor. Hearts and Minds Uplifted: The Power of Falun Dafa. 1st ed. Taipei City, Taiwan: Broad Press International; 2006

[45] McCoy WF, Zhang L, editors. Falun Gong stories: A Journey to Ultimate Health. 1st ed. Golden Lotus Press; 1998

[46] Burgdoff CA. How Falun Gong undermines Li Hongzhi's total rhetoric. Nova Religio: The Journal of Alternative and Emergent Religions. 2003;**6**(2):332-347. DOI: 10.1525/nr.2003.6.2.332

[47] Parker N. What is Falun Gong? An introduction to the practice and how

it developed in China and around the world. Compassion. 2004;**5**:40-43

[48] Lowe S. Chinese and international contexts for the rise of. Falun Gong Nova Religio: The Journal of Alternative and Emergent Religions. 2003;**6**(2):263-276. DOI: 10.1525/nr.2003.6.2.263

[49] Ownby D. Falun Gong and the Future of China. New York: Oxford University Press; 2008

[50] Porter N. Falun Gong in the United States: An Ethnographic Study. Parkland, Florida: Dissertation.com; 2003

[51] Spiegel M. Dangerous Meditation: China's campaign against Falungong. New York: Human Rights Watch; 2002

[52] Penny B. The Falun Gong, buddhism and "buddhist qigong." Asian Studies Review. 2005;**29**(1):35-46. DOI: 10.1080/10357820500139513

[53] Ownby D. Falungong as a Cultural Revitalization Movement: An Historian Looks at Contemporary China. Transnational China Project Commentary. 2000. Retrieved from: http://www.ruf.rice.edu/~tnchina/commentary/ownby1000.html

[54] Ownby D. A history for Falun Gong: Popular religion and the Chinese state since the Ming Dynasty. Nova Religio: The Journal of Alternative and Emergent Religions. 2003a;**6**(2):223-243. DOI: 10.1525/nr.2003.6.2.223

[55] Ownby D. Unofficial Religions in China: Beyond the Party's Rules—Statement of Professor David Ownby. 2005. Retrieved from: https://www.cecc.gov/events/roundtables/unofficial-religions-in-china-beyond-the-partys-rules

[56] Penny B. The life and times of Li Hongzhi: Falun Gong and religious biography. The China Quarterly. 2003;**175**:643-661. DOI: 10.1017/S0305741003000389

[57] Irons E. Falun Gong and the sectarian religion paradigm Nova Religio. The Journal of Alternative and Emergent Religions. 2003;**6**(2):244-262. DOI: 10.1525/nr.2003.6.2.244

[58] Ownby D. The Falun Gong in the new world. European Journal of East Asian Studies. 2003b;**2**(2):303-320. DOI: 10.1163/157006103771378437

[59] Porter N. Professional practitioners and contact persons: Explicating special types of Falun Gong practitioners. Nova Religio: The Journal of Alternative and Emergent Religion. 2005;**9**(2):62-83. DOI: 10.1525/nr.2005.9.2.062

[60] Wessinger C. Nova religio symposium: Falun Gong - introduction and glossary. Nova Religio: The Journal of Alternative and Emergent Religions. 2003;**6**(2):215-222. DOI: 10.1525/nr.2003.6.2.215

[61] Gale DD, Gorman-Yao WM. Falungong: Recent developments in Chinese notions of healing. Journal of Cultural Diversity. 2003;**10**(4):124-127

[62] Ackerman SE. Falun Dafa and the new age movement in Malaysia: Signs of health, symbols of salvation. Social Compass. 2005;**52**(4):495-511

[63] Li H. Zhuan Falun. Gloucester, MA, U.S.: Fair Winds Press; 2001

[64] Penny B. The Religion of Falun Gong. Chicago: The University of Chicago Press; 2012

[65] Falun Dafa Information Center. Ancient Roots, Almost Lost. 2015a. Retrieved from: https://faluninfo.net/falun-gong-story-ancient-roots/

[66] Falun Dafa Information Center. Why Is Falun Gong Persecuted in China? 2015b. Retrieved from: https://

faluninfo.net/why-is-falun-gong-is-persecuted-in-china/

[67] Li H. Falun Gong. Gloucester, MA, U.S.: Fair Winds Press; 2001a

[68] Nania J. Falun Gong, Popular and Serene. The Epoch Times New York Edition. 2013. Retrieved from: http://www.theepochtimes.com/n3/21898-falun-gong-popular-and-serene/

[69] Xie FT, Zhu T. Ancient wisdom for modern predicaments: The truth, deceit, and issues surrounding Falun Gong. In: Paper presented at the American Family Foundation Conference in October 17-18, 2003, published in Cultic Studies Re-view; 2004. Retrieved from: http://franktianxie.blog.epochtimes.com/article/show?articleid=4511

[70] Trey M. With wings, will fly: A spiritually integrated approach with Falun Gong, Paper presented at the International Conference on Spirituality and Psychology, from March 13-15th, 2017. Thailand: Bangkok; 2017b

[71] Trey M. Changing perceptions: An integrated approach with Falun Gong. Presented at The International Conference on Social and Behavioral Sciences, 14-16 August 2017. Singapore. 2017d

[72] Trey M. Changing perceptions: An integrative Approach with Falun Gong. Unpublished paper presented at The International Conference on Social & Behavioral Sciences. Singapore. 2017:14-16

[73] Trey M. Therapy sans therapists: Overcoming anxiety, depression, and post-traumatic stress disorder with Falun Gong. In: Presented at the International Conference on Spirituality and Psychology, from March 13-15th, 2018. Bangkok, Thailand as invited speaker; 2018

[74] Won X. Integrating Falun Gong into Western Counselling and Therapy. Singapore: Epoch Times; 2017

[75] Crankshaw R. I Raced with the Devil and Won. North Charleston, SC: Crankshaw. Createspace Independent Publishing; 2015

[76] Lio M, Hu Y, He M, Huang L, Chen L, Cheng, S. 2003. The effect of practicing qigong on health status: A case study of Falun Dafa practitioners in Taiwan. Unpublished research paper

[77] Research Report from Taiwan Illustrates the Power of Falun Gong in Improving Physical and Emotional Health While Reducing Health Care Expenses. 2003. Retrieved from: http://.clearwisdom.net/emh/articles/2003/1/1/30401.html

[78] Russia: Report on the Healing Effects of Falun Gong from the Moscow Business Committee. 2003. Retrieved from: http://clearharmony.net/articles/200302/10494.html

[79] Dong Y, Huang C, Liao J, Chen A, Liu JG, Hsu KH. An observational cohort study on terminal cancer survivors practicing Falun Gong (FLG) in China. Journal of Clinical Oncology. 2017;**34**(15 suppl):e21568-e21568. Retrieved from: http://ascopubs.org/doi/abs/10.1200/JCO.2016.34.15_suppl. e21568

[80] Baer D. 3 Reasons Everyone at Google Is Meditating. Fast Company. 2013. Retrieved from: http://www.fastcompany.com/3013333/unplug/3-reasons-everyone-at-google-is-meditating

[81] Baer D. Here's What Google Teaches Employees in Its "Search Inside Yourself" Course. Business Insider. 2014. Retrieved from: http://www.businessinsider.com/search-inside-yourself-googles-life-changing-mindfulness-course-2014-8

[82] Essig T. Google Teaches Employees to "Search Inside Yourself." Forbes. 2012. Retrieved from: http://www.forbes. com/sites/toddessig/2012/04/30/google-teaches-employees-to-search-inside-yourself/

[83] Workout M. How Mindfulness Can Help Your Employees: A Special Report for Wellness Directors. 4th ed. New York, NY & Copenhagen, Scandinavia: Mental Workout Inc; 2016

[84] Grepmair L, Mitterlehner F, Loew T, Bachler E, Rother W, Nickel M. Promoting mindfulness in psychotherapists in training influences the treatment results of their patients: A randomized, double-blind, controlled study. Psychotherapy and Psychosomatics. 2007;**76**(6):332-338. DOI: 10.1159/000107560

[85] Schure MB, Christopher J, Christopher S. Mind–body medicine and the art of self-care: Teaching mindfulness to counseling students through yoga, meditation, and qigong. Journal of Counseling & Development. 2008;**86**:47-56. DOI: 10.1002/j.1556-6678.2008.tb00625.x

[86] Li H. Zhuan Falun. (Minghui.org and Falun Dafa Association, Trans.). Taipei, Taiwan: Yih Chyun Book Co. Ltd; 2014

8

Assessing the Effectiveness of Brief and Low Intensity Psychological Interventions for Medically Unexplained Symptoms and Health Anxiety

Orla McDevitt-Petrovic and Karen Kirby

Abstract

This chapter presents a systematic review of the literature to assess the effectiveness of *brief* psychological interventions for medically unexplained symptoms (MUS)/somatic symptom disorder, non-cardiac chest pain, and illness anxiety disorder or health anxiety (HA). Google Scholar, PubMed, and Web of Science were searched as data sources. Reference lists were subsequently examined for other relevant articles. Studies were assessed according to specified inclusion criteria and extracted according to PRISMA guidelines. A total of 23 studies were included in the final synthesis. Significant effects for intervention groups relative to control groups were reported in 19 studies, whilst 4 studies did not determine any signifi-cant benefits of interventions compared with controls. All of the brief interventions (CBT, psychosocial, psychophysiological, psychosomatic, relaxation and group therapy), with the exception of metaphor therapy, showed significant effects relative to controls in at least one study. The evidence suggests that brief psychological interventions, more specifically time limited CBT based interventions may be effective in treating HA and MUS with psychological distress. Findings are comparable with other reviews. Future research may facilitate the piloting of an intervention, and there remains a need to provide more robust evidence of cost effectiveness.

Keywords: LICBT, MUS, HA, depression, anxiety

1. Introduction

1.1 Definitions, diagnostic criteria and comorbidities

There has been considerable dispute around the classification and terminologies used in relation to medically unexplained symptoms (MUS) and associated syndromes [1, 2]. MUS is a general term for syndromes without a known pathological cause. The use of the term itself is also often problematic given the negative connotations. Indeed, many patients prefer the use of alternative terms, for example 'persistent physical symptoms' [3]. The current review assesses the effectiveness of brief interventions for MUS, illness anxiety disorder, somatic symptom disorder, health anxiety (HA) and non-cardiac chest pain (NCCP). Although there may be a degree of overlap within these, it is important to outline what distinguishing features there may be.

Some of the most pronounced revisions within the latest version of the DSM-V relate to MUS [4]. A new category ('Somatic Symptom and Related Disorders') has been created, wherein MUS fits. The category includes diagnoses of Somatic Symptom Disorder (SSD) which replaces the term MUS, and Illness Anxiety Disorder (IAD) which replaces HA. The term hypochondriasis is no longer referred to. The key difference between MUS and SSD is that SSD accounts for cases where symptoms may have an underlying pathology, but there remains an exaggerated response. However, given that SSD also includes cases where there is an absence of pathological cause (i.e. MUS), the term has been included in the current review in addition to a specific SSD and NCCP. The terms IAD and HA are both used to refer to the preoccupation with having a serious illness; somatic symptoms may not be present, or may present in mild form. MUS and IAD may therefore present in isolation or comorbidly; this is determined by the presence (or not) of physical symptoms without pathological cause, and the subsequent response to these.

Up to one third of individuals with physical heath presentations have MUS [5]. The prevalence of MUS within the general population, and more particularly within medical settings, is high [6, 7]. MUS and HA are both associated with increased costs accrued through frequent and inappropriate use of healthcare services, absenteeism and long-term unemployment [8, 9]. It has been estimated that annual healthcare service costs resulting from psychosomatic symptoms are approximately £3 billion in the UK [10].

1.2 The role of depression and anxiety

Pain is one of the most commonly presented MUS [11]. Physical symptoms are highly prevalent in depression and may result in chronic pain and impede treatment effectiveness. Depression and pain are influenced by the same neurochemical processes, therefore both must be treated simultaneously in order to achieve improvements. Previous research has demonstrated that improvements in depressive symptoms was correlated with the improvement of some physical symptoms [12]. The prevalence of depression and anxiety among MUS patients has been estimated at 70% [11]. The division between services for physical health problems and mental health disorders reinforces the notion of body and mind as entirely separate enti-ties, consequently adding to the psychological distress associated with MUS [13]. In relation to NCCP specifically, higher levels of anxiety have been detected among individuals with NCCP compared with health individuals [14]. Given that MUS and pain have high levels of psychiatric comorbidity, it has been suggested that a multidisciplinary intervention strategy may be appropriate [15].

1.3 Psychological interventions: MUS/SSD

Qualitative research has reported that individuals with MUS have a tendency to reject psychological constructs of their problems [16], resulting in an unwillingness to engage in psychological treatments [8, 17, 18]. However other studies have suggested that a significant percentage of these patients would consent to undergo psychological or psychiatric interventions [19]. Evidence suggests that cognitive behaviour therapy (CBT) is beneficial in the treatment of MUS [20, 21]. A systematic review and meta-analysis of non-pharmacological interventions for somatoform disorders and MUS in adults determined that psychological therapies irrespective of modality were more beneficial overall than standard care or waiting lists in relation to reducing symptoms severity [22]. Fourteen from twenty one studies included in the review and subsequent analysis focused on CBT based interventions. CBT was determined to be more effective in reducing the severity of MUS, but there was insufficient evidence to support the efficacy of other modalities. Furthermore, although there is a robust evidence base demonstrating the effectiveness of high intensity CBT for somatoform related disorders, there are limited reviews investigating the effectiveness of low intensity or brief psychological interventions.

A critical review of 31 controlled clinical trials including 1600 patients where CBT was employed as an intervention for somatization and symptoms syndromes, found that CBT contributed to the improvement of physical symptoms in 71% of studies, functional status in 47% and psychological distress in 38% [23] Furthermore, group therapy and brief treatments of 5 sessions were also found to be effective, with benefits maintained for up to one year. The review concluded that CBT is an effective intervention for this patient population, and that benefits were achievable even if psychological distress was not entirely alleviated. Similarly, although the focus was not on brief or low intensity treatments, a randomised clinical trial comparing an intensive psychodynamic therapy and CBT for patients with medically unexplained pain indicated that both groups achieved reductions in psychological distress, catastrophic thinking and depression; and interventions were deemed to be equally effective at a three month follow up [24]. The CBT group however, demonstrated an improvement in self-efficacy that was not observed in the other group.

In relation to low intensity (brief) interventions, patients attending an IAPT pilot site specifically tailored for long term conditions (LTC)/MUS referrals were offered either a low intensity CBT (guided self-help delivered by a Psychological Wellbeing Practitioner) based intervention, or a mindfulness-based stress reduction treatment (brief, low intensity interventions). Subsequent thematic analysis of qualitative interviews indicated that patients typically reported a positive treatment experience, and felt better able to manage symptoms, even if this was not necessarily reflected by psychometric scores on the Patient Health Questionnaire-9 (PHQ9), Generalised Anxiety Disorder-7 (GAD7), and the WSAS. Although these interventions have been determined as appropriate for these patient groups, it has been suggested in terms of evaluation, that routine outcome measures may not entirely capture the true benefits of interventions [25]. It is also important to consider the clinical implications of these initial findings, namely that there were a higher number of LTC referrals compared with MUS. This may be partly explained by previous reports that GPs feel inadequate and discouraged when dealing with MUS cases [26]. Furthermore, as previously highlighted, research has indicated that MUS patients believe there is disparity between their physical symptoms and a psychological intervention [27]. The difference in referral rates between LTC and MUS patients suggest a need for separate dedicated services for each of these patient groups [28].

1.4 Psychological interventions: NCCP

Current reviews of clinical care have highlighted a failure to appropriately manage NCCP despite the substantial prevalence rates [29]. Studies to date have pointed to the efficacy of CBT [30, 31]. The efficacy of CBT as an intervention for NCCP has been evaluated in a number of randomised controlled trials [32]. A comparison of CBT and standard clinical advice among NCCP patients found major reductions in both the frequency and severity of symptoms in the CBT group, and only modest improvements within the control group [13].

Similarly, an RCT with UCP patients and found that those who had completed a course of CBT had a significantly higher treatment response when compared with placebo and medication groups [30]. A LICBT intervention, more specifically 'coping skills' resulted in significant improvement relating to the catastrophizing of pain symptoms and anxiety when compared to a placebo group [33].

Recent research has also emphasised the success of brief cognitive behavioural therapy, with a three session CBT intervention determined as effective for UCP patients in terms of illness perception [34]. A recent study concluded that a brief cognitive behavioural intervention significantly reduced levels of anxiety and depression in patients with NCCP, with a diagnosis of panic and/or a depressive disorder based on Hospital anxiety and depression scale (HADS) scores [35]. Based on these findings, it was recommended that individuals presenting with NCCP should be assessed for psychopathology, and a cognitive behavioural intervention offered in cases where psychological difficulties are detected. Cognitive behavioural interventions as brief as even a single session initiated within two weeks of an emer-gency attendance for the primary complaint of chest pain, have also been found to be effective for panic disorder [36]. Furthermore, it has been recommended that increased efforts should be employed to implement these interventions in the emergency department/primary care setting, considering the high prevalence of panic disorder there.

1.5 Psychological interventions: HA/IAD

A recent systemic review and meta-analysis evaluating CBT for health anxiety found a large effect size for CBT compared with several control conditions including standard care, waiting lists, medications and other psychological therapies [37]. In Van Gils et al. [38], another systematic review and met-analysis suggested self-help was associated with significant reduction in symptom sever-ity and improvement in quality of life measures among individuals with MUS [38]. Low intensity interventions which are brief and facilitate flexible delivery have been determined as effective for identified health anxiety within medical settings [39].

1.6 Aims of the current review

A recent study determined that 58.7% of all chest pain presentations to an ED across a three year period resulted in a diagnosis of NCCP [40]. However, care pathways and guidance on the most appropriate interventions for this patient population are very unclear. To date a consolidated and systematic review has not been carried out. In light of these findings, and given the lack of reviews focused on *brief or low intensity* treatments, the purpose of the current review was to assess the effectiveness of brief interventions which may be suitable for these particular and similar patient populations. Given that there is a high prevalence of MUS within primary care with possible associated anxiety, this review sought to examine evidence for brief interventions which may in principle, improve ease of access to appropriate treatment within a stepped care approach, and be implemented at a reduced cost compared with higher intensity or longer term treatments in second-ary care. To ensure a more robust assessment, conditions which may exist comor-bidly with NCCP were included. Therefore the current review specifically aimed to assess the effectiveness of brief interventions for MUS, illness anxiety disorder,

SSD, HA and NCCP, accounting also for the recent changes in terminologies and diagnostic criteria within the DSM-V.

2. Method

2.1 Eligibility criteria

Studies were assessed for eligibility for inclusion as per the following criteria: (1) written in the English language; (2) published in a journal; (3) included a quantita-tive evaluation of a brief intervention, with brief defined as ten or fewer individual of group based treatment sessions; (4) interventions were aimed at reducing the frequency and/or impact of MUS, HA, SSD, illness anxiety disorder, or NCCP; (5) participants were over 18 years of age; (6) outcome measures indicated the degree of MUS, and/or psychological wellbeing pre and post intervention; and (7) ran-domised controlled trial, with control group(s).

2.2 Search strategy

Three databases, specifically Google Scholar, PubMed, and Web of Science were searched for full-text articles which were published in peer reviewed journals. Combinations of the following keywords were used: brief* and intervention*, treatment*, therapy*. The key search terms were (1) medically unexplained symp-toms (2) health anxiety, (3) somatic symptom disorder, (4) illness anxiety disorder and (5) non-cardiac chest pain. **Table 1** indicates the complete search strategy employed in Google Scholar advanced searches, which was subsequently modified for the remaining searches. The reference lists of the articles selected from database searches were also examined.

2.3 Study selection and data extraction

Studies were selected by (1) screening the titles; (2) screening the abstracts and methodologies; (3) reviewing the complete paper if the title, abstract and method-ologies did not present conclusive evidence that the inclusion criteria were achieved. Studies which did not meet inclusion criteria were subsequently disregarded. Data were extracted according to PRISMA guidelines, onto an Excel workbook which was

Searches
a. brief intervention*
b. brief treatment*
c. or brief therapy*
d. and exact phrase medically unexplained symptoms
e. or somatic symptom disorder (exact)
f. or illness anxiety disorder (exact)
g. or health anxiety (exact)
h. or non-cardiac chest pain (exact)

Table 1.
Search strategy.

used throughout the searches and the review. This was used specifically to record information about study and participant characteristics, details of interventions, outcome measures and analyses.

2.4 Risk of bias

The Cochrane Collaboration Risk of Bias Tool was used in order to assess the risk of bias in the studies selected for the review. This involved screening for bias risk in relation to sequence generation, allocation concealment, blinding of participants and assessors, incomplete data, selective reporting and any other relevant bias. Both authors independently reviewed the selected studies and subsequently agreed on the level of risk of bias as either low, unclear or high.

3. Results

3.1 Study selection

The literature search and search of references from fully screened articles yielded a total of 1674 studies. After removal of duplicates the total was 885. **Figure 1** indicates the process of exclusion and final selection.

3.2 Study characteristics

3.2.1 Location

A summary of the selected studies is presented in **Table 2**. Studies originated in the USA (n = 6), Spain (n = 2), Germany (n = 2), Netherlands (n = 3), UK (n = 4), Iran (n = 2), Norway (n = 1), Sweden (n = 1) and Canada (n = 2). In seven of the studies, the purpose was to evaluate the effect of interventions on medically unexplained symptoms. The remaining studies investigated intervention effects on soma-tisation (n = 3), health anxiety (n = 2), hypochondriasis (n = 2) and non-cardiac chest pain [10]. All studies considered effectiveness in terms of physical symptoms and psychological wellbeing.

3.3 Participants

All of the included studies involved both male and female participants, and ages ranged from 16 to 81. The total number of participants varied in each of the studies. Eleven of the studies included less than 60 participants, 4 studies included between 61 and 100 participants, 3 studies included between 101 and 150 participants, 4 studies included between 151 and 200 participants and one study involved 444 participants.

3.3.1 Sample size

All studies employed selective sampling methods (purposive), whereby potential participants were initially identified by health professionals prior to subsequent additional eligibility screening using diagnostic interview and psychometric questionnaires. Five studies concurrently used opportunistic sampling methods (through public advertising) prior to the additional screening. Six studies provided some details of power calculations made in order to determine optimum sample sizes. The remaining studies did not describe how sample size was calculated.

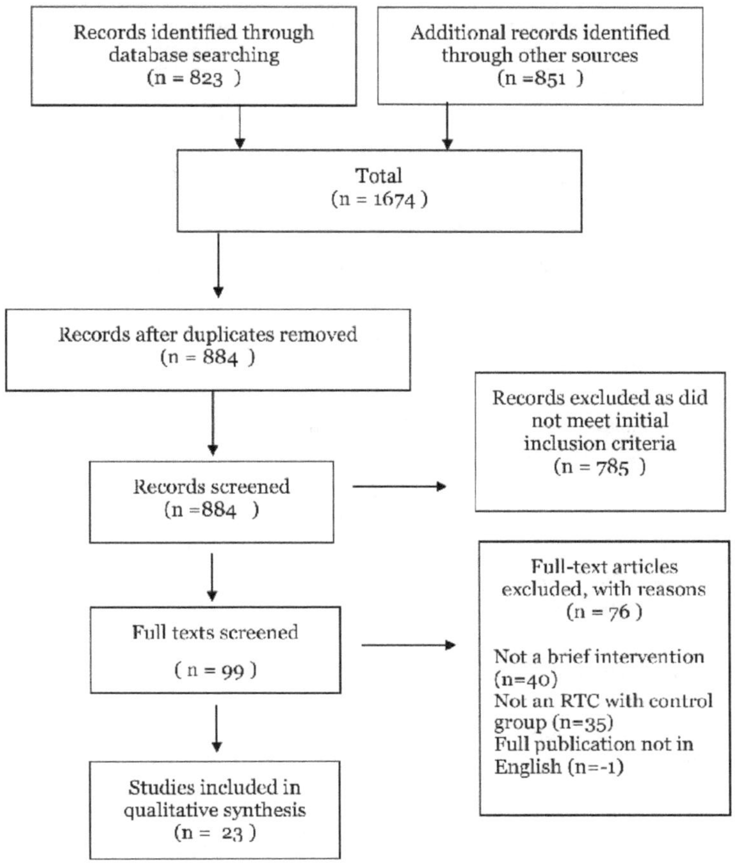

Figure 1.
Prisma flow diagram of search results and selected studies.

3.3.2 Unit of allocation and risk of bias

All of the included studies used random allocation to intervention or control groups. However, one of these studies [41] did not allocate participants in a conven-tional way, given that they were not actually randomly assigned to conditions, but rather the decision was taken by the authors (for ethical reasons) that the order of the three condition cohorts should be randomly predetermined.

3.3.3 Theoretical basis of the interventions

All of the interventions had a psychological basis. Cognitive behavioural therapy formed the theoretical basis of the interventions in 17 of the studies. Two studies described the intervention as psychosocial and communicative. One study described the intervention as psychophysiological, and one study used a brief psychosomatic intervention. Two studies used relaxation and metaphor therapies. Interventions were delivered as individual sessions in the majority of studies (n = 20), and inter-ventions were delivered in a group basis in the remaining studies (see **Table 2**).

3.3.4 Duration

The studies selected for the current review varied in their duration from six months to four years.

Study	Type of intervention	Duration of session	Duration of treatment	Measures
[45]	Time limited CBT-type	45–60 minutes	Maximum of 10 sessions	CGI-S, CGI-I, VAS, MOS-10, HAM-D, HAM-A
[50]	Psychosocial and communication intervention	30 minutes	Maximum of six sessions	MOS, SF-36, CIDI, PRIME-MD, SLE, NAS
[46]	Single session CBT	3–4 hours	One session	BSI-SOM, SOMS-7 BSI-GSI, WI, BDI, KKG-I
[47]	Time limited CBT	45 minutes	Maximum of 5 sessions	PSC-51, HADS, MOS SF-36
[52]	Time limited psychophysiological intervention	Not specified	Maximum of 10 sessions	CGI-S, HAM-A, HAM-D
[53]	Brief multimodal psychodynamic therapy	45 minutes	Maximum of 9 sessions	VAS, NHL, 4DSQ, SF-36 MAF
[55]	Time-limited mindfulness cognitive therapy	2 hours	Maximum of 8 sessions	DSM-IV (structured clinical interview), SHAI, WI, BAI, BDI
[39]	Time limited CBT	Not specified	5–10 sessions	HADS, SFQ-36, EQ-5D
[59]	Brief psychoeducation based on CBT	1 hour	1 face to face session and 2 brief follow-up phone calls	BDI, STAI, SF-36, WI, SCL-90
[41]	Short-term CBT	60–90 minutes	Maximum of 3 sessions	BSQ, SF-36, BDI, HRQOL
[62]	Relaxation training or metaphor therapy	2 hours	Maximum of 4 sessions	BPI, JIBT
[61]	Guided internet therapy (CBT based)	Not specified	Maximum of 4 sessions	CAQ, BSQ, PHQ-9
[35]	Brief CBT	45 minutes	Maximum of 6 sessions	CGI, HADS, MINI, STAI, FQ
[60]	Brief	1 hour	1 session	Chest Pain Interview, ASI, CAQ, SF-36, BSI
[57]	Time limited CBT	90 minutes	Maximum of 6 sessions	WI, HAI, HCQ, SSI, FSQ, SCL-90, SIS
[63]	Metaphor therapy	2 hours	Maximum of 4 sessions	PDS, DASS,
[58]	Brief CBT or pharmacological treatment	1 hour	Maximum of 7 sessions	ADIS-IV, ACQ, ASI, PAS, BDI, CAQ
[49]	Time limited CBT	Not specified	Maximum of 10 sessions	CGI-SD, SF-36, SSS
[51]	Brief psychosocial	20 minutes	Maximum of 6 sessions	HADS, SF-36, GHQ,-12, SOMS
[36]	Brief panic management (PM) or brief CBT	2 hours (PM) 1 hour (CBT)	1 session (PM) 7 sessions (CBT)	ADIS-IV, BSQ, PAS, ASI, CAQ, ACQ
[54]	Short-term group therapy	2 hours	8 sessions	SF-36

Study	Type of intervention	Duration of session	Duration of treatment	Measures
[42]	Short-term group based educational CBT	90 minutes	6 sessions	IAS, SDIH, BDI, FSS, DAS, QOL, DHBQ, NEO-PI
[43]	Short-term group psychological (CBT based) treatment	2 hours	6 sessions	HADS, NHL, SIP, NHP

SSP: *Somatoform Symptoms Scale;* **BSI-GSI**: *Global Severity Index;* **BDI**: *Beck Depression Inventory;* **KKG-I**: *'Internal Control' Multidimensional Self-Report Questionnaire;* **WI**: *Whitely Index;* **PSC-51**: *Physical Symptoms Checklist;* **HADS**: *Hospital Anxiety And Depression Scale;* **NHL**: *Nijmegen Hyperventilation List;* **4DSQ**: *Four-Dimensional Symptom Questionnaire (Distress, Anxiety, Depression, Somatization);* **MAF**: *Measure of General Functioning;* **EQ-5D**: *Health Related Quality Of Life;* **STAI**: *State Trait Anxiety Inventory;* **SCL-90**: *Symptom Checklist;* **BSQ**: *Bodily Sensations Questionnaire;* **HRQOL**: *Health Related Quality of Life;* **BPI**: *Brief Pain Inventory;* **JIBT**: *Jones Irrational Belief Test;* **PHQ-9**: *Patient Health Questionnaire (Depression);* **CAQ**: *Cardiac Anxiety Questionnaire;* **FQ**: *Fear Questionnaire;* **MINI**: *Mini International Neuropsychiatric Interview;* **ASI**: *Anxiety Sensitivity Index;* **HCQ**: *Hypochondrial Cognitions Questionnaire;* **SSI**: *Somatic Symptoms Inventory;* **FSQ**: *Functional Status Questionnaire;* **SIS**: *Severity of Illness Scale;* **PDS**: *Pain Discomfort Scale;* **DASS**: *Depression, Anxiety, Stress Scale;* **PAS**: *Panic, Agoraphobia Scale;* **ADIS-IV**: *Anxiety Disorder Interview Schedule;* **SSS**: *Severity of Somatic Symptom Scale;* **GHQ**: *General Health Questionnaire;* **SUI**: *Summary Utility Index;* **ACQ**: *Agoraphobic Cognitions Questionnaire;* **IAS**: *Illness Attitude Scale;* **SDIH**: *Structured Diagnostic Interview, Hypochondriasis;* **FSS**: *Fear Survey Schedule;* **DAS**: *Dysfunctional Attitude Scale;* **QOL**: *Quality of Life Questionnaire;* **DHBQ**: *Dysfunctional Health Beliefs Questionnaire;* **NEO-PI**: *Personality Inventory;* **SIP**: *Sickness Impact Profile;* **NHP**: *Nottingham Health Profile.*

Table 2.
Key characteristics of selected studies.

3.3.5 Control conditions

The vast majority of the selected studies (n = 21), employed a 'treatment as usual' control condition. The remaining 2 studies [42, 43] employed 'waiting list' control conditions.

3.4 Interventions: Description and impact

3.4.1 MUS/SSD

3.4.1.1 Brief CBT

The cognitive behavioural model considers predisposing, precipitating and perpetuating factors [44]. Psychological distress may be triggered and maintained in individuals with physical health symptoms via a cycle of inaccurate perceptions, avoidance behaviours and subsequent intensification of symptoms. Four of the selected studies included brief CBT based interventions targeting MUS/SSD. One of these, assessed the effectiveness of a 10 session treatment (averaging 50 minutes duration), which had been modified to target somatization problems. More specifically it applied relaxation training, emotional awareness, cognitive restructuring (CR) and communication [45]. Another study facilitated a single session (3–4 hours) which focused primarily on developing psychophysiological explanations of symptoms, relaxation, cognitions and healthcare use [46]. The third of these studies based their brief CBT intervention on the Consequences model within which the focus is on the consequences as opposed to the causes of physical symptoms; applied techniques aim to alter the consequences of symptoms [47, 48]. Participants were offered a maximum of 5, 45 minute sessions. The final study assessing brief CBT for MUS, offered a 10 session manualized intervention adapted for somatization disorder aimed at coping with stress and physical discomfort [49].

Of the five studies which implemented brief CBT interventions targeting MUS/ SSD, significant effects were observed in three whereby the intervention was deemed to be effective relative to control groups. No significant effects were observed in one study. One study reported medium effect sizes, and found that the intervention group had a higher percentage of patients with 'very much' or 'much' improved physical symptoms as reported by blinded evaluators (60% vs. 25.8% odds ratio = 4.1; 95% CI, 1.9–8.8; $p < .001$). There was a significant improvement in the intervention vs. the control group ($p < 0.5$) for depressive symptoms. Effects however were no longer noticeable at six month follow-up [45]. Small to medium effect sizes were observed in another study and a stronger effect size was detected for the intervention group in relation to reduction of doctors' visits ($\eta^2 = 0.031$), and the reduction of somatization severity ($\eta^2 = 0.048$). Although significant improvements in all other measures were observed for both groups, all participants were still highly impaired with the degree of somatization, health anxiety and depression all above clinical thresholds at a six month follow-up. [46]. One study observed large effect sizes and found that somatization symptoms were significantly improved in the intervention group relative to the control group ($p < 0.01$), with the intervention also associated with improved self-reported functioning [49] The remaining study determined that the intervention was not more effective than care as usual, although approximately 30% of participants in both groups demonstrated improvements on the clinically relevant outcomes [47].

3.4.1.2 Brief psychosocial interventions

Two of the included studies used psychosocial and communication interventions targeting MUS/SSD. One study trained GPs to explain symptoms in a physical tangible way as result of hormone imbalance, to subsequently attribute this imbalance to irrational thinking, and to explore psychosocial issues indirectly. Participants were offered six sessions of 30 minutes [50].

Similarly, the second study trained GPs to gather a thorough psychosocial history, evaluate subjective understanding, demonstrate empathy, explain the relationship between symptoms and emotional distress, use symptom diaries, identify stressors and develop new behaviours; six 20 minute sessions were offered [51].

The first study, observed small to medium effect sizes and large effects sizes for bodily pain, social and emotional functioning, and mental health [50]. More specifically, quality of life dimensions in the intervention group were significantly improved relative to the control group in relation to several SF-36 subscales, namely bodily pain ($p < 0.03$), mental health ($p < 0.063$), physical functioning ($p < 0.01$), vitality ($p < 0.039$), social functioning ($p < 0.033$), and utility index ($p < 0.039$). The second study [51] found significant improvements were observed for the intervention group relative to the control group in relation to a reduction of physical symptoms ($p = 0.07$), reduction of depression ($p = 0.211$) and reduction of anxiety ($p = 0.388$). Effect sizes however were modest and were not maintained at six month follow up.

3.4.1.3 Brief psychophysiological interventions

One of the selected studies used a brief psychophysiological intervention targeting MUS/SSD. This was a ten session manualized treatment designed specifically for MUS; it was described as a treatment to assist with stress and physical discomfort, and specific components were emphasised depending on individual symptoms profiles [52].

3.4.1.4 Brief multimodal psychosomatic therapy

One study used a brief multimodal psychosomatic therapy targeting MUS. The treatment is based on the biopsychosocial model and involved relaxation, mindful-ness, CBT techniques and activation therapy; up to 9 sessions of 45 minutes dura-tion were offered [53].

At 12 months post intervention, improvement in perceived symptom severity was observed [adjusted mean difference −2.0, 95% confidence interval (CI) −3.6 to −0.3], in somatization (adjusted mean difference −4.4, 95% CI −7.5 to −1.4) and in symptoms of hyperventilation (adjusted mean difference −5.7, 95% CI −10.5 to −0.8). Although the small sample size was deemed to be efficient, the authors concluded that a larger trial would be helpful and feasible. This pilot trail was not powered to indicate treatment effect size.

3.4.1.5 Brief group therapy

One study, implemented a short-term group therapy for MUS/SSD (8 sessions of 2 hour durations), within which the aims were to develop peer support, share coping strategies and improve perceptions and expressions of emotions [54].

In relation to a brief group therapy, the intervention group demonstrated significant improvements compared with the control group on both physical health ($p < 0.05$), and mental health ($p < 0.01$) at post-treatment and at 12 month follow-up. Treatment effect sizes were not indicated.

3.4.2 HA/IAD

3.4.2.1 Brief CBT

Four of the included studies implemented brief CBT interventions targeting HA/IAD. The first offered 5–10 sessions of brief CBT which had been adapted for HA [39]. Similarly, another of the studies, employed a 6 session individualised intervention which was designed specifically to target and restructure hypochon-drial thoughts [9]. One study implemented a time-limited group mindfulness-based CBT intervention, which was described a skills training programme adapted for HA [55–56]. A group based intervention was also employed in another study. This took the form of an educational course aimed at improving coping skills for HA, focused specifically on selective attention, muscle tension, breathing, environmental factors, stress, mood and explaining somatic symptoms [42].

Four of the included studies implemented brief BCT interventions targeting HA/IAD and all reported significant effects for intervention groups relative to con-trol groups. More specifically, one determined small effect sizes, and found that at 12 month follow-up point, the intervention group demonstrated an improvement in health anxiety symptoms which was 2.98 points greater than the control group and these symptomatic improvements were maintained at 2 years follow up. However, there were no significant differences between groups in relation to social function-ing or health related quality of life [39]. At a 12-month follow-up, another study found significantly lower levels of hypochondriacal symptoms, beliefs, and atti-tudes ($P < .001$) and health-related anxiety ($P = .009$). in the intervention group. Furthermore significantly less impairment of social role functioning ($P = .05$) and intermediate activities of daily living ($P < .001$) were also observed. Effect sizes were reported as small to medium and hypochondriacal somatic symptoms were not improved significantly by treatment. The third of these studies determined medium effect sizes; their intervention group demonstrated significantly lower health anxiety than the control group both immediately following treatment (d = 0.48), and at a 12 month follow-up (d = 0.48) [55]. In the final study significant improvement was observed in the intervention group relative to the control group on all measures including physical symptoms (p = 0.03), dysfunctional health beliefs (p = 0.02), vulnerability (p = 0.03) and lack of control (p = 0.06); effect sizes were not reported [42].

3.4.3 NCCP

3.4.3.1 Brief CBT

Seven of the selected studies involved brief CBT based interventions targeting NCCP. One of these implemented a 7 session treatment which incorporated psychoeducation on chest pain, panic disorder (PD), exposure and CR [58]. Two interventions were evaluated in another study [36], namely a single session panic management intervention and a 7 session CBT treatment for NCCP and PD [36]. Another also trialled a single individualised information session with psychoeducational materials [59] One study used a single session of brief CBT (60 minute duration) which included psychoeducation, breathing exercises and CR [62]. Psychoeducation was again a component of the intervention offered in another of the studies, which also included CR, and strategies to influence avoidance behaviours over 6 sessions of 45 minutes [35]. One study offered a 3 session programme (60–90 minutes) which focuses on the CBT model of panic and exposure therapy [41]. Guided brief CBT was delivered online in another study and involved 4 sessions of psychoeducation, physical activity advice and relaxation [61].

Of the seven selected studies which implemented brief CBT based interventions targeting NCCP, five reported significant effects for interventions relative to control groups and two observed no significance. Large treatment effect sizes were observed in one study; both intervention groups demonstrated significant improvements relative to the control group in relation to the severity of panic disorder (p = 0.12), frequency of panic (p = 0.48), and depressive symptoms (p = 0.27) [58]. Similarly large effect sizes were also observed in another study; both interventions also achieved significant reductions in the severity of panic disorder relative to the control group ($\eta^2 = 0.07$), although no superiority was demonstrated by one intervention as compared with the other [36]. Medium effect sizes with significant improvements for the intervention versus control in relation to frequency and fear of chest pain, and anxiety sensitivity, but not in relation to severity of chest pain, quality of life and psychological distress were determined on one study [60]. In another study, significant improvements were observed for intervention versus control group in relation to reduction of disease severity, anxiety and depression symptoms but effect sizes were not determined [35]. A brief CBT intervention was effective compared to care as usual and reported medium to large effect sizes. Significant differences were observed for fear of bodily sensations, avoidance of physical activities and depression. However, the sample size was small and no power analysis was carried out [41]. Another study concluded that although improvements were demonstrated by both intervention and control groups in relation to cardiac anxiety, fear of bodily sensations and depression, no significant differences were observed between the groups [61]. Similarly, the remaining study found that although both groups achieved slight improvements on the main outcomes, specifically chest pain, mood and limitation of activities, no significant effects were observed [59].

3.4.3.2 Relaxation and metaphor therapy

Two studies evaluated relaxation and metaphor therapies targeting NCCP [62, 63]. Both treatments consisted of 4 2 hour sessions. The relaxation therapy was group based involving learning and practising relaxation and breathing techniques. Metaphor therapy involved challenging and connecting metaphoric stories of hopelessness, with the ultimate goal of challenging unhelpful beliefs.

The first of these reported small to medium effect sizes, and determined significant differences between the relaxation group and both control groups for hopeless-ness (DM = 9.79, $p < 0.05$), pain severity (DM = 1.96, $p < 0.05$), and emotional irresponsibility (DM = 4.80, $p < 0.05$). No significant effects were observed in relation to the metaphor therapy intervention group [62]. The subsequent study assessed the effectiveness of metaphor therapy only, and again determined no significant treatment effects relative to the control group [63].

3.4.3.3 Short-term group therapy

One study implemented a short-term (8 session of 2 hours) group therapy for NCCP within which the focus was on sharing experiences and coping strategies, education on chest pain, relaxation and breathing exercise, physical exercise, CR and graded exposure [43]. Significant improvements were observed in the interven-tion group relative to the control group in relation to chest pain episodes ($p < 0.01$) and anxiety and depression ($p < 0.05$), with benefits maintained at a six month follow-up. Treatment effect sizes were not indicated.

3.5 Delivery of the intervention

Therapists trained specifically in the relevant interventions were used in eleven of the studies. Primary care physicians (GPSs) delivered interventions in four of the studies, and four of the studies used clinical psychologists to deliver treatments Cardiac nurses delivered interventions in two studies.

3.6 Outcome measures

Several combinations of primary and secondary outcome measures including questionnaires and diagnostic interviews were used in the selected studies at pre, post and follow-up points. The measures assessed medically unexplained symptoms, mental health, health related quality life and general functioning. The most frequently used outcome measure was the MOS SF-36 (medical outcomes study 36 item short-form health survey), which was used in ten of the selected studies. A full list of the outcome measures used in each of the included studies is presented in **Table 2**. Intervention effects are presented in **Table 3**.

3.7 Pre, post and follow-up data

The majority of the studies (n = 17) included in the review adapted longitudinal designs and evaluated outcomes at pre and post intervention points and at one or more follow-up points. Six of the included studies evaluated outcomes at pre and post intervention points only and did not use a longitudinal design.

Study	Intervention	Outcomes
[45]	Time limited CBT type therapy delivered in primary care for patients with medically unexplained physical symptoms	The intervention group had a higher percentage of patients with 'very much' or 'much' improved physical symptoms as reported by blinded evaluators (60% vs. 25.8% odds ratio = 4.1; 95% CI, 1.9–8.8; $p < 0.001$). There was a significant improvement in the intervention vs. the control group ($p < 0.5$) for depressive symptoms. Effects were no longer noticeable at six month follow-up. Effect sizes medium.
[50]	A psychosocial and communication intervention delivered by GPs for patients with medically unexplained symptoms.	Improvements in all dimensions of the SF-36 were demonstrated by patients in both groups. The intervention group demonstrated significantly more improvement in bodily pain, mental health, physical functioning, social functioning and vitality ($p < 0.039$). Effect sizes: small to medium (large effect sizes for bodily pain, social and emotional functioning and mental health).
[46]	A one session CBT intervention for medically unexplained symptoms delivered by clinical psychologist	There was a stronger effect size in the intervention group in relation to reduction of doctors' visits ($\eta^2 = 0.031$), and the reduction of somatization severity ($\eta^2 = 0.048$). Although significant improvements in all other measures were observed for both groups, all participants were still highly impaired with the degree of somatization, health anxiety and depression all above clinical thresholds at a six month follow-up. Effect sizes: small to medium
[47]	Cognitive behavioural treatment delivered by family physician for medically unexplained symptoms	The intervention was not more effective than care as usual; approximately 30% of participants in both groups demonstrated improvements on the clinically relevant outcomes. No significance observed: intervention not effective as compared with control group. Effect sizes: N/A.
[52]	Psychophysiological treatment (described to participants as an intervention to assist in coping with physical comfort and distress) delivered by psychologists	There was a significantly greater improvement in the frequency and severity of physical symptoms in the interventions group ($p < 0.05$). Effect sizes also indicated a greater improvement in the interventions group for depression symptoms ($d = 0.81$)
[53]	Brief multimodal psychodynamic therapy for medically unexplained symptoms delivered by trained practitioners.	Significant differences between groups were observed at 12 month follow up; the intervention group demonstrated greater improvement in perceived symptom severity, somatization and hyperventilation. Effect sizes: unknown (trial not powered to indicate treatment effect sizes)
[55]	Time-limited mindfulness-based cognitive therapy for health anxiety delivered by trained practitioners and clinicians.	The intervention group demonstrated significantly lower health anxiety than the control group both immediately following treatment ($d = 0.48$), and at a 12 month follow-up ($d = 0.48$). Effect sizes: medium
[39]	CBT for health anxiety delivered by trained health professionals	At a 12 month follow-up point, the intervention group demonstrated an improvement in health anxiety symptoms which was 2.98 points greater than the control group. Significance observed: intervention effective as compared with control group. Effect sizes small

Study	Intervention	Outcomes
[59]	Brief psychoeducational and cognitive behavioural intervention for non-cardiac chest pain, delivered by cardiac nurses	Although both groups achieved slight improvements on the main outcomes, specifically chest pain, mood and limitation of activities, no significant effects were observed. Effect sizes: NA
[41]	Short-term CBT for non-cardiac chest pain delivered by trained therapists.	The intervention was effective compared to care as usual; significant differences were observed for fear of bodily sensations, avoidance of physical activities and depression. Effect sizes medium to large
[63]	Relaxation training versus metaphor therapy for non-cardiac chest pain delivered by clinical psychologists.	There were significant differences observed between the relaxation group and both control groups for hopelessness (DM = 9.79, $p < 0.05$), pain severity (DM = 1.96, $p < 0.05$), and emotional irresponsibility (DM = 4.80, $p < 0.05$). Effect sizes small to medium.
[61]	Guided internet therapy (CBT based) for non-cardiac chest pain delivered by cardiac nurses	Although improvements were demonstrated by both groups in relation to cardiac anxiety, fear of bodily sensations and depression, no significant differences were observed between the groups. No significance observed. Effect sizes: N/A
[35]	Brief CBT for non-cardiac chest pain with associated depression and panic disorder delivered by clinical psychologists	Significant improvements were observed for intervention versus control group in relation to reduction of disease severity, anxiety and depression symptoms. Effect sizes: unknown (trial not powered to indicate treatment effect sizes.
[60]	Brief CBT for non-cardiac chest pain	Significant improvements were observed for intervention versus control in relation to frequency and fear of chest pain, and anxiety sensitivity, but not in relation to severity of chest pain, quality of life and psychological distress. Effect sizes: medium
[57]	CBT for hypochondriasis delivered by trained therapists	Significant differences were observed for the intervention group versus control group in relation to hypochondrial symptoms, beliefs and attitudes, health anxiety, and social functioning. Effect sizes: small to medium
[63]	Metaphor therapy for non-cardiac chest pain delivered by psychologists	There were no significance differences demonstrated by the intervention group compared with control group on any of the outcome variables (depression, anxiety, stress and pain discomfort). No significance observed: intervention not effective as compared with control group Effect sizes: NA
[58]	Brief CBT or pharmacological treatment for non-cardiac chest pain with associated panic disorder delivered by psychologists.	Both intervention groups demonstrated significant improvement relative to the control group in relation to the severity of panic disorder ($p = 0.12$), frequency of panic ($p = 0.48$), and depressive symptoms ($p = 0.27$). Effect sizes large.
[49]	Time limited CBT for somatization disorder	Somatization symptoms were significantly improved in the intervention group relative to control group ($p < 0.01$). Effect sizes large.

Study	Intervention	Outcomes
[51]	Psychosocial intervention for somatising patients delivered by general practitioners	Significant improvements were observed for the intervention group relative to the control group in relation to a reduction of physical symptoms ($p = 0.07$), reduction of depression ($p = 0.211$) and reduction of anxiety ($p = 0.388$). Effects were not maintained at six month follow up. Effects not maintained at 6 month follow-up. Effect sizes small
[36]	Brief psychological interventions (panic management and CBT) for panic disorder with non-cardiac chest pain delivered by trained therapists.	Both interventions demonstrated significant reductions in the severity of panic disorder relative to the control group ($\eta^2 = 0.07$) although no superiority was demonstrated by one intervention as compared with the other. Effect sizes large (time)
[54]	Short-term group therapy for somatization disorder delivered by trained therapists	The intervention group demonstrated significant improvements relative to the control group on both physical health ($p < 0.05$), and mental health ($p < 0.01$) at post-treatment and at 12 month follow-up. Effect sizes: Unknown (trial not powered to indicate treatment effect sizes
[42]	Short-term group therapy (CBT based) for hypochondriasis delivered by trained therapists	Significant improvements were observed in the intervention group relative to the control group on all measures including physical symptoms ($p = 0.03$), dysfunctional health beliefs ($p = 0.02$), vulnerability ($p = 0.03$) and lack of control ($p = 0.06$). Effect sizes unknown (trial not powered to indicate treatment effect sizes
[43]	Time limited group psychological treatment for non-cardiac chest pain delivered by trained therapists	Significant improvements observed in the intervention group relative to the control group in relation to chest pain episodes ($p < 0.01$) and anxiety and depression ($p < 0.05$), with benefits maintained at a six month follow-up. Effect sizes: Unknown (trial not powered to indicate treatment effect sizes.

Table 3.
Summary of results for included studies.

4. Discussion

4.1 Summary of evidence

This is the first systematic review which examined evidence for brief or time-limited interventions for both MUS/SSD, HA/IAD and NCCP specifically. Significant effects for the intervention groups relative to control groups were reported in 19 studies, and 4 studies did not determine any significant benefits of interventions compared with control groups. Significant effects relative to controls were determined for all of the brief interventions in at least one study (CBT, psycho-social, psychophysiological, psychosomatic, relaxation and group therapy), with the exception of metaphor therapy for which no significant effects were reported. [63]. Of those studies reporting significance, large treatment effects were reported in 3 [39, 49, 58], medium effect sizes were reported by 3 [45, 55, 60], medium to large effects were reported in 2 [34, 52], four studies observed small to medium effect sizes [46, 50, 57, 62], and small effect sizes were determined in 2 [39, 51]. Five studies did not indicate effect sizes (see **Table 3**). All of the studies within which the largest effect sizes were reported, involved brief CBT for either MUS or NCCP [36, 49, 58].

There are several possible explanations for the lack of effect on medically unexplained symptoms and psychological wellbeing in the trials within which no significance was observed. The findings specifically, that time limited CBT delivered by GPs for MUS did not result in significantly better outcomes than care as usual, are consistent with other research which has outlined the limited feasibility and effectiveness of CBT for MUS delivered by primary care doctors [47, 64, 65].

Although it was found that brief online CBT guided by cardiac nurses was feasible for NCCP given that it decreased cardiac anxiety, frequency of chest pain and depression symptoms, no significant differences were observed relative to the control group [61]. These findings were comparable with another study where no significant treatment effects were determined after a brief single session CBT intervention for NCCP again delivered by cardiac nurses [59]. Authors of both studies have highlighted the limitations of small sample sizes and recruitment difficulties, possibly due to the fact that patients found it difficult to reject a physical explanation for the cause of chest pain. As outlined earlier, previous research has suggested that individuals with MUS have a tendency to reject psychological constructs of their problems resulting in an unwillingness to engage in psychological treatments [8, 16–18].

Regarding the use of metaphor therapy for NCCP after which no significant benefits were observed in terms of discomfort, anxiety or depression, the authors suggested that the nature of the intervention itself may not be suitable given that it is dependent on an individual's ability to visualise [62, 63]. However, some evidence exists to support the use of this intervention, and it was a component of a group psychological intervention for NCCP included in the current review within which significant treatment effects were observed [43].

Some included studies reported significant treatment effects compared with controls after brief CBT for MUS/SSD [45, 46, 49]. As previously highlighted, findings in one indicated a more marked reduction in the amount of doctor's visits and in the severity of somatization in the CBT group compared with the standard care group [46]. Although actual treatment effects were smaller for this single session intervention when compared with more intensive CBT approaches, brief interventions still facilitate the treatment of a greater number of MUS patients. It has been suggested that brief intervention could improve the general management of MUS at the primary care level and subsequently aid access to more specialist interventions if clinically required. Furthermore, the importance of early intervention should be highlighted given that the condition becomes much less manageable and complex over time [9]. It has been suggested that a brief treat-ment such as a single session CBT/LICBT intervention could be an appropriate and effective first point of treatment within a stepped care approach in order to improve management of MUS [46, 66].

4.2 Variations in outcomes

Differences in the outcomes observed in the selected studies, may be a result of variations in the components and theoretical frameworks of the interventions, the duration of the interventions, sampling issues, the selection strategies employed to recruit participants, the outcome measures used to determine MUS and psychological wellbeing, the experience levels of persons delivering the interventions, and how data was collected and analysed.

The psychological framework of the interventions evaluated in the selected studies included CBT, psychosocial, psychosomatic, relaxation, metaphor, and gen-eral group therapy. Significant effects at the post-intervention stage (at least), were reported by all included studies except 3 studies which implemented brief CBT, and 2 studies which implemented brief metaphor therapy.

However, 13 studies did determine significant effects for brief CBT, as did both studies which used psychosocial treatments. Furthermore each of the single studies evaluating either psychosomatic, relaxation or general group therapy also reported significance. It is not possible therefore to concretely conclude if one of these brief interventions might offer superior benefits to the other, given the more limited available outcomes from trials assessing interventions other than those which are CBT based. Rather, it may concluded that some evidence exists to support the use of all of the interventions for medically unexplained symptoms and associated psychological distress, with the exception of metaphor therapy. More specifically there is substantial evidence within the current review supporting the use of brief/time-limited CBT, and existing but more limited evidence supporting the use of the remaining included interventions.

Several studies highlighted issues with sampling and sampling size, which might have influenced outcomes. Despite screening 6409 potential participants, only 65 were included in the trial for one study [47]. Some were excluded due to a natural reduction of symptoms or due to the presence of severe and comorbid conditions. Chronic issues with somatization are likely to follow a path of highs and lows in relation to the severity of and response to symptoms, much like depression and anxiety disorders, however, a majority of eligible participants declined the interven-tion as they had 'accepted' symptoms were part of their life.

As indicated earlier, there was a large variation in sample size in the selected studies. Eleven of the studies included 60 or fewer participants, and one study included 444 participants. Given that the power of the study may be affected by a sample which is either too large or small, it is reasonable to suppose that at least some of the included studies may have been under-powered to clearly indicate between-group differences of statistical significance [67, 68].

The selection of an appropriate outcome measure is an important consid-eration which can impact the value of results from clinical studies. Selection of measures has tended to concentrate more on the psychometric properties, but less on the actual suitability of the instruments for their intended purpose. It has been suggested that in addition to an evaluation of basic psychometric proper-ties, researchers should consider that different instruments may capture different aspects of complex phenomena and may therefore not be equally valid for everyone. Furthermore, a good fit between the measure and what the researcher expects to change post treatment is required to facilitate a valid interpretation of the out-comes. As indicated earlier, a considerably large variety of primary and secondary outcome measures were included in the selected studies, and it may be the case that not all of those were the optimum instruments [69].

The interventions evaluated in the selected studies were delivered by either therapists who had been trained specifically in the relevant interventions, GPs, clinical psychologists, or cardiac nurses. Both studies using cardiac nurses reported no significant intervention effects, and 2 of the 4 studies within which interventions were delivered by GPs also reported no significant intervention effects. A systematic review and meta-analysis of randomised controlled tri-als of psychological treatments found psychological interventions were more beneficial when delivered by psychotherapists compared with GPs, and more specifically that psychotherapists had a greater effect on physical symptoms than GPs [70]. An earlier systematic review considered the prevalence of medically unexplained physical symptoms, the extent of comorbidity with psychiatric disorders, the importance of psychological processes and the effectiveness of interventions. It was reported that there was significant overlap between symp-toms and syndromes, and that patients with MUS should therefore be considered as having complex adaptive systems within which cognitive, physiological and environmental factors interact. CBT and antidepressants are effective, however these benefits are heightened when patients feel empowered by their own doctors to address their problems [71]. The importance of the GP role was consequently highlighted i.e. to validate the patient experience, provide positive and empowering explanations of symptoms and to offer evidence based interventions including CBT. Further research has suggested that GP-patient interactions did impact consultation and communication patterns but did not subsequently impact patient outcomes [72].

It is also important to acknowledge that while the current review focused on time-limited intervention, the duration of the course of treatments evaluated in the included studies ranged from a single session to ten sessions, with sessions also varying in length in addition to varying times between sessions, and the point at which follow up data was collected. The potential impact of this on outcomes cannot be disregarded. In order to reach more robust conclusions regarding the confounding factors which impact clinical outcome in MUS, larger sample sizes and longer follow –ups should be employed, given the effects of clustering and generally modest effects observed.

There are other methodological issues to consider including that there a were variety of methodologies employed in relation to data analysis. Not all of the included studies reported specifically how data was cleaned or how missing data was handled, and there is a possibility this may account for variability between outcomes. Furthermore, some studies employed power analysis and reported effect sizes, and some did not. It is therefore recommended that any future trial addresses this methodological weakness in order to improve and determine the most effective treatment.

4.3 Risk of bias

All of the included studies employed random allocation to intervention or control group, although many lacked precise details regarding how this was achieved, and the risk of bias remained unclear in several studies.

4.4 Strengths and limitations

The main strength of this systematic review is the focus on brief interventions which are feasible to offer as part of a stepped care approach. A limitation is that the included studies were screened by only one author (except for risk of bias examina-tion), increasing the possibility that a study might have been missed.

5. Conclusion

The evidence suggests that brief psychological interventions, more specifically time limited BCT based interventions may have small to large effects in reduc-ing the severity of MUS and associated psychological distress. These findings are comparable with other reviews which have assessed the efficacy of higher intensity and/or longer term interventions. Given that there is a broad range of symptom severity and willingness to engage in psychological treatments among MUS patients in primary care, it is reasonable to suggest that a stepped care approach may be suitable thereby facilitating a more specialist intervention in chronic cases [73–75]. However, there remains a need to provide more robust evidence of cost effective-ness is relation to mild and moderate cases for which briefer interventions such as those evaluated here, tend to be recommended.

Author details

Orla McDevitt-Petrovic* and Karen Kirby
School of Psychology, Ulster University, United Kingdom

*Address all correspondence to: om.mcdevitt-petrovic@ulster.ac.uk

References

[1] Salmon P. Conflict, collusion or collaboration in consultations about medically unexplained symptoms: the need for a curriculum of medical explanation. Patient education and counseling. 2007 Aug 1;67(3):246-54.

[2] Creed FH, Davies I, Jackson J, Littlewood A, Chew-Graham C, Tomenson B, Macfarlane G, Barsky A, Katon W, McBeth J. The epidemiology of multiple somatic symptoms. Journal of psychosomatic research. 2012 Apr 1;72(4):311-7.

[3] Marks EM, Hunter MS. Medically unexplained symptoms: an acceptable term?. British journal of pain. 2015 May;9(2):109-14.

[4] American Psychiatric Association. Diagnostic and statistical manual of mental disorders (DSM-5®) (2013) American Psychiatric Pub. https://doi.org/10.1176/appi.books.9780890425596

[5] Kirmayer LJ, Groleau D, Looper KJ, Dao MD. Explaining medically unexplained symptoms. The Canadian journal of psychiatry. 2004 Oct;49(10):663-72.

[6] Creed F, Barsky A. A systematic review of the epidemiology of somatisation disorder and hypochondriasis. Journal of psychosomatic research. 2004 Apr 1;56(4):391-408.

[7] Gureje O, Üstün TB, Simon GE. The syndrome of hypochondriasis: a cross-national study in primary care. Psychological Medicine. 1997 Sep;27(5):1001-10.

[8] Nezu AM, Nezu CM, Lombardo ER. Cognitive-behavior therapy for medically unexplained symptoms: a critical review of the treatment literature. Behavior Therapy. 2001 Jun 1;32(3):537-83.

[9] Barsky AJ, Orav EJ, Bates DW. Somatization increases medical utilization and costs independent of psychiatric and medical comorbidity. Archives of general psychiatry. 2005 Aug 1;62(8):903-10.

[10] Department of Health. No health without mental health: a cross-government mental health outcomes strategy for people of all ages (2011) Retrieved from https://www.gov.uk/government/publications/no-health-without-mental-health-a-cross-government-outcomes-strategy

[11] Department of Health. No health without mental health: a cross-government mental health outcomes strategy for people of all ages (2008) Retrieved from https://www.gov.uk/government/publications/no-health-without-mental-health-a-cross-government-outcomes-strategy

[12] Trivedi MH. The link between depression and physical symptoms. Primary care companion to the Journal of clinical psychiatry. 2004;6(suppl 1):12.

[13] Mayou RA, Bryant BM, Sanders D, Bass C, Klimes I, Forfar C. A controlled trial of cognitive behavioural therapy for non-cardiac chest pain. Psychological medicine. 1997 Sep;27(5):1021-31.

[14] Smeijers L, van de Pas H, Nyklicek I, Notten PJ, Pedersen SS, Kop WJ. The independent association of anxiety with non-cardiac chest pain. Psychology & health. 2014 Mar 4;29(3):253-63.

[15] Von Korff M, Crane P, Lane M, Miglioretti DL, Simon G, Saunders K, Stang P, Brandenburg N, Kessler R. Chronic spinal pain and physical–mental comorbidity in the United States: results from the national comorbidity survey replication. Pain. 2005 Feb 1;113(3):331-9.

[16] Chew-Graham C, Brooks J, Wearden A, Dowrick C, Peters S. Factors influencing engagement of patients in a novel intervention for CFS/ME: a qualitative study. Primary health care research & development. 2011 Apr;12(2):112-22.

[17] Shaw, J., & Creed, F. The cost of somatization. Journal of psychosomatic research, 35(2), 307-312. 1991 https://doi.org/10.1016/0022-3999(91)90085-3

[18] Sumathipala A. What is the evidence for the efficacy of treatments for somatoform disorders? A critical review of previous intervention studies. Psychosomatic medicine. 2007 Nov 1;69(9):889-900.

[19] Speckens AE, Van Hemert AM, Bolk JH, Rooijmans HG, Hengeveld MW. Unexplained physical symptoms: outcome, utilization of medical care and associated factors. Psychological medicine. 1996 Jul;26(4):745-52.

[20] Malouff, J. M., Thorsteinsson, E. B., Rooke, S. E., Bhullar, N., & Schutte, N. S. Efficacy of cognitive behavioral therapy for chronic fatigue syndrome: a meta-analysis. Clinical psychology review, 28(5), 736-745 . 2008 https://doi. org/10.1016/j.cpr.2007.10.004

[21] Moss-Morris R, McAlpine L, Didsbury LP, Spence MJ. A randomized controlled trial of a cognitive behavioural therapy-based self-management intervention for irritable bowel syndrome in primary care. Psychological medicine. 2010;40(1):85.

[22] Van Dessel, N., Den Boeft, M., van der Wouden, J. C., Kleinstäuber, M., Leone, S. S., Terluin, B., ... & van Marwijk, H. (2014). Non-pharmacological interventions for somatoform disorders and medically unexplained physical symptoms (MUPS) in adults. *Cochrane Database Syst Rev*, *11*. doi: 10.1002/14651858. CD011142.pub2.

[23] Kroenke K, Swindle R. Cognitive-behavioral therapy for somatization and symptom syndromes: a critical review of controlled clinical trials. Psychotherapy and psychosomatics. 2000;69(4):205-15.

[24] Chavooshi B, Mohammadkhani P, Dolatshahee B. Telemedicine vs. in-person delivery of intensive short-term dynamic psychotherapy for patients with medically unexplained pain: A 12-month randomized, controlled trial. Journal of telemedicine and telecare. 2017 Jan;23(1):133-41.

[25] Gerskowitch C, Norman I, Rimes KA. Patients with medically unexplained physical symptoms experience of receiving treatment in a primary-care psychological therapies service: a qualitative study. The Cognitive Behaviour Therapist. 2015;8.

[26] Wileman L, May C, Chew-Graham CA. Medically unexplained symptoms and the problem of power in the primary care consultation: a qualitative study. Family Practice. 2002 Apr 1;19(2):178-82.

[27] Unigwe, C., Rowett, M. and Udo, I. Reflections of the management of medically unexplained symptoms. British Journal of Psychiatry Bulletin,. 2014.38, 252. https://dx.doi. org/10.1192%2Fpb.38.5.252

[28] Kellett S, Webb K, Wilkinson N, Bliss P, Ayers T, Hardy G. Developing services for patients with depression or anxiety in the context of long-term physical health conditions and medically unexplained symptoms: evaluation of an IAPT pathfinder site. Behavioural and cognitive psychotherapy. 2016 Sep 1;44(5):553.

[29] Chambers JB, Marks EM, Russell V, Hunter MS. A multi-disciplinary, biopsychosocial treatment for non-cardiac chest pain. International journal of clinical practice. 2015 Sep;69(9):922-7.

[30] Spinhoven P, Van der Does AW, Van Dijk E, Van Rood YR. Heart-focused anxiety as a mediating variable in the treatment of noncardiac chest pain by cognitive-behavioral therapy and paroxetine. Journal of psychosomatic research. 2010 Sep 1;69(3):227-35.

[31] Marchand A, Belleville G, Fleet R, Dupuis G, Bacon SL, Poitras J, Chauny JM, Vadeboncoeur A, Lavoie KL. Treatment of panic in chest pain patients from emergency departments: efficacy of different interventions focusing on panic management. General hospital psychiatry. 2012 Nov 1;34(6):671-80.

[32] George N, Abdallah J, Maradey-Romero C, Gerson L, Fass R. the current treatment of non-cardiac chest pain. Alimentary pharmacology & therapeutics. 2016 Jan;43(2):213-39.

[33] Keefe FJ, Shelby RA, Somers TJ, Varia I, Blazing M, Waters SJ, McKee D, Silva S, She L, Blumenthal JA, O'Connor J. Effects of coping skills training and sertraline in patients with non-cardiac chest pain: a randomized controlled study. PAIN®. 2011 Apr 1;152(4):730-41.

[34] Jonsbu E, Martinsen EW, Morken G, Moum T, Dammen T. Change and impact of illness perceptions among patients with non-cardiac chest pain or benign palpitations following three sessions of CBT. Behavioural and cognitive psychotherapy. 2013 Jul;41(4):398-407.

[35] Beek, M. H. C. T., Oude Voshaar, R. C., Beek, A. M., Zijderveld, G. A., Visser, S., Speckens, A. E. M., & Balkom, A. J. L. M. A brief cognitive behavioural intervention for treating depression and panic disorder in patients with non-cardiac chest pain: a 24 week randomised controlled trial. Depression and anxiety . 2013. 30(7), 670-678. https://doi.org/10.1002/da.22106

[36] Lessard MJ, Marchand A, Pelland MÈ, Belleville G, Vadeboncoeur A, Chauny JM, Poitras J, Dupuis G, Fleet R, Foldes-Busque G, Lavoie KL. Comparing two brief psychological interventions to usual care in panic disorder patients presenting to the emergency department with chest pain. Behavioural and cognitive psychotherapy. 2012 Mar 1;40(2):129.

[37] Cooper, K., Gregory, J. D., Walker, I., Lambe, S., & Salkovskis, P. M. Cognitive behaviour therapy for health anxiety: a systematic review and meta-analysis. 2017. Behavioural and cognitive psychotherapy, 45(2), 110-123. https://doi.org/10.1017/S1352465816000527

[38] van Gils, A., Schoevers, R. A., Bonvanie, I. J., Gelauff, J. M., Roest, A. M., & Rosmalen, J. G. (2016). Self-help for medically unexplained symptoms: a systematic review and meta-analysis. Psychosomatic medicine. 2016 *78*(6), 728-739. doi: 10.1097/PSY.0000000000000325

[39] Tyrer, P., Cooper, S., Salkovskis, P., Tyrer, H., Crawford, M., Byford, S., ... & Murphy, D. Clinical and cost-effectiveness of cognitive behaviour therapy for health anxiety in medical patients: a multicentre randomised controlled trial. The Lancet. 2014. 383(9913), 219-225. doi: 10.1016/S0140-6736(13)61905-4. Epub 2013 Oct 18.

[40] McDevitt-Petrovic O, Kirby K, Shevlin M. The prevalence of non-cardiac chest pain (NCCP) using emergency department (ED) data: a Northern Ireland based study. BMC health services research. 2017 Dec 1;17(1):549.

[41] Jonsbu E, Dammen T, Morken G, Moum T, Martinsen EW. Short-term cognitive behavioral therapy for non-cardiac chest pain and benign palpitations: a randomized controlled trial. Journal of psychosomatic research. 2011 Feb 1;70(2):117-23.

[42] Avia MD, Ruiz MA, Olivares ME, Crespo M, Guisado AB, Sánchez A,

Varela A. The meaning of psychological symptoms: effectiveness of a group intervention with hypochondriacal patients. Behaviour Research and Therapy. 1996 Jan 1;34(1):23-31.

[43] Potts SG, Lewin R, Fox KA, Johnstone EC. Group psychological treatment for chest pain with normal coronary arteries. Qjm. 1999 Feb 1;92(2):81-6.

[44] Beck, A. T. Cognitive Therapy and the Emotional Disorders. New York: Penguin. 1976. https://www.penguin.co.uk/books/151/15136/cognitive-therapy-and-the-emotional-disorders/9780140156898.html

[45] Escobar JI, Gara MA, Diaz-Martinez AM, Interian A, Warman M, Allen LA, Woolfolk RL, Jahn E, Rodgers D. Effectiveness of a time-limited cognitive behavior therapy–type intervention among primary care patients with medically unexplained symptoms. The Annals of Family Medicine. 2007 Jul 1;5(4):328-35.

[46] Martin A, Rauh E, Fichter M, Rief W. A one-session treatment for patients suffering from medically unexplained symptoms in primary care: a randomized clinical trial. Psychosomatics. 2007 Jul 1;48(4):294-303.

[47] Arnold, I. A., De Waal, M. W., Eekhof, J. A., Assendelft, W. J., Spinhoven, P., & Van Hemert, A. M. Medically unexplained physical symptoms in primary care: a controlled study on the effectiveness of cognitive-behavioral treatment by the family physician. Psychosomatics. 2009 50(5), 515-524. doi: 10.1176/appi.psy.50.5.515.

[48] Speckens AE, van Hemert AM, Bolk JH, Hawton KE, Rooijmans HG. The acceptability of psychological treatment in patients with medically unexplained physical symptoms. Journal of psychosomatic research. 1995 Oct 1;39(7):855-63.

[49] Allen LA, Woolfolk RL, Escobar JI, Gara MA, Hamer RM. Cognitive-behavioral therapy for somatization disorder: a randomized controlled trial. Archives of Internal Medicine. 2006 Jul 24;166(14):1512-8.

[50] Aiarzaguena JM, Grandes G, Gaminde I, Salazar A, Sanchez A, Arino J. A randomized controlled clinical trial of a psychosocial and communication intervention carried out by GPs for patients with medically unexplained symptoms. Psychological medicine. 2007 Feb 1;37(2):283.

[51] Larisch A, Schweickhardt A, Wirsching M, Fritzsche K. Psychosocial interventions for somatizing patients by the general practitioner: a randomized controlled trial. Journal of psychosomatic research. 2004 Dec 1;57(6):507-14.

[52] Katsamanis M, Lehrer PM, Escobar JI, Gara MA, Kotay A, Liu R. Psychophysiologic treatment for patients with medically unexplained symptoms: a randomized controlled trial. Psychosomatics. 2011 May 1;52(3):218-29.

[53] Wortman MS, Lucassen PL, van Ravesteijn HJ, Bor H, Assendelft PJ, Lucas C, Olde Hartman TC. Brief multimodal psychosomatic therapy in patients with medically unexplained symptoms: feasibility and treatment effects. Family practice. 2016 Aug 1;33(4):346-53.

[54] Kashner TM, Rost K, Cohen B, Anderson M, Smith Jr GR. Enhancing the health of somatization disorder patients: Effectiveness of short-term group therapy. Psychosomatics. 1995 Sep 1;36(5):462-70.

[55] McManus F, Surawy C, Muse K, Vazquez-Montes M, Williams JM. A randomized clinical trial of mindfulness-based cognitive therapy versus unrestricted services for health anxiety (hypochondriasis). Journal of

consulting and clinical psychology. 2012 Oct;80(5):817.

[56] McManus F, Muse K, Surawy C. Mindfulness-based Cognitive Therapy (MBCT) For Severe Health Anxiety. Healthcare, Counselling and Psychotherapy Journal. 2011:19-23.

[57] Barsky AJ, Ahern DK. Cognitive behavior therapy for hypochondriasis: a randomized controlled trial. Jama. 2004 Mar 24;291(12):1464-70.

[58] Pelland MÈ, Marchand A, Lessard MJ, Belleville G, Chauny JM, Vadeboncoeur A, Poitras J, Foldes-Busque G, Bacon SL, Lavoie KL. Efficacy of 2 interventions for panic disorder in patients presenting to the ED with chest pain. The American journal of emergency medicine. 2011 Nov 1;29(9):1051-61.

[59] Sanders D, Bass C, Mayou RA, Goodwin S, Bryant BM, Tyndel S. Non-cardiac chest pain: why was a brief intervention apparently ineffective?. Psychological medicine. 1997 Sep;27(5): 1033-40.

[60] Esler, J. L., Barlow, D. H., Woolard, R. H., Nicholson, R. A., Nash, J. M., & Erogul, M. H. A brief cognitive-behavioral intervention for patients with noncardiac chest pain. Behavior Therapy,. 2003 34(2), 129-148. https://doi.org/10.1016/0005-7894(03)80009-6

[61] Mourad G, Strömberg A, Jonsbu E, Gustafsson M, Johansson P, Jaarsma T. Guided Internet-delivered cognitive behavioural therapy in patients with non-cardiac chest pain–a pilot randomized controlled study. Trials. 2016 Dec 1;17(1):352.

[62] Bahremand M, Moradi G, Saeidi M, Mohammadi S, Komasi S. Reducing irrational beliefs and pain severity in patients suffering from non-cardiac chest pain (NCCP): a comparison of relaxation training and metaphor therapy. The Korean Journal of Pain. 2015 Apr;28(2):88.

[63] Bahremand M, Saeidi M, Komasi S. How effective is the use of metaphor therapy on reducing psychological symptoms and pain discomfort in patients with non-cardiac chest pain: a randomized, controlled trial. Journal of Cardio-Thoracic Medicine. 2016;4(2):444-9.

[64] Smith RC, Lyles JS, Gardiner JC, et al: Primary care clinicians treat patients with medically unexplained symptoms: a randomized controlled trial. J Gen Intern Med 2006; 21:671-677

[65] Huibers MJ, Beurskens AJ, Bleijenberg G, et al: The effective-ness of psychosocial interventions delivered by general practitioners. Cochrane Database Syst Rev 2003(2):CD003494

[66] Rief W, Nanke A, Emmerich J, Bender A, Zech T. Causal illness attributions in somatoform disorders: associations with comorbidity and illness behavior. Journal of psychosomatic research. 2004 Oct 1;57(4):367-71.

[67] Machin D, Campbell MJ, Tan SB, Tan SH. Sample sizes for clinical, laboratory and epidemiology studies. John Wiley & Sons; 2018 Aug 20.

[68] Button KS, Ioannidis JP, Mokrysz C, Nosek BA, Flint J, Robinson ES, Munafò MR. Power failure: why small sample size undermines the reliability of neuroscience. Nature reviews neuroscience. 2013 May;14(5):365-76.

[69] Coster WJ. Making the best match: selecting outcome measures for clinical trials and outcome studies. American Journal of Occupational Therapy. 2013 Mar 1;67(2):162-70.

[70] Gerger H, Hlavica M, Gaab J, Munder T, Barth J. Does it matter who

provides psychological interventions for medically unexplained symptoms? A meta-analysis. Psychotherapy and Psychosomatics. 2015;84(4):217-26.

[71] Burton C. Beyond somatisation: a review of the understanding and treatment of medically unexplained physical symptoms (MUPS). British Journal of General Practice. 2003 Mar 1;53(488):231-9.

[72] Morriss R, Dowrick C, Salmon P, Peters S, Dunn G, Rogers A, Lewis B, Charles-Jones H, Hogg J, Clifford R, Rigby C. Cluster randomised controlled trial of training practices in reattribution for medically unexplained symptoms. The British Journal of Psychiatry. 2007 Dec;191(6):536-42.

[73] Looper KJ, Kirmayer LJ. Behavioral medicine approaches to somatoform disorders. Journal of consulting and clinical psychology. 2002 Jun;70(3):810.

[74] Smith, R. C., Lein, C., Collins, C., Lyles, J. S., Given, B., Dwamena, F. C., ... & Given, C. W. Treating patients with medically unexplained symptoms in primary care. *Journal of General Internal Medicine*, 18 2003. (6), 478-489. https://doi.org/10.1046/j.1525-1497.2003.20815.x

[75] Williams GC, Halvari H, Niemiec CP, Sørebø Ø, Olafsen AH, Westbye C. Managerial support for basic psychological needs, somatic symptom burden and work-related correlates: A self-determination theory perspective. Work & Stress. 2014 Oct 2;28(4):404-19.

9

Emotional Eating and Obesity

Ignacio Jáuregui-Lobera and Marian Montes-Martínez

Abstract

The first time that terms such as food addiction and addictive eating were mentioned was in 1956, in an article by T.G. Randolph. Recently, from a psychosomatic point of view, some authors have linked obesity and food addiction. Along with the concept of food addiction (derived from the similarities between the consumption of certain foods and "substance addictions"), a couple of questions seem to arise: What if it's not just the particular food (the substance) that we are addicted to? Could it be that we are addicted to something else that makes us eat it? Thus, the concept of eating addiction has its own set of particulars. It brings the attention back to the individual and not the external substance (the food or ingredient). The focus on confronting the obesity problem should be moved away from the food itself (the addictive substance) to the person's act of eating (the addictive behavior). Undoubtedly, there are many links between emotions and overweight/obesity. This chapter aims to review the current state of this field of study which is the emotional basis of obesity (at least a particular case of obesity and weight-related disorders).

Keywords: food addiction, eating addiction, emotional eating, stress, negative emotions, posttraumatic stress disorder, overweight, obesity

1. Introduction

Some time ago, in a wonderful article by Adriaanse et al. [1], a question was suggested, "Emotional eating: Eating when emotional or emotional about eating?" Due the increasing number of people who are overweight and the increase in the worldwide prevalence of obesity over the past decades [2], some etiological factors have been proposed. Summarizing, both environmental and personal factors seem to be involved. With respect to the first, a "toxic food environment" was mentioned by Wadden et al. [3], and other authors have thought that tempting palatable foods available everywhere might be a relevant factor to explain the epidemic figures of overweight [4]. Along with food, personal factors must be considered. How does a person respond individually to food? Are there different possible responses depend-ing on specific foods? Are there individuals prone to develop food addiction or addictive eating?

The first time that terms such as food addiction and addictive eating were mentioned was in 1956, in an article by T.G. Randolph [2]. Recently, from a psychosomatic point of view, some authors have linked obesity and food addiction [5, 6]. Along with the concept of "food addiction" (derived from the similarities between the consumption of certain foods and "substance addictions"), a couple of ques-tions seem to arise: What if it is not just the particular food (the substance) that we are addicted to? Could it be that we are addicted to something else that makes us eat it? Thus, the concept of eating addiction has its own set of peculiarities. It brings the attention back to the individual and not the external substance (the food or ingredi-ent). The focus on confronting the obesity problem should be moved away from the food itself (the addictive substance) to the person's act of eating (the addictive behavior). Undoubtedly, there are many links between emotions and overweight/obesity.

It is well known that calorie-restricted diets are clearly ineffective for patients with overweight beyond the short term. In the long term, the most amount of weight lost is usually regained, with some patients even ending up weighing more than before the diet [7–9]. It is usual to think about emotional eating just linked to the abandon of restricted diets. Nevertheless, emotional eating may also occur, independently or regardless of dieting. Several authors have referred to emotional eating as an outcome of poor interoceptive awareness, a confusion of internal states of hunger and satiety and physiological symptoms associated with emotions, alexithymia, or poor emotion regulation strategies [9, 10]. Emotional eating has also been associated with a reversed stress response of the hypothalamic pituitary adrenal (HPA) axis (a blunted instead of the typical elevated cortisol response to stress) [11, 12].

2. When does emotional eating appear?

The prevalence of emotional eating in childhood is usually very low. In this regard, what tends to occur when food intake is linked to negative emotions/stress in children? The usual, natural response is that they tend to lose appetite. Then, in the transition from childhood to adulthood, emotional eating emerges in the form of overeating. Puberty (with its hormonal changes) would be the base for this phenomenon in adolescence [9]. As we referred, a common explanation for the increase in obesity over recent decades is the environment and, in particular, the availability of highly varied, palatable, and fattening foods—which have been considered to be addictive [13–16]. The point is that many individuals manage to resist these temptations and maintain a healthy weight, but others (e.g., overweight and obese individuals) have been shown to have preference for energy-dense foods compared to healthy-weight people [17–19]. In sum, not all children would become emotional eaters during adolescence.

Some research has shown that when food is eaten to satisfy one's feelings instead of satisfying hunger, it might result in emotional eating, which increases the risk of obesity. The study of emotional eating is complex because it is influenced by several risk factors, and some of these factors have been studied from a psychological point of view, such as self-regulation, effects of stress on eating behavior, parenting and emotional eating, and parental bonding and coping.

Considering self-regulation, emotional eating, as a learned response, is suggested to be associated with depressive feelings and inadequate parenting in adoles-cence [20], and it seems that self-regulation plays an important role in this respect. Galloway et al. [21] investigated the association between feeding practices used in childhood, eating behaviors, and weight status in early adulthood, and they found a significant positive correlation between practices based on controlling child feed-ing, emotional eating, and body mass index among children. Moreover, controlling child feeding practices are linked with poorer self-regulation of food intake [22]. On the one hand, the probability of eating in the absence of hunger is increased by restrictive feeding practices [23]. On the other hand, children's natural ability to self-regulate would be interfered by eating under pressure [24].

Although research shows that children tend to have poorer self-regulation because of immaturity of the brain [25], proper parenting such as being a positive role model [26] is a crucial factor to consider a successful self-regulation.

The effects of stress on eating behavior might be summarized, highlighting that the response to stressful circumstances is usually loss of appetite. Therefore, emotional eating would be an atypical response to this factor [27]. Besides, it can influence preference for sweet and fatty foods, among other unhealthy foods [11]. Studies have found that stressful circumstances such as examinations or times of high workloads are associated with greater energy and fat intake [28], so that emotion regulation through eating is experienced in a student population during stress under real life conditions with distraction as a possible mediating mechanism [29].

Other fields of study are the parenting styles and their influence on eating. In this regard, studies have found that authoritative parenting style is associated with higher levels of emotional eating in children and adolescents [30] as well as less maternal support, more maternal psychological control, and less maternal behavioral control [31], which is, on the other hand, associated with alexithymia [32]. Emotional awareness among obese children has been associated with other parenting styles such as overprotection and, in turn, emotional awareness with emotional eating [33]. In addition, the ability to cope with challenging situations, which determines children's well-being and success in college, seems to be positively associated with parental bonding [34]. Besides, the use of problem solving, active distraction, social-support seeking, and less passive resignation of failure has been linked with maternal bonding [35].

3. Food addiction, eating addiction, and emotional eating

If we focus on specific foods, the person's act of eating, and emotions linked to eating, it seems that two aspects of self-regulatory failure that are particularly pertinent in both substance use and overeating are impulsivity and reward sensitivity [36–38]. With respect to impulsivity (a multifaceted construct, it can be defined broadly as "the tendency to think and act without sufficient forethought, which often results in behavior that is discordant with one's long-term goals") [39], it has been implicated in overeating and obesity [40–43]. Regarding reward sensitivity, a heightened general sensitivity to reward has also been linked to overeating [44–46]. Nevertheless, the causal direction between reward sensitivity and overeating remains uncertain. On the one hand, increasing reward sensitivity may lead to overeating by increasing motivation toward pleasurable activities, such as consuming energy-dense foods that elicit dopamine and opioid activation. On the other hand, decreased reward sensitivity may cause individuals to seek out rewarding activities as a form of "self-medication" in order to boost dopamine functioning (i.e., addictive behavior would be the result of a "reward deficiency syndrome") [47, 48].

It seems that we face two possibilities: (a) an increased reward sensitivity might lead to overeating (which will produce an activation of dopamine and opioids) via increased motivation to obtain gratification; and (b) a decreased reward sensitivity might push individuals to seek "something" capable to stimulate dopamine functioning. Burger and Stice have proposed several theories about the way these two causal directions would combine to explain obesity [49]. Thus, high sensitivity to reward might initially cause individuals to over-consume palatable foods. Nevertheless, this sensitivity would be modified over time as the brain's reward system adapts and shows divergent changes in food motivation ("wanting") versus hedonic pleasure ("liking"). The point is that with repeated exposures to palatable foods, the hedonic pleasure derived from the ingestion would decrease due to neural habituation, while the anticipation of reward would increase. As a result, the indi-vidual is experiencing less pleasure from the food ("liking"), but simultaneously he/she experiences an increased desire ("wanting") for the food, driving further food seeking and consumption [50–55].

Impulsivity, reward sensitivity, and the experience of intense craving (the intense desire to consume a specific food) [56, 57] would be the three facets of food addiction in the field of overeating, overweight, and obesity. Chocolate, carbohydrates, and salty snack are the most commonly craved foods [58–62]. Studies on cue-reactivity research have repeatedly shown similarities between drug and food craving. In both cases craving is more likely to occur in the presence of substance-related stimuli. Thus, substance cues or food cues tend to increase the craving [63].

4. Between personal risk factors and overweight/obesity: emotional eating as mediator?

One might emphasize dispositional factors (biological or psychological), which would lead to overweight or obesity, or focus the attention on food properties (to some extent "addictive") or the mere fact of eating (eating behavior, eating addiction). Alternatively, the mediation of emotions might be considered (emotional eating).

The tendency to eat in response to negative emotions or stress is an atypical stress response, as the typical stress response consists of not eating because the physiological stress reactions mimic the internal sensations associated with feeding-induced satiety [27] (see for empirical support [64]). Emotional eating, as "disinhibitor," requires prior inhibition (i.e., restraint) by definition. However, it has not yet been resolved whether restraint eating is a cause of the consequence of emotional eating [65, 66], and this may also differ in various subgroups [67]. Nevertheless, as it was mentioned above, emotional eating may also occur, independently of food restrictions. We noted that emotional eating tends to co-occur with external eating (i.e., overeating in response to food-related cues such as the sight and smell of attractive food) [68]. In addition, Slochower [69] reported that nega-tive emotions and food cues were shown to operate conjointly to elicit overeating in female students with obesity—the participants only overate in the high anxiety-high food salience condition, but not when the anxiety and/or the food salience was low.

With respect to "negative emotions," feeling depressed is normally associated with loss of appetite and subsequent weight loss. There exists, however, a subtype of depression that is characterized by the atypical features of increased appetite and subsequent weight gain [70]. Emotional eating has been considered a marker of this depression subtype [71] because it shares with this subtype the atypical feature of increased appetite in response to distress such as feelings of depression (for support, see [72]). In various cross-sectional studies, emotional eating was indeed found to act as a mediator between depression and obesity [73–76].

Generally speaking, life adverse experiences are defined as all kinds of traumatic experiences occurring in childhood, adolescence, and adulthood, which include emotional abuse, physical abuse, sexual abuse, sexual harassment, rape, bullying by peers, witnessing domestic violence, and serious accidents that threatened the lives of subjects. As an example of traumatic experiences, abuse-related PTSD symptoms are associated with hyperactivation of HPA axis and with subsequent increases in peripheral cortisol, which in turn have been linked to accumulation of fat in adipose tissues and, consequently, an increase in abdominal obesity [77, 78]. In line with these findings, the hyperactivation of HPA axis with an exaggerated cortisol response to stress has been observed in obese patients [79] and was also put in relation with stress-induced eating [80], with night eating syndrome (NES) [81] and with waist adiposity in binge eating disorder (BED) patients [82].

Stress, depression, life adverse experiences, abuse-related PTSD, etc. might be potential risk factors for obesity via emotional eating. Some studies have focused their interest on the relationship between trauma, dissociation, and binge eating disorder. Generally, it is concluded that dissociation may play an important mediating role between the presence of early trauma and the development of eating disorders (e.g., [83]). In this regard, it has been hypothesized that when negative emotional states are activated, a shift toward lower levels of cognition and self-awareness is initiated, which involves cognitive processes similar to dissociation. This mechanism tends to remove the inhibitions, thereby facilitating the start of binge eating or overeating, both in clinical (e.g., [84]) and in nonclinical subjects [85]. Several studies seem to support the hypothesis that dissociation may have a mediating role in the abuse and binge eating link [86, 87].

Along with dissociation, other authors have proposed some specific psychological variables that function as mediators in the relationship between childhood abuse, obesity, and bingeing, such as depression [88], trait anger [89], and perceived stress [90]. With respect to depression, Moyer et al. [88] even suggested that depression may be the only significant variable in the link between childhood abuse and adult obesity. Depression has been consistently associated with obesity and central obesity [91]. Once again, a possible way to interpret the link between childhood abuse, depression, and obesity is emotional eating. Regarding trait anger, (a) it seems to be related to the increase of visceral adipose tissue [92]; and (b) it is associated with emotional eating [93].

Considering adverse experiences, the following ideas seem to be relevant:

- Subjects with adverse childhood experiences have a higher risk of developing maladaptive coping strategies, including stress-induced emotional eating [94].
- Perceived stress may explain the link between child abuse and the development of obesity in adulthood [90].
- Activation of the stress response can lead to emotional dysregulation that has been associated with increased appetite, a preference for foods high in sugar and fat [11, 95–97], fat visceral accumulation, and obesity in adults [97–99] and adolescents [98, 99].
- Some authors have reported that overweight subjects tend to gain weight when stressed [11] and that obese individuals increase their food intake after having experienced negative emotions and perceived stress [100, 101].
- Laboratory studies have demonstrated that acute physical or emotional distress was followed by high cortisol reactivity, which induces increased intake of "comfort" foods [102–104].
- Stress-related adaptation involves the concept of allostasis, which is the ability to achieve the physiological balance through the change of the internal envi-ronment [96, 105, 106].
- Conditions of repeated or incontrollable chronic stress are followed by higher cortisol response and tend to activate a state of allostatic load, resulting in neu-ral and emotional dysregulation, which contribute to maladaptive behaviors such as repeated consumption of high caloric food [96], lack of control over eating, and binge eating [82, 107, 108].

Overall these abovementioned results suggest that psychophysiological responses to stress may influence subsequently eating behavior and hence may also mediate between the trauma and eating disorder link.

5. Posttraumatic stress disorder (PTSD): a psychosomatic paradigm of emotional eating?

It is well known that PTSD is usually associated with significantly higher rates of substance use disorders, other comorbid psychiatric disorders, and a variety of self-destructive and impulsive behaviors, including suicide [109–111]. It has been suggested that the ingestion, and especially over-ingestion, of fatty or sugary energy sources may be just another strategy that traumatized individuals use to numb themselves from their unpleasant feeling states and memories [112]. Thus, certain foods might act just like other substances that alter brain chemistry and, hence, consciousness. As we mentioned above, Randolph first described the phenomenon of food addiction and linked it with addictive drinking in 1956 [2]. Since then, the notion that certain foods can act like other addicting substances in the brain (despite having other peripheral metabolic effects that substances of abuse do not necessarily have) has been accepted. In fact, food intake and drug use both cause dopamine release in parts of the brain that mediate pleasure and emotion. The degree of subjective reward or experience of pleasure is clearly linked with the amount of dopamine release. Comparing similarities between action of certain foods and other substances of abuse, it must be noted that (a) food can stimulate the opiate system and there are similarities in use and withdrawal patterns of sugar and of classic drugs of abuse; (b) similar patterns of brain activation occur in response to food and drug cues; and (c) people may gain weight when they stop smoking or drinking.

It has been proposed that certain foods can be addicting to certain people, especially traumatized people. Part of the people exposed to alcohol, nicotine, drugs of abuse, etc. are prone to be attracted for these substances/behaviors, and finally they are at high risk to develop addictions. The point is how can we determine if someone will go on to develop an addiction to food or to any substance or behavior? From a genetic perspective, it has been proven that people with reduced dopamine type 2 receptor availability have a predisposition toward obesity and substance dependence. Other risk factors are environmental. In this regard, a history of psycho-trauma would be an example and leads to the self-medication hypothesis of PTSD. This way, victims of interpersonal violence may select highly palatable foods containing high concentrations of sugar, fat, salt, or caffeine, sometimes to the point of addiction, in an attempt to dampen arousal and facilitate numbing and avoidance specific symptoms to PTSD [112].

Hirth et al. [113] observed an association between PTSD symptoms and drinking more than one serving of soda per day as well as consumption of fast food more often. The participants of this study may have eaten more fast food to reduce

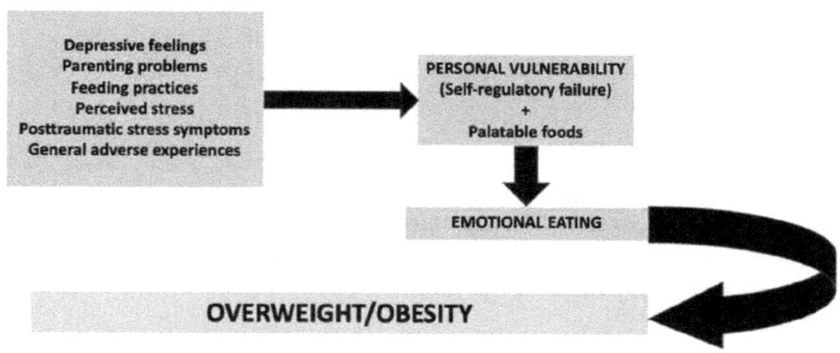

Figure 1.
Negative emotions, emotional eating, and weight gain.

trauma-induced PTSD symptoms, using that food as self-medication. Both fast food consumption and sugary soda consumption are usually associated with weight gain. PTSD symptoms may initiate a process of overindulging in unhealthy food and beverages in an attempt to compensate for the way trauma-induced memories make trauma victims feel. Through this process overeating behavior would lead to overweight/obesity. The problem would get worse when patients with PTSD symptoms try to reduce the effects of bingeing with unhealthy dieting behaviors and possibly develop eating pathology, consistent with the model of Stice and Shaw [114]. The results reported by Hirth et al. are consistent with theories that unhealthy dieting behaviors, such as vomiting and laxative abuse, are linked to PTSD [115, 116]. In sum, PTSD symptoms are associated with specific food and drink choices, and PTSD symptoms are also associated with unhealthy eating behaviors, which would be the gate to develop overweight/obesity and eating disorders. **Figure 1** tries to summarize the model which links negative emotions with weight gain.

6. Conclusions

In accordance with our review, we found that in spite of the fact that there are many risk factors involved in the increase in prevalence of obesity all around the world over the past few years, from those related to environmental and personal factors, particularly emotional eating plays a crucial and complex role in it. In the meantime, emotional eating is as well influenced by several risk factors: from social and physical environment to genetics, psychology, and food preferences. In addition, concepts such as food addiction and addictive eating were profoundly analyzed in order to explain the person's behavior toward food, and we concluded that there are many links between emotions and overweight/obesity. From our exploration we concluded that the epidemic of overweight and obesity is not only a matter of palatable and addictive foods available everywhere but also the individual responses to food.

Undoubtedly, we explored that emotional eating emerges in response to negative emotions, but it was also important to examine how self-regulation, effects of stress, parenting, and parental bonding and coping would have an effect on the act of eating and subsequently on emotional eating and its correlation with the body mass index. Although it is well known that the typical response of stress on eat-ing behavior is usually loss of appetite, we found that stressful circumstances are associated with greater energy and fat intake.

Considering the field of study focused on overeating, it was seen that impulsivity, reward sensitivity, and the experience of intense craving result from self-regula-tion failures regarding both substance use and overeating. Nevertheless, some more research is needed in order to prove the causal direction between reward sensitivity and overeating.

Another important factor to consider in order to self-regulate successfully among children is the proper parenting styles, which would influence positively on eating behavior. Authoritative parenting style, less maternal support, the lack of parental bond, and overprotection would disrupt the well-being of children and the ability to cope with challenging situations. Subsequently, these factors would interfere with their attitudes toward the act of eating.

On the other hand, regarding negative emotions and feeling depressed, it is known that they are associated with loss of appetite and, as a result, weight loss. However, research showed that emotional eating would act as a mediator for a specific subtype of depression and it would have just the opposite effect on eating behavior, increasing weight as a result. In this regard, life adverse experiences, childhood trauma, and abuse-related PTSD, among other traumatic and stressful situations, were associated with dissociation, which plays an important role in the development of eating disorders, emotional eating, and obesity. In the field of over-ingestion of specific kinds of foods, such as sugary and fatty sources, these foods were proposed to be addicting to traumatized people. The genetic hypothesis proved the link between reduced dopamine type 2 receptor availability and the predisposition toward obesity and substance dependence. On the other hand, the PTSD hypothesis showed the over-ingestion of palatable foods in traumatized people derives from an attempt to lessen arousal and to avoid specific symptoms derived from PTSD, that is, emotional eating as self-medication.

In conclusion, in order to face the obesity problem, the addictive behavior should be the focus of research and treatment and not the addictive substance as traditionally has been considered.

Conflict of interest

The authors declare no conflict of interest.

Author details

Ignacio Jáuregui-Lobera* and Marian Montes-Martínez
Behavioral Sciences Institute, Seville, Spain

*Address all correspondence to: ijl@tcasevilla.com

References

[1] Adriaanse MA, de Ridder DTD, Evers C. Emotional eating: Eating when emotional or emotional about eating? Psychology & Health. 2011;**26**(1):23-39

[2] Randolph TG. The descriptive features of food addiction; addictive eating and drinking. Quarterly Journal of Studies on Alcohol. 1956;**17**:198-224

[3] Wadden TA, Brownell KD, Foster GD. Obesity: Responding to the global epidemic. Journal of Consulting and Clinical Psychology. 2002;**70**:510-525

[4] Van den Bos R, de Ridder DTD. Evolved to satisfy our immediate needs: Self-control and the rewarding properties of food. Appetite. 2006;**47**:24-29

[5] Avena NM, Bocarsly ME, Hoebel BG. Animal models of sugar and fat binge-ing: Relationship to food addiction and increased body weight. Methods in Molecular Biology. 2012;**829**:351-365

[6] Pedram P, Wadden D, Amini P, Gulliver W, Randell E, Cahill F, et al. Food addiction: Its prevalence and significant association with obesity in the general population. PLoS One. 2013;**8**:e74832

[7] Langeveld M, De Vries H. The long-term effect of energy restricted diets for treating obesity. Obesity. 2015;**23**:1529-1538

[8] Mann T, Tomiyama J, Wesling E, Lew A, Samuels B, Chatman J. Medicare's search for effective obesity treatments. Diets are not the answer. American Psychologist. 2007;**62**:220-233

[9] Van Strien T. Causes of emotional eating and matched treatment of obesity. Current Diabetes Reports. 2018;**18**:35

[10] Bruch H. Eating Disorders. New York: Basic Books; 1973

[11] Dallman MF. Stress-induced obesity and the emotional nervous system. Trends in Endocrinology and Metabolism. 2010;**21**:159-165

[12] Van Strien T, Roelofs K, de Weerth C. Cortisol reactivity and distress-induced emotional eating. Psychoneuroendocrinology. 2013;**38**:677-684

[13] Cummins S, Macintyre S. Food environments and obesity—Neighbourhood or nation? International Journal of Epidemiology. 2006;**35**:100-104

[14] Jeffery RW, Utter J. The changing environment and population obesity in the United States. Obesity Research. 2003;**11**:12S-22S

[15] Levitsky DA. The non-regulation of food intake in humans: Hope for reversing the epidemic of obesity. Physiology & Behavior. 2005;**86**:623-632

[16] Schulte EM, Avena NM, Gearhardt AN. Which foods may be addictive? The roles of processing, fat content, and glycemic load. PLoS One. 2015;**10**:e0117959

[17] Blundell JE, Burley VJ, Cotton JR, Lawton CL. Dietary fat and the control of energy intake: Evaluating the effects of fat on meal size and postmeal satiety. American Journal of Clinical Nutrition. 1993;**57**:772S-778S

[18] Drewnowski A, Brunzell J, Sande K, Iverius P, Greenwood M. Sweet tooth reconsidered: Taste responsiveness in human obesity. Physiology & Behavior. 1985;**35**:617-622

[19] Drewnowski A, Kurth C, Holden-Wiltse J, Saari J. Food

preferences in human obesity: Carbohydrates versus fats. Appetite. 1992;**18**:207-221

[20] Snoek HM, van Strien T, Janssens JM, Engels RC. Emotional, external, restrained eating and overweight in Dutch adolescents. Scandinavian Journal of Psychology. 2007;**48**(1):23-32

[21] Galloway AT, Farrow CV, Martz DM. Retrospective reports of child feeding practices, current eating behaviors, and BMI in college students. Obesity. 2010;**18**(7):1330-1335

[22] Constanza PR, Woody EZ. Domain-specific parenting styles and their impact on the child's development of particular deviance: The example of obesity and proneness. Journal of Social and Clinical Psychology. 1985;**3**:425

[23] Birch LL, Fisher JO, Davison KK. Learning to overeat: Maternal use of restrictive feeding practices promotes girls' eating in the absence of hunger. American Journal of Clinical Nutrition. 2003;**78**:215-220

[24] Johnson SL, Birch LL. Parents' and children's adiposity and eating style. Pediatrics. 1994;**94**(5):653-661

[25] McRae K, Gross JJ, Weber J, Robertson ER, Sokol-Hessner P, Ray RD, et al. The development of emotion regulation: An fMRI study of cognitive reappraisal in children, adolescents and young adults. Social and Cognition Affective Neuroscience. 2012;**7**(1):11-22

[26] Ho AY. Risk factors of emotional eating in undergraduates [Dissertation]. Cleveland, Ohio: Case Western Reserve University; 2014

[27] Gold PW, Chrousos GP. Organization of the stress system and its dysregulation in melancholic and atypical depression: High vs low CRH/NE states. Molecular Psychiatry. 2002;**7**:254-275

[28] McCann BS, Warnick GR, Knopp RH. Changes in plasma lipids and dietary intake accompanying shifts in perceived workload and stress. Psychosomatic Medicine. 1990;**51**(1):97-108

[29] Macht M, Haupt C, Ellgring H. The perceived function of eating is changed during examination stress: A field study. Eating Behaviors. 2005;**6**(2):109-111

[30] Topham GL, Hubbs-Tait L, Rutledge JM, Page MC, Kennedy TS, Shriver LH, et al. Parenting styles, parental response to child emotion, and family emotional responsiveness are related to child emotional eating. Appetite. 2011;**56**(2):261-264

[31] Snoek HM, Engels RC, Janssens JM, van Strien T. Parental behaviour and adolescents' emotional eating. Appetite. 2007;**49**(1):223-230

[32] De Panfilis C, Rabbaglio P, Rossi C, Zita G, Maggini C. Body image disturbance, parental bonding and alexithymia in patients with eating disorders. Psychopathology. 2003;**36**(5):239-246

[33] Rommel D, Nandrino JL, Ducro C, Andrieux S, Delecourt F, Antoine P. Impact of emotional awareness and parental bonding on emotional eating in obese women. Appetite. 2012;**59**(1):21-26

[34] Adlaf EM, Gliksman L, Demers A, Newton-Taylor B. The prevalence of elevated psychological distress among Canadian undergraduates: Findings from the 1998 Canadian campus survey. Journal of American College Health. 2001;**50**(2):67-72

[35] Matheson K, Kelly O, Cole B, Tannenbaum B, Dodd C, Anisman H. Parental bonding and depressive affect: The mediating role of coping resources. The British Journal of Social Psychology. 2005;**44**(Pt3):371-395

[36] Dawe S, Loxton NJ. The role of impulsivity in the development of substance use and eating disorders. Neuroscience & Biobehavioral Reviews. 2004;**28**:343-351

[37] Gullo M, Dawe S. Impulsivity and adolescent substance use: Rashly dismissed as "all-bad"? Neuroscience & Biobehavioral Reviews. 2008;**32**:1507-1518

[38] Schulte EM, Grilo CM, Gearhardt AN. Shared and unique mechanisms underlying binge eating disorder and addictive disorders. Clinical Psychology Review. 2016;**44**:125-139

[39] Adams RC, Sedgmond J, Maizey L, Chambers CD, Lawrence NS. Food addiction: Implications for the diagnosis and treatment of overeating. Nutrients. 2019;**11**(9):E2086

[40] Emery RL, Levine MD. Questionnaire and behavioral task measures of impulsivity are differentially associated with body mass index: A comprehensive meta-analysis. Psychological Bulletin. 2017;**143**:868-902

[41] Guerrieri R, Nederkoorn C, Jansen A. The interaction between impulsivity and a varied food environment: Its influence on food intake and overweight. International Journal of Obesity. 2008;**32**:708-714

[42] Jentsch JD, Pennington ZT. Reward, interrupted: Inhibitory control and its relevance to addictions. Neuropharmacology. 2014;**76**:479-486

[43] Meule A. Impulsivity and overeating: A closer look at the subscales of the Barratt impulsiveness scale. Frontiers in Psychology. 2013;**4**:177

[44] Appelhans BM, Woolf K, Pagoto SL, Schneider KL, Whited MC, Liebman R. Inhibiting food reward: Delay discounting, food reward sensitivity, and palatable food intake in overweight and obese women. Obesity. 2011;**19**:2175-2182

[45] Dissabandara LO, Loxton NJ, Dias SR, Dodd PR, Daglish M, Stadlin A. Dependent heroin use and associated risky behaviour: The role of rash impulsiveness and reward sensitivity. Addictive Behaviors. 2014;**39**:71-76

[46] Franken IH, Muris P. Individual differences in reward sensitivity are related to food craving and relative body weight in healthy women. Appetite. 2005;**45**:198-201

[47] Blum K, Braverman ER, Holder JM, Lubar JF, Monastra VJ, Miller D, et al. The reward deficiency syndrome: A biogenetic model for the diagnosis and treatment of impulsive, addictive and compulsive behaviors. Journal of Psychoactive Drugs. 2000;**32**:1-112

[48] Bowirrat A, Oscar-Berman M. Relationship between dopaminergic neurotransmission, alcoholism, and reward deficiency syndrome. Neuropsychiatric Genetics, Part B of the American Journal of Medical Genetics. 2005;**132**:29-37

[49] Burger KS, Stice E. Variability in reward responsivity and obesity: Evidence from brain imaging studies. Current Drug Abuse Reviews. 2011;**4**:182-189

[50] Robinson T. The neural basis of drug craving: An incentive-sensitization theory of addiction. Brain Research Reviews. 1993;**18**:247-291

[51] Robinson TE, Berridge KC. Incentive-sensitization and addiction. Addiction. 2001;**96**:103-114

[52] Robinson TE, Berridge KC. Addiction. Annual Review of Psychology. 2003;**54**:25-53

[53] Berridge KC. 'Liking' and 'wanting' food rewards: Brain substrates and roles in eating disorders. Physiology & Behavior. 2009;**97**:537-550

[54] Berridge KC, Ho CY, Richard JM, Di Feliceantonio AG. The tempted brain eats: Pleasure and desire circuits in obesity and eating disorders. Brain Research. 2010;**1350**:43-64

[55] Hetherington M, Pirie L, Nabb S. Stimulus satiation: Effects of repeated exposure to foods on pleasantness and intake. Appetite. 2002;**38**:19-28

[56] Kekic M, McClelland J, Campbell I, Nestler S, Rubia K, David AS, et al. The effects of prefrontal cortex transcranial direct current stimulation (tDCS) on food craving and temporal discounting in women with frequent food cravings. Appetite. 2014;**78**:55-62

[57] Weingarten HP, Elston D. The phenomenology of food cravings. Appetite. 1990;**15**:231-246

[58] Cocores JA, Gold MS. The salted food addiction hypothesis may explain overeating and the obesity epidemic. Medical Hypotheses. 2009;**73**:892-899

[59] Corsica JA, Spring BJ. Carbohydrate craving: A double-blind, placebo-controlled test of the self-medication hypothesis. Eating Behaviors. 2008;**9**:447-454

[60] Hill AJ, Heaton-Brown L. The experience of food craving: A prospective investigation in healthy women. Journal of Psychosomatic Research. 1994;**38**:801-814

[61] Massey A, Hill AJ. Dieting and food craving. A descriptive, quasi-prospective study. Appetite. 2012;**58**:781-785

[62] Rozin P, Levine E, Stoess C. Chocolate craving and liking. Appetite. 1991;**17**:199-212

[63] Jáuregui-Lobera I, Bolaños-Ríos P, Valero E, Ruiz-Prieto I. Induction of food craving experience; the role of mental imagery, dietary restraint, mood and coping strategies. Nutrición Hospitalaria. 2012;**27**(6):1928-1935

[64] Van Strien T, Ouwens MA, Engel C, de Weerth C. Hunger, inhibitory control and distress-induced emotional eating. Appetite. 2014;**79**:124-133

[65] Polivy J, Herman CP. Dieting and bingeing. A causal analysis. American Psychologist. 1985;**40**(2):193-201

[66] Van Strien T, Herman CP, Verheijden MW. Eating style, overeating and overweight in a representative Dutch sample: Does external eating play a role? Appetite. 2009;**52**:380-387

[67] Van Strien T, Engels RCME, Van Leeuwe J, Snoek HM. The Stice model of overeating: Tests in clinical and non-clinical samples. Appetite. 2005;**4**:205-213

[68] Van Strien T. Nederlandse Vragenlijst voor eetgedrag (NVE). Handleiding. [Dutch Eating Behaviour Questionnaire. Manual]. Amsterdam: Hogrefe; 2015

[69] Slochower JA. Excessive Eating. The Role of Emotions and the Environment. New York: Human Sciences Press, Inc.; 1983

[70] American Psychiatric Association. Diagnostic and Statistical Manual of Mental Disorders. 5. (DSM-5). Washington, DC: American Psychiatric Publication; 2013

[71] Van Strien T, van der Zwaluw CS, Engels RCME. Emotional eating in adolescents: A gene (SLC6A4/5-HTT)-depressive feelings interaction analysis. Journal of Psychiatric Research. 2010;**44**(15):1035-1042

[72] Paans NPG, Bot M, Van Strien T, Brouwer IA, Visser M,

Penninx WJH. Eating styles in major depressive disorder: Results from a large-scale study. Journal of Psychiatric Research. 2018;**97**:38-46

[73] Clum GA, Rice JC, Broussard M, Johnson CC, Webber LS. Associations between depressive symptoms, self-efficacy, eating styles, exercise and body mass index in women. Journal of Behavioral Medicine. 2014;**37**(4):577-586

[74] Goldschmidt AB, Crosby RD, Engel SG, Crow SJ, Cao L, Peterson CB, et al. Affect and eating behavior in obese adults with and without elevated depression symptoms. International Journal of Eating Disorders. 2014;**47**(3):281-286

[75] Konttinen H, Männistö S, Sarlio-Lähteenkorva S, Silventoinen K, Haukkala A. Emotional eating, depressive symptoms and self-reported food consumption. A population-based study. Appetite. 2010;**54**(3):473-479

[76] Van Strien T, Winkens LHH, Broman Toft M, Pedersen S, Brouwer IA, et al. The mediation effect of emotional eating between depression and body mass index in Denmark and Spain. Appetite. 2016;**105**:500-508

[77] Glaser D. Child abuse and neglect and the brain—A review. Journal of Child Psychology and Psychiatry. 2000;**41**(1):97-116

[78] Pasquali R, Vicennati V, Cacciari M, Pagotto U. The hypothalamic-pituitary-adrenal axis activity in obesity and the metabolic syndrome. Annals of New York Academy of Sciences. 2006;**1083**:111-128

[79] Marin P, Darin N, Amemiya T, Andersson B, Jern S, Bjorntorp P. Cortisol secretion in relation to body fat distribution in obese premenopausal women. Metabolism. 1992;**41**:882-886

[80] Vicennati V, Pasqui F, Cavazza C, Pagotto U, Pasquali R. Stress-related development of obesity and cortisol in women. Obesity. 2009;**17**(9):1678-1683

[81] Birketvedt GS, Florholmen J, Sundsfjord J, Osterud B, Dingers D, Bilker W, et al. Behavioral and neuroendocrine characteristics of the night-eating syndrome. The Journal of the American Medical Association. 1999;282:657-663

[82] Gluck ME, Geliebter A, Lorence M. Cortisol stress response is positively correlated with central obesity in obese women with binge eating disorder (BED) before and after cognitive-behavioral treatment. Annals of New York Academy of Sciences. 2004;**1032**:202-207

[83] Treuer T, Koperdak M, Rozsa S, Furedi J. The impact of physical and sexual abuse on body image in eating disorders. European Eating Disorders Review. 2005;**13**:106-111

[84] Engelberg MJ, Steiger H, Gauvin L, Wonderlich SA. Binge antecedents in bulimic syndromes: An examination of dissociation and negative affect. International Journal of Eating Disorders. 2007;**40**:531-536

[85] Lyubomirsky S, Casper RC, Sousa L. What triggers abnormal eating in bulimic and non-bulimic women? The role of dissociative experiences, negative affect, and psychopathology. Psychology of Women Quarterly. 2001;**25**:223-232

[86] Rodriguez-Srednicki O. Childhood sexual abuse, dissociation and adult self-destructive behavior. Journal of Child Sexual Abuse. 2001;**10**(3):75-90

[87] La Mela C, Maglietta M, Castellini G, Amoroso L, Lucarelli S. Dissociation in eating disorders: Relationship between dissociative experiences and binge-eating episodes. Comprehensive Psychiatry. 2010;**51**(4):393-400

[88] Moyer D, Di Pietro L, Berkowitz R, Sunkard AJ. Childhood sexual abuse and precursors of binge eating in an adolescent female population. International Journal of Eating Disorders. 1997;**21**(1):23-30

[89] Midei AJ, Matthews KA, Bromberger J. Childhood abuse is associated with adiposity in mid-life women/possible pathways through trait anger and reproductive hormones. Psychosomatic Medicine. 2010;**72** (2) :215-223

[90] Alvarez J, Pavao J, Baumrind N, Kimerling N. The relationship between child abuse and adult obesity among California women. American Journal of Preventive Medicine. 2007;**33**(1):28-33

[91] Katz JR, Taylor NF, Goodrick S, Perry L, Yudkin JS, Coppack SW. Central obesity, depression and the hypothalamo-pituitary-adrenal axis in men and postmenopausal women. International Journal of Obesity and Related Metabolic Disorders: Journal of the International Association for the Study of Obesity. 2000;**24**(2):246-251

[92] Räikkönen K, Matthews KA, Kuller LH. Anthropometric and psychosocial determinants of visceral obesity in healthy postmenopausal women. International Journal of Obesity and Related Metabolic Disorders: Journal of the International Association for the Study of Obesity. 1999;**23**(8):775-782

[93] Appelhans BM, Whited MC, Schneider KL, Oleski J, Pagoto SL. Response style and vulnerability to anger-induced eating in obese adults. Eating Behaviors. 2011;**12**(1):9-14

[94] Evers C, Stok FM, de Ridder DT. Feeding your feelings: Emotion regulation strategies and emotional eating. Personality and Social Psychology Bulletin. 2010;**36**:792-804

[95] Adam TC, Epel ES. Stress, eating and the reward system. Physiology & Behavior. 2007;**91**(4):449-458

[96] McEwen BS. Physiology and neurobiology of stress and adaptation: Central role of the brain. Physiological Reviews. 2007;**87**(3):873-904

[97] Torres SJ, Nowson CA. Relationship between stress, eating behavior, and obesity. Nutrition. 2007;**23**(11):887-894

[98] Cohen S, Janicki-Deverts D, Miller GE. Psychological stress and disease. Journal of the American Medical Association. 2007;**298**(14):1685-1687

[99] De Vriendt T, Clays E, Maes L, De Bourdeaudhuij I, Vicente-Rodriguez G, Moreno LA, et al. European adolescents' level of perceived stress and its relationship with body adiposity—The HELENA study. The European Journal of Public Health. 2012;**22**(4):519-524

[100] Barrington WE, Beresford SA, McGregor BA, White E. Perceived stress and eating behaviors by sex, obesity status, and stress vulnerability: Findings from the vitamins and lifestyle (vital) study. Journal of the Academy of Nutrition and Dietetics. 2014;**114**(11):1791-1799

[101] Telch CF, Agras WS. Do emotional states influence binge eating in the obese? International Journal of Eating Disorders. 1996;**20**(3):271-279

[102] Epel E, Lapidus R, McEwen B, Brownell K. Stress may add bite to appetite in women: A laboratory study of stress-induced cortisol and eating behavior. Psychoneuroendocrinology. 2001;**26**(1):37-49

[103] Garg N, Wansink B, Inman JJ. The influence of incidental affect on consumers' food intake. Journal of Marketing. 2007;**71**(1):194-206

[104] Newman E, O'Connor DB, Conner M. Daily hassles and eating behaviour: The role of cortisol reactivity status. Psychoneuroendocrinology.2007;**32**(2): 125-132

[105] Seeman TE, Singer BH, Rowe JW, Horwitz RI, McEwen BS. Price of adaptation allostatic load and its health consequences: MacArthur studies of successful aging. Archives of Internal Medicine. 1997;**157**(19):2259-2268

[106] Sinha R, Jastreboff AM. Stress as a common risk factor for obesity and addiction. Biological Psychiatry. 2013;**73**(9):827-835

[107] Gluck ME, Geliebter A, Hung J, Yahav E. Cortisol, hunger, and desire to binge eat following a cold stress test in obese women with binge eating disorder. Psychosomatic Medicine. 2004;**66**:876-881

[108] Groesz LM, McCoy S, Carl J, Saslow L, Stewart J, Adler N, et al. What is eating you? Stress and the drive to eat. Appetite. 2012;**58**(2):717-721

[109] Brewerton TD. Eating disorders, victimization and PTSD: Principles of treatment. In: Brewerton TD, editor. Clinical Handbook of Eating Disorders: An Integrated Approach. New York: Marcel Dekker; 2004. pp. 509-545

[110] Dansky BS, Brewerton TD, Kilpatrick DG. Comorbidity of bulimia nervosa and alcohol use disorders: Results from the National Women's study. International Journal of Eating Disorders. 2000;**27**:180-190

[111] Brady K, Killeen TK, Brewerton TD, Sylverini S. Comorbidity of psychiatric disorders and posttraumatic disorder. Journal of Clinical Psychiatry. 2000;**61**(Suppl 7):22-32

[112] Brewerton TD. Posttraumatic stress disorder and disordered eating: Food addiction as self-medication. Journal of Women's Health. 2011;**20**(8):1-2

[113] Hirth J, Mahbubur R, Berenson AB. The association of posttraumatic stress disorder with fast food and soda consumption and unhealthy weight loss behaviors among young women. Journal of Women's Health. 2011;**20**:8

[114] Stice E, Shaw HE. Role of body dissatisfaction in the onset and maintenance of eating pathology: A synthesis of research findings. Journal of Psychosomatic Research. 2002;**53**:985-993

[115] Brewerton TD. Eating disorders, trauma, and comorbidity: Focus on PTSD. Eating Disorders. 2007;**15**:285-304

[116] Gleaves DH, Ebarenz KP, May MC. Scope and significance of posttraumatic symptomatology among women hospitalized for an eating disorder. International Journal of Eating Disorders. 1998;**24**:147-156

10

Psychosomatic Pain

Ertuğrul Allahverdi

Abstract

Disorders that are not clearly attributable to an organic disease are called somatoform disorders. Their symptoms are called psychosomatic symptoms and include insomnia, fatigue, and weakness. These disorders can also be associated with heartburn, depression, irregular heartbeat, dizziness, pain, cardiovascular problems, gastrointestinal discomfort, erectile dysfunction, a sensation of pressure in the throat, chest problems, hallucinations, and double vision. Somatoform disorders can be an expression of untreated mental pain and life experiences, resulting from serious loss, profound personal injury, or disrespect. Such symptoms occur in almost all humans, but these disorders can have a serious effect in 4–20% of the population.

Keywords: psychosomatic, pain, chronic pain, stress

1. Introduction

Psychosomatic pain: "A combination of symptoms of physical pain in various body areas that occur during any life period, where treatment is sought for the pain by going to many health clinics, and resulting in disruption of social and/or occupa-tional activities" [1–3].

"Soma" means the body. "Psychosomatic" diseases in psychiatry are mainly due to psychological causes that are not based on an organic etiology or physical disorders.

It is currently believed that conscious or unconscious emotions, thoughts, and behaviors are also effective in psychosomatic disease in biological organisms and should be evaluated together with the dual thoughts related to the body and mind status. The patient may use more atypical and exaggerated expressive words from time to time when defining psychogenic pain. The localization and periodicity of the patient's pain can also be persistently atypical. The pain of the patient usually begins after some important life events and stresses. The emotional burden of the factors stimulating and triggering pain is reflected in the patient's voluntary posture and the relevant muscle groups. A psychological dimension, depression and anxiety are usually noted among the accompanying symptoms. It is noteworthy that the characteristics of the pain do not conform to anatomical facts and physiological functioning. Besides, the response to analgesics is also often atypical. Accompanying symptoms such as anger, impatience, helplessness, boredom, and restlessness must be considered in patients with psychological pain.

Both psychosocial and biological factors always play a role in the development and pathophysiological mechanism of psychogenic pain [1–4].

The *Diagnostic and Statistical Manual of Mental Disorders* (DSM-IV) reference book of diagnostic criteria in psychiatry explains psychosomatic diseases as follows [1–3]:

"A combination of multiple physical symptoms that occur within a period of time, with continuing search for treatment, and resulting in deterioration of social or professional life."

The following criteria must be present to make a diagnosis of a psychosomatic disorder according to the DSM-IV:

- *Having at least four separate pains* (headache, abdominal pain, pain in the arms and legs, back pain, etc.)
- *Two gastrointestinal tract symptoms* (nausea, bloating, vomiting without pregnancy, diarrhea, gastric irritation)
- *One sexual function or genital system symptom* (menstrual irregularity, impotence in men, sexual aversion to women and men, etc.)
- *One neurological symptom* (impaired balance, regional paralysis or decreased strength, difficulty swallowing, double vision, deafness, loss of consciousness, etc.)
- *Lack of an organic disorder to explain these symptoms as a result of medical examination, laboratory investigations, and imaging methods*
- *No addiction to alcohol, drugs, or other substances*
- *Insecure and skeptical approach to psychiatric examination*
- Stress is one of the major causes of psychosomatic diseases. Stress causes many bodily functions to deteriorate or not work properly.
- The most common trigger of psychosomatic diseases is loss and separation.

The American Board of Medical Specialties and the American Psychiatry and Neurology Board have approved specialization in psychosomatic medicine in 2003. This decision has emphasized the importance of this field and also reintroduced the widespread use of the "psychosomatic" term [1–3].

The Diagnostic Criteria for Psychosomatic Research (DCPR) are considered to be more explanatory than the DSM-IV [1–3].

2. DCPR definition criteria

Persistent somatization subjects with a psychosomatic disorder are believed to have a higher incidence of other nonfunctional system (chronic fatigue) syndromes in the future with this approach, and these are called "multisomatoform disorder," "pure somatization," or "chronic somatization." The functional somatic symptoms secondary to a psychiatric disorder are as follows:

a. **Conversion symptoms**

b. **Anniversary reaction:** the anniversary reaction defines the somatic, emotional, and behavioral responses at the anniversary of the period where a loss has been suffered.

2.1 Abnormal behavior

a. **Health anxiety:** the health anxiety concept includes many different types of beliefs and fears related to illness and pain.

b. **Fear of illness:** fear of illness is the unsupported and persistent fear that a specific illness (such as AIDS or cancer) is present despite examination results and assurances to be contrary, as defined in the DCPR.

c. **Denial of illness:** the denial concept as specified in psychoanalytic theory is an ego defense mechanism against unpleasant thoughts. Denial has later been included in the emotion-focused coping strategies when faced with stressful conditions.

d. **Fear of death (thanatophobia):** this is a sudden feeling or belief that the subject is about to die despite the lack of a medical reason. It must not be confused with the fear of unavoidable death.

3. The psychological aspect of disease: psychological factors influencing medical conditions

Demoralization (lack of resistance): hopelessness is the most important aspect. There is a loss of the feeling of usefulness/effectiveness. Mood reactivity is usually preserved.

Alexithymia: alexithymia is a personality type that is characterized by difficulty in recognizing emotions, difficulty communicating, and a cognitive structure and operative thought that focuses on external focus and external center adaptation.

Type A behavior: Type A behavior leads to taking care of more work in continually shorter times. Coronary disorders are more common in these subjects. They have irritable mood and are impatient and agitated.

Irritable mood: irritable mood is characterized by decreased anger control and usually results in verbal or behavioral bursts of anger.

It is important to have knowledge about the pain and its variety before psychosomatic pain, because pain can cause psychosomatic problems as well as result.

Pain is thought to be an important clinical and socioeconomic problem all around the world. We investigated the incidence, prevalence, and economic burden of pain conditions in children, adolescents, and adults based on the electronic scanning of databases for articles published between 2000 and 2014 in this review. Differences in methodology and the epidemiological studies make it difficult to give precise predictions of prevalence and incidence; however, the economic burden of psychosomatic pain is clearly high. There is a need to develop concepts and methods to examine pain from a population perspective and to advance the development of pain prevention and management strategies. Family physicians and clinicians have great responsibilities in the diagnosis and treatment of pain and especially psychosomatic pain within this context. The participation of physicians in multidisciplinary training and studies is also a fundamental principle [3, 5].

It is appropriate to explain psychosomatic pain primarily in accordance with general principles. Pain is a defining characteristic in the diagnosis of many diseases. It can serve as an index of the symptoms and activity of the disease or diseases and as a prognostic indicator and a predictor of the use of health care for the underlying etiology [1, 2]. The International Association for the Study of Pain (IASP) and the World Health Organization (WHO) describe pain as “an unpleasant sensory and emotional experience associated with or described in relation to real or potential tissue damage or associated with such damage," "an unpleasant sensory and emotional experience associated with existing or possible tissue damage or associated with such damage," and "a protection mechanism" [2].

An overview of the epidemiology and economic burden of pain conditions in children, adolescents, and adults is summarized below under the relevant headings. The incidence and prevalence of pain conditions as well as the risk factors and the effect of pain on individuals have also been described. The wide range of pain con-ditions in clinical and research areas include pain in children and adolescents, spinal pain, neuropathic pain, musculoskeletal pain, and fibromyalgia/chronic diffuse pain. In addition to the factors associated with the prevalence of pain, the indi-vidual, economic, and social burden of pain conditions should also be considered.

4. Classification of pain

1. According to neurophysiological mechanisms
    a. Nociceptive
    b. Somatic
    c. Visceral
    d. Neuropathic (non-nociceptive) central or peripheral
    e. Psychogenic
2. According to the duration
    a. Acute
    b. Chronic
3. According to the etiologic factors
    a. Cancer pain
    b. Postherpetic neuralgia
    c. Pain due to sickle cell anemia
    d. Arthritis pain
4. According to the pain region
    a. Headache
    b. Facial pain
    c. Low back pain
    d. Pelvic pain

Before making a diagnosis of **psychogenic pain**, somatic pathology must be definitely eliminated. A diagnostic nerve block can be used for the diagnosis, and psychological or psychiatric conditions should be evaluated as a factor in pain etiology using the criteria in the DSM-IV and DCPR classifications. One must know the general pain definitions, classifications, and criteria well to be able act objectively when dealing with the diagnosis and criteria of psychosomatic pain. Psychosomatic pain is often found in the etiology together with the definitions provided below [1–3, 5].

5. Pain incidence and definition

Describing the epidemiology of pain is difficult because of the subjective nature of symptoms and the lack of consensus on the definitions of specific diagnoses and conditions. It is problematic to identify pain areas, especially with musculoskeletal pain. Many pain conditions are episodic, and the majority of patients express recurrent symptoms at varying intervals and durations during periods with and without pain. The actual incidence of most pain conditions may therefore remain unknown.

Similarly, study results vary due to differences in the identification of diffuse pain cases and the specific diagnosis. While case definitions may also vary depending on the duration, intensity, or psychological burden of pain in the patient, the diagnoses are based on subjective patient experience, clinical tests, or results of imaging and pathological studies. It may be difficult to compare studies reporting different periods of prevalence (e.g., timepoint, weekly, monthly, lifetime) [5].

6. The incidence and distribution of pain

6.1 Pain in children and adolescents

Pain conditions in children and adolescents have gradually become the focus of the scientific literature in recent years. The occurrence of pain in children evidence as indicates childhood or adolescence pain can predict adulthood pain. Children with pain discontinue their education or become withdrawn. Physical inactivity is a possible result. Low back pain, headache, and abdominal pain are the most common types of childhood and adolescence pain.

The reported 1-year incidence of low back pain in children and adolescents varies from 11.8 to 33.0% (median, 22.4%), while the 1-month prevalence varies from 9.8 to 36.0% (median, 22.9%). Since there are a lower number of studies on the prevalence of neck pain (49.0%) and upper back pain (30.0%), some doubt remains about the accuracy of these predictions. A systematic review of chronic pain epidemiology in children and adolescents (pain continuing for more than 3 months) has reported that the 1-month prevalence of chronic back pain was between 18.0 and 24.0% (median, 21.0%) [6–9]. In addition to these predic-tions obtained from systematic reviews, the 1-month prevalence of low back pain was reported to be 37.0% in more than 400,000 children and adolescents aged 11–15 years [10–14].

The predicted 1-month headache prevalence in children and adolescents is 26.0–69.0% (median, 47.5%) in systematic investigations. Swain et al. have reported this figure to be 54.1% in a survey based on 312 schools [15]. Recurrent abdominal pain (at least three episodes that limit the child's functions for at least 3 months) is the focus of most childhood and adolescence pain studies [16]. Recurrent abdominal pain prevalence has been reported as 0.3–19.0% (median, 8.4%) [17] and 3.8–41.2%

(median, 12.0%) [7]. Childhood and adolescence monthly multiple pain prevalence was 12.1–35.7% (median, 23.9%).

Further studies on pain epidemiology in children and adolescents are still required to evaluate the effect of age on the pain prevalence. The effects of the increased pain rates in childhood and adolescence and of the transition to adolescence on the incidence and prevalence of pain conditions are not clear at present [17].

6.2 Spinal pain

Spinal pain, and especially low back pain, is a common problem that most people experience at a certain point in their lives. The lifetime prevalence of low back pain is reported to be between 51.0 and 84.0%. There are many studies on the epidemiology of low back pain compared to other pain conditions.

Predictions for the 1-year first low back pain events varied between 6.3 and 15.4% (median, 10.9%) in one review [18] and between 13.5 and 26.2% (median, 19.9%) in others [11, 16, 18–22]. Predictions of the 1-year incidence of low back pain events (including patients with previous episodes) vary between 1.5 and 38.9% (median, 20.2%). Many people who experience activity-limiting low back pain recover quickly [23], but some have recurrent pains [24]. Predictions for the 1-year recurrence vary between 24.0 and 80.0% (median, 52.0%) [18].

Important information is present on the prevalence of low back pain. The 1-month prevalence is predicted to be between 24.0 and 49.5% (median, 36.8%) [25]. The prevalence of thoracic spine pain varies between 1.4 and 34.8% (median, 18.1%) [26], while the 1-month prevalence of neck pain varies between 15.4 and 45.3% (median, 30.4%) [27].

Chronic low back pain (CLBP) is usually defined as low back pain continuing for more than 12 weeks [28]. The prevalence of CLBP in the general European popula-tion has been predicted as 5.9–18.1% (median, 12%).

6.3 Neuropathic pain and sciatica

Neuropathic pain has been defined by the International Association for the Study of Pain as “pain caused by a lesion or disease of the somatosensory nervous system” [29]. It is differentiated from other inflammatory conditions by characteristic signs and symptoms such as “burning” or “freezing,” numbness, tingling, or “pins and needles” sensations [29]. There are only a few studies on the incidence and prevalence of neuropathic pain in the population.

Chronic pain with neuropathic features has a prevalence of 0.9–17.9% (median, 9.4%) [13]. Prevalence in cancer is 19.0–39.1% (median, 29.1%) [14]. The incidence is 3.9–42.0 per postherpetic neuralgia, 12.6–28.9 for trigeminal neuralgia, 0.2–0.4 for glossopharyngeal neuralgia, and 15.3–72.3 for painful diabetic periph-eral neuropathy, respectively, all per 100.000 person years [13].

Sciatica is also called radiculopathy, nerve root compression-irritation, nerve root pain, or lumbosacral radicular syndrome [30]. The pain is believed to arise in the lumbar spine but is felt in the leg pain by the patline. The 1-year sciatica incidence is reported as 9.3% [30]. The 1-month sciatica prevalence varies between 0.4 and 16.4% (median, 8.4%) [31].

6.4 Musculoskeletal pain

Musculoskeletal system disorders are among the most common causes of disability and incapacity, especially in the elderly [32]. Upper extremity pain is also common; monthly shoulder pain symptoms are present in 18.6–31.0% (median, 24.8%) of adults [33]. Monthly knee pain prevalence in adults is 13.0–28.0% (median, 20.5%) [34]. The prevalence was 28.0, 15.0, and 14.0% for foot ankle and toe pain in a review combining the reported figures [35].

6.5 Fibromyalgia and chronic diffuse pain

Chronic diffuse pain is defined as the presence of chronic pain with diffuse localization [36]. The American College of Rheumatology defines chronic diffuse pain as bilateral axial skeleton pain continuing for 3 months or more in its 1990 guidelines [37]. Fibromyalgia diagnostic criteria have been defined using the same definition [38]. Some fibromyalgia prevalence figures are 2.0–5.0% in the USA, 0.7% in Denmark, and 10.5% in Norwegian women. Fibromyalgia is a clinical diagnosis similar to other chronic pain conditions, and the lack of a clear definition therefore limits the comparison of prevalence predictions. The diagnostic criteria for fibromyalgia in the American College of Rheumatology's 2010 Criteria include the evaluation of diffuse pain together with the other symptoms (such as fatigue and cognitive symptoms) to develop a more specific case definition [38]. Future studies on the epidemiology of fibromyalgia are likely to increase the accuracy of current prevalence predictions by using this definition [39].

7. Prevalence tendencies over time

Only a few studies have evaluated the prevalence of pain conditions, and most have focused on the prevalence of low back pain. Palmer et al. [40] reported that the 1-year prevalence of low back pain increased by 12.7% over a 10-year period from 1987 to 1997, and this increase was associated with gender, age group, social class, and residence area. A contrasting decrease in the 1-month prevalence from 26.1 to 22.6% has been reported over a 7-year period in another study [41]. The chronic low back pain frequency In the USA has increased from 3.9 in 1992 to 10.2% in 2006 [42].

8. The effects of pain on health

Pain, and especially chronic pain, creates a significant burden for patients and their families. It adversely affects the general health perception, significantly inhibits daily activities, is associated with depressive symptoms, and significantly and negatively affects the relationships and interactions with others. The World Health Organization Global Burden of Disease uses the term "disability" to assess the potential for non-mortality-related disease. They define disability as any short- or long-term loss of health [43]. Disability-adjusted life years (DALYs) and years lived with disability (YLDs) are needed to measure and compare the limita-tions of a wide range of disorders associated with pain. Pain-related disorders that are characterized or defined by the presence of pain (low back pain, neck pain, other musculoskeletal disorders, migraine, and falls) constitute 5 of the top 10 conditions responsible for YLDs in the world. Acute low back pain has caused 83 million DALYs, and according to the effects of the chronic types of back pain, this constitutes 10.7% of all YLDs [43]. Neck pain and migraine/headache each account for about 24 million DALYs. Other musculoskeletal disorders are responsible for 28 million DALYs and traumas due to falls for 19 million DALYs. Other important con-tributions include osteoarthritis (17 million DALYs) and accident-related injuries

(13 million DALYs) [44]. These results for 1990 and 2010 supersede all previously published Global Burden of Disease results.

9. Risk factors for pain

It is difficult to determine the factors initiating pain episodes in the population as studies only specify an estimate due to the differences in the methodology and reporting. It is necessary to focus on the main risk categories such as age, gender, social group, and individual factors. Generally, there is no evidence for the risk factors of pain. Future studies that evaluate all aspects of the pain experience from both the individual and the population point of view are needed. These studies must employ multidimensional methods in the case of psychosomatic pain.

10. Age and gender

Studies on pain in children and adolescents have shown that females generally suffer more pain than males. The relationship between pain and gender is clear in adults. Females report more severe pain, more frequent pain, and longer-lasting pain than males in most studies. However, it is not known whether this gender difference is due to underlying biological pain mechanisms or the effects of psycho-logical and social factors.

As regards age, the prevalence of some pain disorders such as back pain increases from childhood to adolescence. The effect of age is not relevant on the pain preva-lence in the elderly as some studies report that it increases, while others report it decreases with age. The effect also varies by gender and the pain location [41]. It is believed that musculoskeletal pain is most common in adults in the employment age and the prevalence therefore decreases from the middle of the sixth decade [41]. However, recent studies have shown that pain continues to be a widespread and serious problem in the elderly. The prevalence of chronic pain in the active elderly (>65 years) varies between 25.0 and 76.0%, while it is much higher in the sedentary elderly at between 83.0 and 93.0% [41].

11. Social factors

The role of social factors continuously increases throughout life [45]. The socioeconomic status is usually measured by the complex created by education, income, and occupation. Many studies in children and adolescents have evaluated the relationship between pain and socioeconomic status, but there is some evidence of a conflict between these studies [7]. An inverse relationship is present between the socioeconomic status and pain prevalence in adults. The data show that lower educational status, low income, and being unemployed are related to increased pain prevalence [5].

More recently, pain prevalence studies have been conducted in populations of various cultural, ethnic, and socioeconomic statuses. Native Americans, Alaska Natives, and Aboriginal Canadians have been found to have a higher prevalence of pain than the general population of the United States [45]. Studies in Africa have found the 1-year prevalence of pain to be 33.0% in adolescents and 50.0% in adults [46]. This value is higher than reported in studies conducted in most Western countries (mean prevalence of 38.1%) [25]. However, it is difficult to make a definite comparison due to the differences in methodology. Another study based on the World Bank Human Development Index has reported the prevalence of chronic pain to be 24.8% in less developed countries and 28.1% in more developed countries [47].

12. Individual factors

Various individual risk factors have been associated with the development of pain disorders. The demands of employment, lack of job security, an immobile job position, dissatisfaction with work, low levels of social support at work, and vibrating bodily work conditions have been associated with various occupational factors that lead to musculoskeletal pain. Individual lifestyle factors that create health problems such as smoking and obesity can also play a role in the development of pain disorders [34]. The psychosocial variables believed to influence the pain prevalence include stress, anxiety, lack of sleep, depression, low self-confidence, and the presence of chronic health problems (irregular heartbeat, dizziness, pain, cardiovascular problems, gastrointestinal discomfort, erectile dysfunction, feeling of lump or pressure in the throat, chest problems, hallucinations, and double vision).

Pain and disorders that are not clearly attributable to an organic disease are called somatoform disorders. These disorders can be an expression of untreated mental pain and life experiences resulting from serious loss, profound personal injury, and disrespect. These symptoms occur in almost all humans, but they can become a serious problem in 4–20% of the population [1–3, 5–9, 48].

Genetic research on pain is increasing, and chronic pain is being seen as a classic example of the gene–environment interaction [49]. It is generally believed that the first trigger of chronic pain syndromes are inflammatory processes or nerve trauma. Once chronic pain develops, the pain intensity and response to analgesics are also quite variable. However, evidence is lacking regarding the influence of genetic effects and the interaction with psychosocial environmental factors as regards the development of chronic pain. Patients with chronic pain feel that the cause is life challenges, but the disease also makes life more difficult. This contradictory approach is related to the importance attributed to the pain. A person with intrapsychic conflict may not have to express the problem verbally and may have to use the organs to do so (alexithymia).

The presence of enhancers in the environment: one example is caring for one's wife when she has pain but not caring when she does not. Other examples are as follows: finding comfort by suffering pain for a bad action; excessive interest in pain and then relaxing when the test results are normal (somatization); and feeling sure an illness is present and changing physicians frequently (hypochondriasis).

Type A persons (hasty, impatient, hyperactive) perceive pain more easily than type B persons (calm, cool), probably due to autonomic hyperactivity. The risk of hypertension and coronary heart disease is 3–5 times higher in type A persons [50, 51].

13. The financial effects of pain

13.1 Total cost

The cumulative cost of chronic pain to the patient, the health-care system, and the economy is huge. In Australia, with a population of 22.7 million, the total annual cost of chronic pain was estimated as 34.3 billion dollars in 2007 or 10.847 dollars per person [52]. The total cost in Europe is estimated as 1.5–3.0% of the European GDP [53]. In the USA, approximately 100 million adults have been affected by chronic pain in 2008, including joint pain and arthritis [54]. The total cost in 2010 was 560–635 billion dollars. The annual cost of pain is higher than that of heart disease (309 billion dollars), cancer (243 billion dollars), and diabetes (188 billion dollars) [53, 55–60].

The term psychosomatic means the person. It combines two basic components, including the mind and the body. The reason is that physical complaints are at the forefront. However the research will investigate if there are any physical symptoms to explain such bodily complaints.

There is no medical illness, and this is a definable psychiatric disorder.

14. Examples of psychological problems seen with psychosomatic pain disorders

1. **Somatoform disorders:** (a) somatization disorder, (b) conversion disorder, (c) pain disorder, (d) hypochondriasis, and (e) body dysmorphic disorder

2. **Mood disorders:** (a) generalized anxiety disorder (objective anxiety, neurotic anxiety, or traumatic anxiety and moral anxiety), b) panic disorder, (c) agoraphobia, (d) dysthymic disorder, and (e) major depressive disorder

Pain experts still do not know whether pain is one of the senses or an experience. The fact that pain can be learned and that it can be affected by beliefs, expectations, and emotional states is quite important in its diagnosis and treatment. It is known that psychological disorders increase pain, while extreme fear, stress, and shock decrease pain. Many studies have reported that cultural norms and expectations play a major role in feeling pain and the related behavior.

The gate control system that monitors pain is especially influenced by neurotransmitter modulation that is associated with cortical stimulants in anxious subjects. The lack of an adequate 5-hydroxyl tryptamine (5HT) level in the synapse disturbs pain perception and decreases the pain threshold and pain tolerance [50, 51].

The physical and psychological problems of the person described under the following titles also play a role in psychosomatic pain.

Emotional crises. Emotional crises and chronic distress can lead to various psychosomatic complaints. The whole organism can be affected and the effects are therefore not listed here.

Somatoform pain disorder. Somatoform pain disorder is characterized by intense and agonizing pain that is subjectively felt in a part of the body for at least 6 months and that cannot be reasonably explained by a physical disorder or physiological event. The onset of the pain is related to a significant problem that has created serious emotional and/or psychosocial stress, conflict, or trauma. The increased interest in the person and the medical care received are the possible gains from the disorder. When compared with somatization disorders, these pains are long-lasting, and the patient focuses on them. The differential diagnosis of pain syndromes requires differentiation of organic physical pain from histrionic processing.

Dissociative disorder. The absence or modification of physical functions without a physical cause is usually the result of an intrapsychic conflict and can lead to psychogenic paralysis, coordination disorders, tremors, and myoclonus (muscle twitching).

Major depression. Major depression affects the entire body including the metabolism and the musculoskeletal system. Inactivity or pain syndromes may be present. The pain, lack of exercise, social withdrawal, smoking habits, and malnutrition lead to significant difficulties in the patient's life.

The patient comes to the doctor because of the somatic complaints as he/she has usually not noticed the depression: it is therefore not an independent disease. It is possible to determine the real psychic etiology during the examination if retrospective evaluations are also performed. Neurobiological studies have demonstrated that somatic symptoms are associated with brain dysfunction that is also responsible for depression. Psychological pain and emotional pain have been shown to cause activation of the same sites as physical pain stimuli on MR investigations.

Evaluation of the stress axis. The documentation of neuroendocrine abnormal-ities in cases of depression and pain have revealed the parallel course of the func-tional changes in depression and pain and the hypothalamus-hypophysis-adrenal axis with excess production of corticotropin-releasing hormone (CRH). It is also known that a deficiency in the serotonin and norepinephrine monoamines can play an important role in the decreased inhibition of pain pathways and the development of somatic symptoms in depression [50, 51].

Comorbid symptoms. Masked depression can have various symptoms. Urogenital system symptoms include dysuria, painful urination and defecation, signs of urinary and fecal incontinence, functional prostate problems (prostatitis), and bladder dysfunction in women without additional genital muscle weakness. There may also be upper abdominal discomfort, bloating, colic-like abdominal discomfort, stomach pain, and constipation [51].

Weakened immune system. Negative emotions such as fear and anger permanently weaken our immune system and defense. The risk of catching infections such as influenza increases many times, and wounds heal slower and in a worse manner.

Sleep disorders. Sleep problems are common when pain is present. Lack of sleep affects both the social life and performance of the patient. Fatigue can lead to depression and accidents. Sleep disorders have various signs such as difficulty falling asleep, waking up frequently and quickly, long period of staying awake during the night, being irritable, superficial sleep, loud and irregular snoring, leg restlessness, waking up early in the morning, and disturbing thoughts. Anger and hopelessness can also have a strong effect on sleep disorders.

It has recently been found that our brain is active in a very special manner during sleep. The brain sends impulses, produces active substances, and is involved in coding and storing data 24 h a day with its 100 billion nerve cells, and it is the organ that benefits most from a good night's sleep. This has been demonstrated with decreased brain capacity when we get little sleep. The first sign of cerebral fatigue is difficulty with concentrating and performing coordinated tasks such as driving or tasks that require a great deal of attention. We then become irritated and feel pain because of the related fatigue.

Sleep apnea. Snoring during sleep is present in 10–30% of adults and it is usually not dangerous. However, pauses in respiration during sleep are an indicator of sleep apnea syndrome, which affects approximately 3 million people in Germany alone. The most common type of the disorder is "obstructive sleep apnea." The pharyngeal muscles relax excessively and do not let air pass, leading to a pause in the respiration during sleep. This breathing problem goes on for about 2 min, usually with explo-sive snoring, and the subject then starts to breath normally again. In severe cases, these periods of paused respiration can recur hundreds of times every night. These patients are usually prone to falling asleep during the day, and the muscles can be weak and painful.

The most important diagnostic step in the diagnosis of sleep apnea syndrome is talking to the patient and family. In case of increased sleep apnea suspicion, the next step is a sleep laboratory investigation. Electrodes record the ECG, blood pres-sure, and brain waves; observe movements of the eyes and legs; measure the oxygen content of the blood; and record each snoring and breathing sound during this test.

Lungs: shortness of breath. Our breathing becomes quite shallow in case of stress, depression, or sadness. The lungs receive less oxygen and can provide less oxygen to the blood, increasing the risk of infection. Pneumonia is five times more common in the elderly than in healthy subjects.

Coronary heart disease and somatization disorder. Somatization disorder and pain syndromes develop after a heart attack in approximately 30% of all patients. A heart attack is experienced as a "spontaneous infarction." Physician appointments are frequently avoided and the recommended medication is not used. This increases the risk of new infarction development two to four times when added to the biologi-cal changes in the metabolism.

The infarction risk is increased several times (deaths due to a heart attack are four to five times more common in depression patients). The more severe the somatization disorders, the worse the prognosis of a heart disorder. Factors such as emotional stress, dissatisfaction with work and the partner, anxiety, and long-term stress increase the heart attack risk more than classical risk factors such as smoking and high blood pressure.

Hair problems. The reason for white hair is mineral deficiency in the hair and scalp, and there can be several causes: decreased nutrition due to age, acidity or nutritional disorder, and psychological reasons. Mineral intake is decreased with fear or stress, resulting in hair loss or white hair.

Skin disorders and skin structure problems. The metabolism slows down and the body functions deteriorate during stress. Free radicals that attack the skin cells and slow down the regeneration of the natural protective layer are created. The skin ages faster and spots develop. The face appears stressed.

Gastric disorders. Gastric absorption becomes difficult in patients with repressed emotions, anger, or anxiety. The stomach becomes tense with stress and anger, leading to increased gastric acid secretion. This in turn causes heartburn and can result in gastric ulcer, bloating, nausea, and cramps. Many subjects suffer from irritable stomach or irritable colon. Psychological components also play a role. Excitement and anxiety increase irritable stomach or irritable colon symptoms.

15. Examples of psychosomatic comorbidity in orthopedics

It is very important to investigate the relationship of psychosomatic pain in many patients admitted between orthopedics and traumatology clinics. In this context;

Osteoarthritis (arthrosis). Depression leads to a long period of internal stress and increased muscle tension, causing a predisposition to motility disorders, immobility, and arthritis. The patient usually sees an orthopedist before going to a neurologist.

Fractures and depression. Patients suffering from depression for a long time can be exposed to fractures more commonly as the mineral content of bone is decreased. Heavy psychological burdens can significantly decrease the blood oxygen content in the elderly as the breathing becomes superficial. The cells cannot receive adequate nutrition and renewal deteriorates. Inflammation and arthritis can develop in the joints.

Orthopedic pain syndromes. Orthopedic surgeons believe that back pain is the result of emotional problems, not organic ones, in most cases. If job dissatisfaction is high, the person feels overwhelmed and does not seek solutions to change the cir-cumstances, leading to a high risk of pain as the spinal system reacts very strongly to mental stress.

Neuropathic pain. Approximately 6% of Germans are affected by neuropathic pain. At least 20% of the patients at pain centers suffer from neuropathic pain syndromes. Peripheral neuropathies can commonly develop after postherpetic neuralgia or trauma. Generalized neuropathies include those due to chemotherapy and diabetic neuropathies.

Nociceptor pain. Nociception is the perception of pain. The responsible receptors are called nociceptors. Nociceptors are present in all the pain-sensitive tissues of the body as the free nerve ends of sensitive neurons of the spinal cord. Nociceptors trigger various types of pain according to their localizations:

- **Surface pain** is perceived superficially by the skin nociceptors. The pain can be clearly localized to the damaged region.

- **Severe pain** can be **muscle pain** or **bone pain** (localized in the periosteum) according to the localization of the nociceptors. It is poorly localized as deep pain due to the different fiber characteristics and the various projection areas of pain fibers.

- **Internal organ pain** develops following stimulation of nociceptive receptors in the internal organs. Classic examples are renal or biliary colic due to smooth muscle stretching.

Myofascial pain. Myofascial pain has local causes. Individual muscles are affected more intensely by chronic pain than muscle groups. Individual muscles contain trigger points that signify very sensitive areas. Overloading of the muscle can prevent excess calcium intake and the related muscle relaxation and therefore create localized oxygen deprivation.

Long-term contraction treatment becomes difficult in the case of myofascial pain. The sensitivity leads to the corresponding areas creating a perception of pain even with mild contact, and these areas are therefore called trigger points.

Excessive stress on such muscles can be the result of muscle damage, inadequate nutrition, hormonal imbalances, immobility, muscle weakness, hypothermia, contractions, and neurological damage.

Myofascial pain mainly develops in the **facial muscles, the neck muscles, the shoulder, and the pelvis region**. The trigger points can be activated spontaneously or with light pressure to make the diagnosis [61].

Psychotherapy in the treatment of pain can be explained as follows:

Patients with psychosomatic pain may have had a very disturbing experience in the past. This event can create links with the memory and senses, and the traumatic disorder may occur at any time when the present experience is once again domi-nant. Psychological stress may also cause physical illnesses. Within the soul-soma-soul sequence, an ever-growing chain of causes can be present. Life-threatening diseases such as cancer or myocardial infarction and the relevant medical interven-tions can also lead to mental trauma.

Traumas, undesirable social experiences, accidents, or stressful experiences have been scientifically proven to be the most common triggers and the causes of many physical disorders, pain, and other illnesses without a physical cause.

Changes related to psychological trauma in the brain can now be scientifically demonstrated by imaging (such as fMRI, a magnetic resonance method) and other diagnostic methods. Brain structure and brain metabolism are altered by the corresponding changes in the autonomic nervous system during the stress process. The entire spectrum of mental trauma should be considered. Psychotherapy for psychosomatic pain due to trauma is performed in three stages and with multiple sessions.

There are some fundamental differences between type I and type II trauma.

Type I trauma is a one-time event such as a traffic accident. The result is a short-term mental balance disorder such as adaptation disorder or posttraumatic stress disorder (PTSD). The patient will not forget the accident and will, for example, be afraid of driving. However, the disorder is also accompanied by physical symptoms (sweating, palpitation, sleep disorders, etc.).

Recurrent trauma (type II trauma) can lead to complicated disorders from all types of neurosis to emotional disorders, anxiety disorders, and phobias, in addition to personality disorders and changes or dependence on psychotropic drugs. Type II trauma can develop after life-threatening disorders such as cancer or myocardial infarction or as a result of chronic diseases. Intensive or long-term medical treat-ment can lead to helplessness in patients with psychosomatic pain.

The results of type II trauma include the consequences of childhood and long-term adult violence. This violence can also be mental as seen with coldness, extreme violence and indifference, emotional wounds, and frequently repeated trauma, especially in childhood. Type II traumas can lead to complex symptoms as in borderline disorder with comorbidities.

A three-stage model is used for the treatment of disorders that are psychosomatic or accompanied by pain. These stages consist of **stabilization**, **confrontation**, and **integration**.

It is not mandatory to include each stage in every treatment process. Stabilization is the foundation of all treatment steps. It can be integrated into other therapeutic methods such as specific interventions for trauma, behavioral therapy, systemic treatment, or deep psychology-associated therapies.

Stabilization stage. Sufficient time is allocated to get to know the patient and to create the basis of trauma therapy while building a mutually trusting relationship.

The stabilization stage creates a foundation for a common understanding of the clinical picture. An objective viewpoint is obtained about the emotions as much as possible. Anxiety and depression are responses to psychologically disturbing experiences and the emotional dissociations within the patient or those around him/her. An emergency state plan is developed together with the patient at this stage. Relaxation techniques such as meditation or Jacobson's progressive muscle relaxation are then used as guides for self-passivation techniques, and the patient thus learns the relevant methods to use the powers of healing within.

Confrontation stage. Behavioral therapy for the confrontation state has been specifically designed to treat phobias and anxiety. Cognitive behavioral therapy and especially systematic desensitization techniques are used. The aim is to re-evaluate the traumatizing event.

Special therapeutic procedures for trauma are also used such as eye movement desensitization and reprocessing (EMDR), imagery rescripting and reprocessing therapy (IRRT), and psychodynamic imaginative trauma therapy (PITT).

Eye movement desensitization and reprocessing has been developed by the American psychologist Francine Shapiro (* 1948). The literary translation indic-ates "eye movement, desensitization and reprocessing." This method is not hy-pnosis. When the patient focuses on an especially stressful stage of the emotionally traumatic experience, the therapist slowly asks the patient to perform rhythmic eye movements by slowly moving his fingers and gives the patient confidence. This stimulates cerebral processes. The aim is to decrease and even eliminate the fears produced by the memories. More than 20 controlled studies have shown the long-term effect of EMDR. EMDR is also included in guidelines as a preferred procedure.

Imagery rescripting and reprocessing therapy has been developed by the American clinical psychologist Mervin Smucker (* 1949). A traumatizing experience is created together with the therapies as though it had happened today. The patient imagines how he dealt with it in the past and how he is dealing with it now. The patients no longer view themselves as helpless victims and feel they are the designers of the condition who can act and maintain control even in the most difficult situations. We can think about it as deleting an old text and then writing over it.

Psychodynamic imaginative trauma therapy has been developed by psychoanalyst Luise Reddemann (* 1943). PITT is based on the idea that people have self-regulating powers to cope with disturbing events even after terrible experiences. Establishing a supportive therapeutic relationship is very important for such self-understanding, and it is also important for helping oneself. At the heart of PITT's therapeutic approach is the "internal phase" that the person is currently acting on.

In this mental "imaginary" game, the patient confronts the previous ego states with the therapist's support. Understanding the multiple egos in the consciousness comes from a scientific and philosophical tradition that has been present in all cultures for a thousand years, and the treatment relies on a systemic approach to therapy. With PITT, you can experience the injustice you have experienced and the area where you feel helpless from a safe distance. The patient learns to accept this part of his personality and to relax and make others relax at the same time. The patient also learns to heal his/her emotional wounds and therefore regains his/her confidence.

Symbol work: the study of symbols has been developed by psychotherapist Maria-Elisabeth Wollschläger and theologian Gerhard Wollschläger in the 1970s. If you associate a certain feeling with an object such as a chair, a doll, or something else, that item becomes the symbol of your senses. Symbol work is used in places where the traumatizing event can leave you speechless and where you cannot find the words to describe your mental wounds, what happened to you, and your anger, grief, or helplessness. By transferring your emotions to objects or using the object to present them, you can activate the brain areas responsible for mental processing. Conditions of loss, for example, can increase a person's confidence in his/her abili-ties. You regain your ability to move and to understand that what you are doing has a meaning, enabling further progress (self-efficacy).

Integration stage. This is the moment the joy of living and the relevant control are regained and understood.

The aim of this stage is to gradually integrate the traumatic experiences of the patient into his/her consciousness. These events are parts of the person's life, and control over life and social integration can be achieved once again by confronting these events [4, 61–64].

16. Conclusion

Our understanding of the epidemiology of psychosomatic pain is limited to a small number of studies that provide estimates of the prevalence in the general population. These studies are usually difficult and costly to conduct and require very large samples. The way data is collected and reported may also have an impact on the estimates with various results obtained from studies that depend on surveys, interviews, or clinical investigations. Large-scale population-based studies can provide richer data related to the age and gender distribution of pain, and assessments over extended periods of time can provide comprehensive information about the incidence and risk factors. Epidemiological studies in various cultural, social, and ethnic groups can clarify the effects and also the interactions between the indi-vidual and population-based risk factors. Physicians should be able to understand the information related to psychosomatic pain, search the relevant information available, and perform research on the subject themselves.

> *"The biggest misconception of today is the separation of the mind and body by physicians."* - *Socrates*

> *"What influences us is not the events themselves but the meanings we assign to them."* - *Epictetus*

Author details

Ertuğrul Allahverdi
Department of Orthopedics and Traumatology, School of Medicine, Kafkas University, Kars, Turkey

*Address all correspondence to: ertugrulallahverdi@hotmail.com

References

[1] Güleç MY. Temperament and character in psychosomatic disorders. Current Approaches in Psychiatry. 2009;**1**:201-214

[2] Porcelli P, Rafanelli C. Criteria for psychosomatic research (*DCPR*) in the medical setting. Current Psychiatry Reports. 2010;**12**(3):246-254

[3] Aral G, Arslan FC. A new operational guide against to traditional classification systems in Consultation-Liaison psychiatry: Diagnostic criteria for psychosomatic research (DCPR). Klinik Psikiyatri Dergisi.

[4] Lazarus RS. From psychological stress to the emotions: A history of changing books. Annual Review of Psychology. 1993;**44**:1-22

[5] Henschke N, Kamper SJ, Maher CG. The epidemiology and economic consequences of pain. Mayo Clinic Proceedings. 2015;**90**(1):139-147.

[6] McBeth J, Jones K. Epidemiology of chronic musculoskeletal pain. Best Practice & Research. Clinical Rheumatology. 2007;**21**:403-425

[7] King S, Chambers CT, Huguet A, et al. The epidemiology of chronic pain in children and adolescents revisited: A systematic review. Pain. 2011;**152**:2729-2738

[8] Jeffries LJ, Milanese SF, Grimmer-Somers KA. Epidemiology of adolescent spinal pain: A systematic overview of the research literature. Spine (Phila Pa 1976).

[9] Palermo TM. Impact of recurrent and chronic pain on child and family daily functioning: A critical review of the literature. Journal of Developmental and Behavioral Pediatrics. 2000;**21**:58-69

[10] Hestbaek L, Leboeuf-Yde C, Kyvik KO, Manniche C. The course of low back pain from adolescence to adulthood: Eight-year follow-up of 9600 twins. Spine (Phila Pa 1976). 2006; **31**:468-472

[11] Juniper M, Le TK, Mladsi D. The epidemiology, economic burden, and pharmacological treatment of chronic low back pain in France, Germany, Italy, Spain and the UK: A literature-based review. Expert Opinion on Pharmacotherapy. 2009;**10**:2581-2592

[12] Reid KJ, Harker J, Bala MM, et al. Epidemiology of chronic non-cancer pain in Europe: Narrative review of prevalence, pain treatments and pain impact. Current Medical Research and Opinion. 2011;**27**:449-462

[13] van Hecke O, Austin SK, Khan RA, Smith BH, Torrance N. Neuropathic pain in the general population: A systematic review of epidemiological studies. Pain. 2014;**155**:654-662

[14] Bennett MI, Rayment C, Hjermstad M, Aass N, Caraceni A, Kaasa S. Prevalence and aetiology of neuropathic pain in cancer patients: A systematic review.

[15] Swain MS, Henschke N, Kamper SJ, Gobina I, Ottová-Jordan V, Maher CG. An international survey of pain in adolescents. BMC Public Health. 2014; **14**:447

[16] Apley J, Naish N. Recurrent abdominal pains: A field survey of 1,000 school children. Archives of Disease in Childhood. 1958;**33**:165-170

[17] Fearon P, Hotopf M. Relation between headache in childhood and physical and psychiatric symptoms in adulthood: National birth cohort study. BMJ. 2001;**322**:1145

[18] Carragee EJ, Alamin TF, Miller JL, Carragee JM. Discographic, MRI and psychosocial determinants of low back pain disability and remission: A prospective study in subjects with benign persistent back pain. The Spine Journal. 2005 Jan-Feb;5(1):24-35

[19] Calvo-Muñoz I, Gómez-Conesa A, Sánchez-Meca J. Prevalence of low back pain in children and adolescents: A meta-analysis. BMC Pediatrics. 2013;**13**:14

[20] Taylor JB, Goode AP, George SZ, Cook CE. Incidence and risk factors for first-time incident low back pain: A systematic review and meta-analysis.

[21] Briggs AM, Smith AJ, Straker LM, Bragge P. Thoracic spine pain in the general population: Prevalence, incidence and associated factors in children, adolescents and adults; a systematic review.

[22] Hogg-Johnson S, van der Velde G, Carroll LJ, et al. The burden and determinants of neck pain in the general population.

[23] Henschke N, Maher CG, Refshauge KM, et al. Prognosis in patients with recent onset low back pain in Australian primary care: Inception cohort study.

[24] Pengel LH, Herbert RD, Maher CG, Refshauge KM. Acute low back pain: Systematic review of its prognosis. BMJ. 2003;**327**:32

[25] Hoy D, Brooks P, Blyth F, Buchbinder R. The epidemiology of low back pain. Best Practice & Research. Clinical Rheumatology. 2010;**24**:769-781

[26] Briggs AM, Smith AJ, Straker LM, Bragge P. Thoracic spine pain in the general population: Prevalence, incidence and associated factors in children, adolescents and adults; a systematic review. BMC Musculoskeletal Disorders. 2009;**10**:77

[27] Hogg-Johnson S, van der Velde G, Carroll LJ, et al. The burden and determinants of neck pain in the general population. European Spine Journal. 2008;**17**:39-51

[28] Furlan AD, Pennick V,Bombardier C, van Tulder M, Editorial Board, Cochrane Back Review Group. Updated method guidelines for syst-ematic reviews in the Cochrane Back Review Group. Spine (Phila Pa 1976). 2009;**34**:1929-1941

[29] Berk HÖS. Kronik Ağrı Yaşantısı Ve Ağrı İnançları: Ağrı İnançları Ölçeğinin Türkçe Geçerlik Ve Güvenirlik Çalişması [PhD thesis]. Turkey: Istanbul University; 2006

[30] Cook CE, Taylor J, Wright A, Milosavljevic S, Goode A, Whitford M. Risk factors for first time incidence sciatica: A systematic review. Physiotherapy Research International. 2014; **19**(2):65-78.

[31] Konstantinou K, Dunn KM. Sciatica: Review of epidemiological studies and prevalence estimates. Spine (Phila Pa 1976). 2008;**33**(22):2464-2472.

[32] Coggon D, Ntani G, Palmer KT, et al. Disabling musculoskeletal pain in working populations: Is it the job, the person, or the culture? Pain. 2013;**154**: 856-863

[33] Luime JJ, Koes BW, Hendriksen IJ, et al. Prevalence and incidence of shoulder pain in the general population: A systematic review. Scandinavian Journal of Rheumatology. 2004;**33**: 73-81

[34] Peat G, McCarney R, Croft P. Knee pain and osteoarthritis in older adults:

A review of community burden and current use of primary health care. Annals of the Rheumatic Diseases. 2001;**60**:91-97

[35] Thomas MJ, Roddy E, Zhang W, Menz HB, Hannan MT, Peat GM. The population prevalence of foot and ankle pain in middle and old age: A systematic review.

[36] Cimmino MA, Ferrone C, Cutolo M. Epidemiology of chronic musculoskeletal pain. Best Practice & Research: Clinical Rheumatology. 2011;**25**:173-183

[37] Arnold LM, Clauw DJ, McCarberg BH, Fibro Collaborative. Improving the recognition and diagnosis of fibromyalgia. Mayo Clinic Proceedings. 2011;**86**:457-464

[38] Freburger JK, Holmes GM, Agans RP, et al. The rising prevalence of chronic low back pain. Archives of Internal Medicine. 2009;**169**:251-258

[39] Froud R, Patterson S, Eldridge S, et al. A systematic review and meta-synthesis of the impact of low back pain on people's lives. BMC Musculoskeletal Disorders. 2014;**15**:50

[40] Palmer KT, Walsh K, Bendall H, Cooper C, Coggon D. Back pain in Britain: Comparison of two prevalence surveys at an interval of 10 years. BMJ. 2000;**320**:1577-1578

[41] Macfarlane GJ, McBeth J, Garrow A, Silman AJ. Life is as much a pain as it ever was. BMJ. 2000;**321**:897

[42] Froud R, Patterson S, Eldridge S, et al. A systematic review and meta-synthesis of the impact of low back pain on people's lives. BMC Musculoskeletal Disorders. 2014;**15**:50

[43] Murray CJ, Vos T, Lozano R, et al. Disability-adjusted life years (DALYs) for 291 diseases and injuries in 21 regions, 1990-2010: analysis for the Global Burden of Disease Study 2010. Lancet. 2012;**380**: 2197-2223

[44] Macfarlane TV, Glenny AM, Worthington HV. Systematic review of population-based epidemiological studies of oro-facial pain. Journal of Dentistry. 2001;**29**:451-467

[45] Jimenez N, Garroutte E, Kundu A, Morales L, Buchwald D. A review of the experience, epidemiology, and management of pain among American Indian, Alaska Native, and Aboriginal Canadian peoples. The Journal of Pain. 2011;**12**:511-522

[46] Louw QA, Morris LD, Grimmer-Somers K. The prevalence of low back pain in Africa: A systematic review. BMC Musculoskeletal Disorders. 2007; **8**:105

[47] Elzahaf RA, Tashani OA, Unsworth BA, Johnson MI. The prevalence of chronic pain with an analysis of countries with a Human Development Index less than 0.9: A systematic review without meta-analysis. Current Medical Research and Opinion. 2012;**28**:1221-1229

[48] Hush JM, Nicholas M, Catherine M. Embedding the IASP pain curriculum into a 3-year pre-licensure physical therapy program: Redesigning pain education for future clinicians. Pain Reports. 2018;**3**(2):e645

[49] Côté P, van der Velde G, Cassidy JD, Carroll LJ, Hogg-Johnson S, Holm LW, et al. The burden and determinants of neck pain in workers: Results of the bone and joint decade 2000-2010 task force on neck pain and its associated disorders. Spine (Phila Pa 1976).

[50] Morris CG. Psikolojiyi Anlamak/ Understanding Psychology. Third Edition. Türk Psikologlar Derneği Yay. No: 23 2002-Ankara

[51] Lopez-lber JJ. Masked depression. British Journal of Psychiatry. 1972;**120**:254-257

[52] Limited AEP. The High Price of Pain: The Economic Impact of Persistent Pain in Australia. Sydney, Australia: Access Economics Pty Limited; 2007

[53] Phillips CJ. Economic burden of chronic pain. Expert Review of Pharmacoeconomics & Outcomes Research. 2006;**6**:591-601

[54] Gaskin DJ, Richard P. The economic costs of pain in the United States. The Journal of Pain. 2012; **13**:715-724

[55] Reid KJ, Harker J, Bala MM, et al. Epidemiology of chronic non-cancer pain in Europe: Narrative review of prevalence, pain treatments and pain impact. Current Medical Research and Opinion. 2011;**27**:449-462

[56] Mogil JS. Pain genetics: Past, present and future. Trends in Genetics. 2012;**28**:258-266

[57] Engbers LH, Vollenbroek-Hutten MM, van Harten WH. A comparison of patient characteristics and rehabilitation treatment content of chronic low back pain (CLBP) and stroke patients across six European countries. Health Policy. 2005;**71**: 359-373

[58] Dagenais S, Caro J, Haldeman S. A systematic review of low back pain cost of illness studies in the United States and internationally. The Spine Journal. 2008;**8**:8-20

[59] Schofield DJ, Shrestha RN, Passey ME, Earnest A, Fletcher SL. Chronic disease and labour force participation among older Australians. The Medical Journal of Australia. 2008.

[60] Vet HC, Heymans MW, Dunn KM, et al. Episodes of low back pain: A proposal for uniform definitions to be used in research. Spine (Phila Pa 1976). 2002;**27**:2409-2416

[61] Emre M, Mathies H, Radvila A. Psychogenic aspects of muscle spasms and pain. Muscle spasms and pain. The Parthenon Publishing Group, New Jersey. 1988;**5**:43-46

[62] Ettlin T, Kischka U. Psychosomatic Rehabilitation: An Overview. Therapeutische Umschau. German. 2019; **76**(8):460-464.

[63] Gomez J. “Pain” Liaison Psychiatry, Mental Health Problems in the General Hospital. London: The Free Press; 1987.

[64] Schmidt AJM. Cognitive factors in the performance level of chronic low back pain patients. Journal of Psychosomatic Research. 1985;**29**: 183-189

11

Assessment and Treatment of Combat-Related Posttraumatic Stress Disorder: Results from STRONG STAR and the Consortium to Alleviate PTSD

Alan L. Peterson, Barbara L. Niles,
Stacey Young-McCaughan and Terence M. Keane

Abstract

Extensive research has been conducted since 11 September 2001 to develop and evaluate evidence-based treatments for combat-related posttraumatic stress disorder (PTSD) in active duty United States military personnel treated in the combat theater and in garrison. This chapter reviews the results of 20 PTSD clinical trials funded by the United States Department of Defense and Department of Veterans Affairs on the treatment of combat-related PTSD. All of the studies were conducted under the leadership and management of two research consortia: the South Texas Research Organizational Network Guiding Studies on Trauma and Resilience (STRONG STAR) Consortium and the Consortium to Alleviate PTSD.

Keywords: posttraumatic stress disorder, PTSD, acute stress disorder, combat and operational stress reactions

1. Introduction

Posttraumatic stress disorder (PTSD) is a common psychiatric disorder that occurs in about 7% of the adult population after exposure to a significant traumatic event [1, 2]. Combat-related PTSD occurs as a result of exposure to military combat or other traumas experienced during military deployments. The rate of combat-related PTSD in active duty military personnel and veterans who have deployed to a combat theater of operations is about double the rate of PTSD seen in civilians. [3–6]. Prior to the terrorist attacks on the United States on September 11, 2001, most research on PTSD had been conducted with civilian and veteran populations, with a striking absence of clinical trials conducted in active duty military popula-tions with combat-related PTSD. The need for such studies was acute because, although there are many similarities in the assessment and treatment of PTSD in civilian, veteran, and military samples, active duty personnel represent a distinct population with specific characteristics and needs. In the early- and mid-2000s, it was unclear whether methods and treatments developed for civilians would suc-cessfully translate to military personnel returning from warzones.

Combat-related PTSD in service members differs from PTSD in other populations. As compared to most civilian populations [7–9], considerable research suggests that combat-related PTSD in service members and veterans is more difficult to treat and results in a smaller percentage of patients achieving significant reductions in symptoms [10–13]. In addition, the types of traumatic events experienced in warzones are often different than for civilians [14–16] and the frequency, intensity, and duration of trauma exposure are often greater.

There are also several factors that distinguish PTSD in active duty military populations from PTSD in veteran populations and that may affect treatment and assessment. Veterans have completed their military service, are not at risk for additional combat deployments, and may receive disability compensation for their PTSD symptoms and diagnoses. Active duty military personnel with PTSD who wish to continue their military careers are faced with unique obstacles and chal-lenges. Many service members actively avoid seeking treatment for PTSD because of the negative stigma associated with mental health treatment and concerns that a PTSD diagnosis might affect career advancement and lead to a premature discharge. Notably, U.S. military personnel who complete a minimum of 20 years of active duty service are eligible to retire at a relatively young age with a sizeable lifelong retirement pension that is often more than half of their active duty base pay in addition to other retirement benefits such a lifetime medical coverage. With few exceptions, military personnel who serve less than 20 years active service receive no military pension or benefits. As a result, there is a strong desire and incentive for many military personnel to serve on active duty for at least 20 years to be eligible for full military retirement benefits, and many are reluctant to seek care that may jeopardize this.

Assessment of PTSD relies on accurate report of symptoms, and the particular circumstances of active duty service members who do seek out treatment may impact how symptoms are reported. Many on active duty have a strong desire to be treated into remission so they can remain fully fit to continue their military service. However, there are undoubtedly some service members who actively seek a diagnosis of PTSD that will lead to separation from active duty and some compensation through a military medical disability. Despite considerable clinical and research efforts, the ability to distinguish between service members seeking continued active duty service versus those who seek a medical separation has remained difficult, and the current method is to simply ask service members their career intentions. In either instance, the service member's future career objective is challenging, but critical for the clinician to assess.

To address the lack of research on combat-related PTSD in active duty military personnel, the U.S. Congress allocated funding to Department of Defense (DoD) in 2007 through the Congressionally Directed Medical Research Programs to establish a Multidisciplinary PTSD Research Consortium. After a competitive peer-reviewed process, the STRONG STAR (South Texas Research Organizational Network Guiding Studies on Trauma And Resilience) Consortium was awarded DoD research funding in 2008 to establish a nationwide PTSD research consortium. STRONG STAR is a multidisciplinary and multi-institutional research consortium focused on the detection, diagnosis, prevention, and treatment of combat PTSD and related conditions (e.g., traumatic brain injury, sleep disorders, chronic pain, substance use disorders, suicide, etc.) in active-duty military personnel and veterans, www.STRONGSTAR.org.

The initial STRONG STAR funding supported 14 research projects and 4 research cores. STRONG STAR investigators subsequently secured additional investigator-initiated, peer-reviewed research funding through the DoD, the Department of Veterans Affairs (VA), the National Institutes of Health, and private organizations to support over 40 additional STRONG STAR-affiliated projects. In 2013, STRONG STAR investigators partnered with the VA's National Center for PTSD and were selected for joint funding by the DoD and VA to establish the Consortium to Alleviate PTSD (CAP). The CAP extended the STRONG STAR Consortium with 11 additional research projects: www.ConsortiumToAlleviatePTSD.org.

This chapter first reviews the assessment measures used to assess PTSD in the STRONG STAR and CAP studies. Next, the results of 20 STRONG STAR and CAP PTSD clinical trials evaluating a variety of treatments for combat-related PTSD in active duty military personnel and veterans are summarized.

2. The assessment of PTSD in military populations

2.1 Clinician-Administered PTSD Scale for *DSM-5*

The Clinician-Administered PTSD Scale for *DSM-5* (CAPS-5) [17, 18] is the gold-standard structured clinical diagnostic interview for assessing PTSD. The CAPS-5 is a 30-item structured clinical interview designed to be administered by a trained clinical interviewer and requires about 45–60 minutes to administer. Administration of the CAPS-5 requires the initial identification of a *DSM-5* Criterion A index traumatic event. It uses a 5-point ordinal rating scale to assess symptom the severity of the 20 PTSD symptoms included in the *DSM-5*. The CAPS-5 score can range from 0–80 with higher scores representing greater symptom severity. However, a diagnosis of PTSD is made only if the individual is experiencing ≥1 intrusion, ≥1 avoidance, ≥2 negative cognitions and mood, and ≥ 2 arousal and reactivity symptom all at a severity rating of ≥2. The CAPS-5 has strong inter-rater reliability (N = 78; *Cohen's kappa* = .90), and the correlation of severity scores between raters is excellent (r = .98) [19].

2.2 PTSD Checklist for *DSM-5*

The PTSD Checklist for *DSM-5* (PCL-5) [20] is a self-report measure of the 20 PTSD symptoms included in the *DSM-5*. Similar to the CAPS-5, it uses a 5-point ordinal rating scale to measure symptom severity with a range from 0–80. The PCL-5 can be scored in several ways, and interpretation should be made by a clinician. Initial research suggests that total scores between 31 and 33 on the PCL-5 are indicative of probable PTSD. A provisional diagnosis of PTSD can be made by summing each of the five *DSM-5* symptoms clusters with items endorsed as a 2 (Moderately) or higher and then following the *DSM-5* diagnostic guidelines. The PCL-5 has excellent psychometric characteristics for screening and as a secondary indicator of PTSD symptom severity [21, 22].

2.3 Primary Care PTSD Screen for *DSM-5*

The Primary Care PTSD Screen for *DSM-5* (PC-PTSD-5) [23] is a 5-item measure to screen for PTSD symptoms and was designed to be administered in primary care settings. The measure begins with one item to evaluate previous exposure to a potentially traumatic event. It then includes five additional yes-no items related to key PTSD symptoms. Validation studies suggest that a cut-off point of 3 on the PC-PTSD-5 is optimally sensitive for probable PTSD. Individuals who screen posi-tive should be further evaluated with the PCL-5 or CAPS-5.

2.4 Assessment of trauma types in military personnel

Due to the unique aspects of combat- or deployment-related PTSD, the STRONG STAR investigators developed a scheme for categorizing traumatic military events [14–16]. The categorization of Criterion-A event descriptions is completed by CAPS-5 trained diagnostic interviewers. The traumatic military events are then categorized into six types of military-related Criterion-A events including (1) life-threat to self, (2) life-threat to others, (3) traumatic loss, (4) exposure to the after-math of violence, (5) moral injury by self, and (6) moral injury by others. Research is ongoing to determine if different military trauma types respond differently to evidence-based treatments for combat-related PTSD.

2.5 The use of common data elements for PTSD research

A recent development to standardize the assessment and outcome measures that are used in PTSD research is to administer what are called *Common Data Elements*, or *CDEs* [24]. When different measures are used across studies, it makes it difficult to interpret the findings. The use of CDEs helps allow for the comparison of find-ings across different research studies. A major benefit of research studies conducted as part of the STRONG STAR Consortium and the Consortium to Alleviate PTSD is the use of CDEs for PTSD research [19]. This strategy also increases the possible use of future metanalytic strategies to understand the impact of various psychothera-peutic approaches in the treatment of PTSD.

3. The treatment of combat-related PTSD in military populations

At the time of the initial funding of the STRONG STAR Consortium by the DoD in 2008, no clinical trials existed to evaluate any form of treatment for combat-related PTSD in active duty military forces. Precious few randomized trials for PTSD treatment in veterans were in the published scientific literature. As a result, STRONG STAR investigators evaluated the published literature on the treatment of PTSD in civilian and veteran populations to help guide the initial studies of combat-related PTSD in active duty military personnel. The 2008 publication by the Institute of Medicine [3] titled the *Treatment of Posttraumatic Stress Disorder: An Assessment of the Evidence* provided an excellent state-of-the science review of the research literature at the time. That IOM committee report reviewed 52 psycho-therapy studies and 37 pharmacotherapy studies and concluded, *"The committee finds that the evidence is sufficient to conclude the efficacy of exposure therapies in the treatment of PTSD"* [3].

Two cognitive-behavioral treatments were highlighted as the treatments with the strongest scientific support for their efficacy—Prolonged Exposure (PE) [25, 26] and Cognitive Processing Therapy (CPT) [27–29]. As a result, PE and CPT were the two treatments identified as leading candidates to be evaluated in randomized clinical trials in active duty military populations with combat-related PTSD.

Prolonged Exposure [30, 31] is a cognitive-behavioral therapy that includes four primary components: (1) imaginal exposure, or the repeated revisiting of the trauma memories, (2) in vivo exposure, or repeated exposure to avoided situations, (3) psychoeducation about common reactions to trauma, and (4) relaxed breathing. The standard treatment program includes 10 to 12 individual treatment sessions of 90 minutes each conducted once or twice a week.

Cognitive Processing Therapy is another cognitive-behavioral therapy that is usually delivered in 12 treatment sessions over the course of 6 weeks, with each session lasting 1 hour [32]. CPT begins with psychoeducation about PTSD symptoms and making connections between events, thoughts, and feelings. Patients write an "impact statement" in which they describe why they think the traumatic event happened and how the event has affected their view of themselves, others, and the world. Throughout CPT, unhelpful cognitions are identified and challenged through Socratic questioning until more helpful and accurate beliefs can replace distorted cognitions. The final five sessions of CPT focus on cognitions related to safety, trust, power, esteem, and intimacy.

A summary of the STRONG STAR and CAP clinical trials is provided in **Table 1**.

3.1 Treating combat-related PTSD in the combat theater

The first clinical case series to report on the treatment of combat-related PTSD in the combat theater [33, 34] used a modified version of Prolonged Exposure [25] that was adapted for the deployed environment. The results showed that PE could be safely and effectively delivered in the deployed environment to allow service members to return to combat duties and complete their deployments. The promising results from this case series led to the funding of a larger nonrandomized clinical trial as part of the STRONG STAR Consortium to evaluate the use of PE and CPT in Iraq and Afghanistan for the treatment of 12 service members with combat-related PTSD [35]. All patients were treated by military behavioral health provid-ers deployed to the combat theater using modified versions of PE ($n = 6$) or CPT ($n = 6$). Because this study was conducted prior to the publication of the PCL-5, the PTSD Checklist-Military Version (PCL-M) was used [36, 37], which was based on *DSM-IV* criteria and asks about symptoms in response to "stressful military experiences." The results showed that both treatments demonstrated clinically significant change in PTSD symptoms on the PCL-M.

Despite the small sample size ($N = 12$), this prospective, nonrandomized trial is the largest study to date to evaluate the treatment of combat-related PTSD in the deployed combat theater. Previous military operational guidelines limited the use of trauma-focused treatments such as PE and CPT and recommended not treating PTSD until military service members returned from their deployments [38]. These recent findings should be considered in future military guidelines on the treatment of combat operational stress reactions and combat-related PTSD in the military combat theater.

3.2 Treating combat-related PTSD in military personnel in garrison

3.2.1 Prolonged Exposure Therapy

The first study to evaluate the efficacy of PE for the treatment of combat-related PTSD in active duty military personnel treated in garrison (i.e., at their non-deployed, home duty location) included 366 active duty US Army soldiers treated at Fort Hood, in Killeen, Texas. The study [39] was a 4-armed RCT to evaluate: (1) the standard delivery format of PE, which was referred to as Spaced PE ($n = 109$; 10 weekly 90-minute PE sessions); (2) a non-trauma focused active comparison condi-tion called Present Centered Therapy (PCT; $n = 107$; 10 weekly 90-minute PCT sessions); (3) a compressed, daily format of PE called Massed PE ($n = 110$; 10 daily 90-minute PE sessions over 2 weeks); and a minimal-contact control condition ($n = 40$) involving brief, weekly phone calls from therapists to be used as a compari-son condition for the Massed PE arm. The results demonstrated significant reduc-tions in PTSD symptoms in all three active treatment arms. The Massed PE format had equivalent efficacy as the Spaced PE arm, although there were fewer dropouts

Principal Investigator/ DoD Award Number	Project Title	Interventions	Project Description	Research Participants
Jeffrey Cigrang W81XWH-08-02-0109	Brief Cognitive-Behavioral Treatment of Combat-Related PTSD in Primary Care Settings: A Pilot Study	Prolonged Exposure for Primary Care	Nonrandomized pilot clinical trial of brief cognitive-behavioral therapy (CBT) for PTSD in primary care	*N* = 24 Active Duty Military
Jeffrey Cigrang W81XWH-08-02-0109	Brief Cognitive-Behavioral Treatment of Combat-Related PTSD in Primary Care Settings: A Randomized Controlled Trial	Prolonged Exposure for Primary Care	RCT of brief cognitive-behavioral therapy for PTSD in primary care vs. wait list	*N* = 67 Active Duty Military
Edna Foa W81XWH-08-02-0111	Prolonged Exposure for PTSD in OIF/OEF Personnel: Massed versus Spaced Trials	Prolonged Exposure; Present-Centered Therapy	Four-armed RCT of spaced (weekly) PE, massed (daily) PE, present-centered therapy (PCT), or a minimal-contact control condition	*N* = 366 Active Duty Military
Edna Foa W81XWH-15-1-0555	60- Versus 90-Minute Prolonged Exposure for PTSD: A Randomized Control Trial in Active Duty Military Personnel	Prolonged Exposure	Two-armed RCT noninferiority trial	*N* = 140 Active Duty Military
Peter Fox W81XWH-13-2-0065	Image-guided, Robotically Delivered TMS for PTSD	Transcranial Magnetic Stimulation	Double-blind RCT of image-guided, robotically delivered transcranial magnetic stimulation versus sham	*N* = 119 (*n* = 114 Active Duty Military; *n* = 5 Veterans)
Steffany Fredman W81XWH-13-2-0065	Multi-Couple Group Intervention for PTSD	Cognitive-Behavioral Conjoint Therapy	Non-randomized clinical trial of abbreviated, intensive, multi-couple group Cognitive Behavioral Conjoint Therapy for PTSD	*N* = 24 Couples (*n* = 17 Active Duty Military; *n* = 7 Veterans

Principal Investigator/ DoD Award Number	Project Title	Interventions	Project Description	Research Participants
John Krystal W81XWH-13-2-0065	Ketamine for Antidepressant-Resistant PTSD	Ketamine	RCT of 0.2 mg/kg ketamine, 0.5 mg/kg ketamine, or saline placebo delivered twice per week for 4 weeks	*N* = 156 (*n* = 54 Active Duty Military; *n* = 102 Veterans)
Brian Marx W81XWH-16-2-0003	Decreasing Suicide Risk among Service Members with Posttraumatic Stress Using Written Exposure Therapy	Written Exposure Therapy for Suicide	Recruitment in Progress	Recruitment target *N* = 140 Active Duty Military
Donald McGeary W81XWH-13-2-0065	RCT of Cognitive Behavioral Therapy for PTS and Headache	Cognitive Behavior Therapy for Headache Cognitive Processing Therapy	RCT of CBT for headaches, CPT, Treatment as Usual	*N* = 193 (*n* = 3 Active Duty Military; *n* = 69 Veterans)
Carmen McLean W81XWH-14-1-0008	A Randomized Clinical Trial of Internet-Delivered PE for PTSD	Prolonged Exposure; Present-Centered Therapy	Two-armed RCT of Web-PE versus PCT	*N* = 40 (37 Active Duty Military; 3 Veterans)
Carmen McLean W81XWH-14-1-0008	A Nonrandomized Trial of Internet-Delivered PE for PTSD	Prolonged Exposure	Open clinical trial of Web-PE	*N* = 34 (2 Active Duty Military; 32 Veterans)
Candice Monson W81XWH-08-02-0115	Individual Prolonged Exposure versus Couples' Cognitive-Behavioral Therapy for Combat-Related PTSD	Cognitive Behavioral Conjoint Therapy; Prolonged Exposure	Two-armed RCT of Cognitive Behavioral Conjoint Therapy versus PE	*N* = 116 (58 Active Duty Military; 58 Military Spouses)
Alan Peterson W81XWH-08-02-0109	Outcomes of PE and CPT for Combat Operational Stress Reactions in Deployed Settings	Prolonged Exposure; Cognitive Processing Therapy	Nonrandomized clinical trial of PE and CPT delivered during a military deployment	*N* = 12 Active Duty Military
Alan Peterson W81XWH-12-2-0073	Clinical Effectiveness Trial of In-Home CPT for Combat-Related PTSD	Cognitive Processing Therapy	Three-armed RCT of In-Office, Telebehavioral Health, and In-Home CPT	*N* = 120 (*n* = 24 Active Duty Military; *n* = 96 Veterans

Principal Investigator/ DoD Award Number	Project Title	Interventions	Project Description	Research Participants
Alan Peterson W81XWH-13-2-0065	Project Remission: Maximizing Outcomes with Intensive PTSD Treatment	Prolonged Exposure	RCT of 15 daily Massed-PE or Intensive Outpatient Program-PE sessions over 3 weeks	N = 234 (n = 145 Active Duty Military; n = 144 Veterans)
Patricia Resick W81XWH-08-02-0116	Group Cognitive Processing Therapy versus Group Present Centered Therapy for Combat-Related PTSD	Cognitive Processing Therapy; Present-Centered Therapy	Two-armed RCT of group CPT versus group PCT	N = 108 Active Duty Military
Patricia Resick W81XWH-08-02-0116	Individual versus Group Cognitive Processing Therapy for Combat-Related PTSD	Cognitive Processing Therapy	Two-armed RCT of individually delivered CPT versus group-delivered CPT	N = 268 Active Duty Military
Patricia Resick W81XWH-13-02-0012 Alan Peterson W81XWH-13-02-0013	Variable-Length CPT for Combat-Related PTSD	Cognitive Processing Therapy	Non-randomized clinical trial of variable-lengths of CPT	N = 130
Denise Sloan W81XWH-15-1-0391	Brief Treatment for PTSD: Enhancing Treatment Engagement and Retention	Written Exposure Therapy	Two-armed RCT comparing WET versus CPT	N = 170 Active Duty Military
Daniel Taylor W81XWH-13-2-0065	Treatment of Comorbid Sleep Disorders and PTSD	Cognitive Processing Therapy; Cognitive-Behavioral Therapy for Insomnia	RCT of CPT, CPT followed by CBT-I, or CBT-I followed by CPT	N = 94 (n = 87 Active Duty Military; n = 7 Veterans)

Notes: CBTi = Cognitive-Behavioral Therapy for Insomnia; CPT = Cognitive Processing Therapy; CAP = Consortium to Alleviate PTSD; DoD = Department of Defense; PTSD = posttraumatic stress disorder; PCT = Present-Centered Therapy; PE = Prolonged Exposure; RCT = randomized clinical trial; STRONG STAR = South Texas Research Organizational Network Guiding Studies on Trauma and Resilience; WET = Written Exposure Therapy.

Table 1.
Summary of STRONG STAR and CAP PTSD clinical trials.

from treatment with the Massed PE format (13.6%) as compared to the Spaced PE format (24.8%), and there were fewer adverse events with the Massed PE format (25.3%) as compared to the Spaced PE format (54.1%). These results provide strong support for the compressed, Massed PE treatment format for active duty military personnel; with close coordination with military leadership, it is much easier to schedule and complete a full dose of treatment over a 2-week period as compared to weekly treatment formats that often require 3–4 months to complete.

The promising findings from the Massed PE arm of the study by Foa, McLean, and colleagues [39] led to the funding of a Consortium to Alleviate PTSD (CAP) project to further enhance the Massed PE treatment and to compare it to an Intensive Outpatient Program based on PE (IOP PE). The CAP study [40] randomized 234 active duty service members and veterans to either 15 sessions of daily Massed PE or IOP PE treatment over a 3-week period. The IOP PE arm included eight enhancements to the Massed PE protocol that targeted many of the unique aspects of combat-related PTSD. The enhancements included (1) a team-based treatment approach, rather than relying on one therapist; (2) completion of daily homework assignments at the clinic; (3) 15- to 30-minute, in-person feedback sessions after daily homework assignments; (4) active involvement of the spouse or other support person for in vivo exposures; (5) targeting the patients' top three most distressing traumas during imaginal exposure; (6) starting imaginal exposure with the least distressing trauma and progressing to the most distressing trauma; (7) a brief review of all other potentially traumatic events that occurred during previous deployments; and (8) the completion of three posttreatment booster sessions. The final results of this study have not yet been published, but preliminary results [41] indicate that both treatments resulted in large reductions in PTSD symptoms at the conclusion of treatment, but only those randomized to the IOP PE maintained the large treatment gains over the 6-month follow-up period. The reduction of PTSD symptoms and maintenance of treatment gains with the IOP PE arm are among the strongest treatment outcomes to date for combat-related PTSD.

Another adaptation of the standard, weekly, 90-minute outpatient format for PE was a series of STRONG STAR studies designed to adapt PE for use in military primary care clinics. The first project was a pilot study ($N = 24$) to develop and test an abbreviated PE protocol adapted for primary care (called PE for Primary Care) consisting of four to six 30-minute treatment sessions conducted by a behavioral health consultant embedded in an integrated primary care clinic. The results showed that PTSD severity was significantly reduced and 50% of the patients no longer met criteria for PTSD after treatment [42, 43].

The results of the pilot project were then used in a subsequent RCT in which 67 service members were randomized to receive the PE for Primary Care treatment or a minimal contact control condition followed by treatment after 6 weeks [44]. The results indicated that the immediate treatment group had large reductions in PTSD severity as compared to the minimal contact control. Similar improvements were found in the delayed treatment group when they received the PE for Primary Care treatment, and the treatment benefits persisted through the 6-month follow-up point for all participants. These finding suggest that an abbreviated version of PE delivered in integrated primary care clinics is effective for the treatment of PTSD and may help reduce barriers and stigma found in specialty care settings.

Another adaptation of the standard outpatient PE protocol was the development of a web-based version of PE [45] to help improve accessibility of effective and efficient evidence-based treatments for PTSD. Web-PE was first compared to in-person Present-Centered Therapy in an RCT with 40 military personnel with PTSD at Fort Hood, Texas. Due to recruitment challenges in the RCT, the efficacy of the Web-PE treatment was then evaluated in an open trial with 34 service members and veterans recruited nationwide. The results of the RCT showed that both Web-PE and PCT significantly reduced interviewer-assessed and self-reported symptoms of PTSD, with no significant differences between the groups and a medium effect size for Web-PE [46]. The open trial of Web-PE showed significant reductions in self-reported PTSD symptoms with a large effect size. These results suggest that Web-PE is a potential alternative to standard, in-person PE, although the benefits in reducing PTSD symptoms are likely to be greater in patients who are specifically seeking a web-based treatment.

A significant limitation of the outpatient version of PE for the treatment of military personnel in garrison is that delivering the standard 90-minute PE sessions is difficult in many military mental health settings. To address this challenge, an RCT was conducted to evaluate the efficacy of 60-minute versus 90-minute PE sessions [47]. The preliminary results indicate that the shorter sessions possess equal efficacy, thereby increasing the potential feasibility of using the 60-minute format in military mental health settings [48].

3.2.2 Cognitive Processing Therapy

The first study to evaluate the efficacy of CPT for the treatment of combat-related PTSD in active duty military personnel treated in garrison included 108 active duty US Army soldiers treated at Fort Hood, in Killeen, Texas [49]. The study was an RCT to compare group CPT to group Present-Centered Therapy (PCT). Participants were randomized to attend twice weekly 90-minute group treatments of CPT or PCT. The results indicated that both treatments resulted in large reduc-tions in both clinician-administered and self-report measures of PTSD symptoms, but the group CPT treatment resulted in larger reductions [49].

As a follow-on study to the group CPT versus group PCT, another RCT ($N = 268$) was conducted at Fort Hood to compare CPT delivered in a group format to CPT delivered in an individual format [50]. The study was designed as a noninferiority trial and hypothesized that group CPT would function as well as individual CPT in reducing symptoms. If proved true, group CPT would be more efficient to deliver to a larger proportion of active duty military patients with the need for fewer therapists. The results, however, did not support this hypothesis. Individual CPT was found to be significantly more effective in reducing PTSD symptoms compared to group CPT. The findings suggest that the effective treatment of PTSD with CPT requires a focus on the specific traumas and related cognitions that are unique to individual patients. However, even among those receiving individual CPT, approximately one-half still had clinically significant PTSD symptoms, indicating that additional improvements are needed for existing treatments.

To address these concerns, a study was conducted modeled after a study conducted with civilians that demonstrated treatment outcomes could be improved by varying the number of CPT sessions based on patient response to treatment. The study was conducted using a nonrandomized, within-group design treating 127 active duty military personnel [51]. Patients received variable-length CPT which could end before 12 sessions or extend up to 24 sessions over 18 weeks if patient and therapist agreed a good end state had been reached (PCL-5 $\leq$ 19). The results indicated that the variable-length CPT outcomes were superior to the previous fixed-length CPT studies conducted with military personnel in proportion to diag-nostic remission on the CAPS-5 (65% vs. 40%) and clinically significant symptom improvement on the PCL-5 (76% vs. 46%) [52].

Another method to address some of the potential limitations of the standard CPT protocol is to evaluate different delivery settings for CPT. To evaluate these factors, an RCT was conducted to determine if CPT delivered face-to-face in a patient's home (In-Home CPT) or by telehealth to their home (Telehealth CPT) would result in increased acceptability, fewer dropouts, and better outcomes for service members and veterans than standard In-Office CPT [53]. This study used an equipoise stratified randomization design in which participants could opt out of one delivery modality and still be randomized to one of the other two.

The results showed that 57% of participants declined one of the treatment arms (In-Home = 30%; In-Office = 1 6%; Telehealth = 11%) However dropout from treatment was lowest when therapy was delivered In-Home (21%) as compared to Telehealth (33%) and In-Office (44%) [54]. Significant reductions in PTSD symp-toms occurred across all three treatments, and a remarkable 56% of participants no longer met diagnostic criteria for PTSD at the end of treatment. Treatment outcomes were better when patients received more treatment, and improvements were considerably better when CPT was delivered In-Home or by Telehealth. An additional advantage of the Telehealth CPT is that it reduced the average patient and therapist time commitment by 50% as compared to the In-Office or In-Home treatments. CPT delivered by telehealth is also an efficient and effective treatment modality for PTSD in active duty military. This is an important scientific observa-tion considering recent limitations to in-person care resulting from the COVID-19 pandemic.

Although CPT was designed for the treatment of PTSD related to sexual assault in civilians, there is increasing evidence that it may also be helpful for PTSD that is comorbid with other deployment-related disorders such as posttraumatic headache and insomnia. One CAP 3-armed RCT (N = 193) compared CPT, Cognitive-Behavioral Therapy for Headache, and treatment as usual for veterans and active duty service members with comorbid posttraumatic and PTSD symptoms [55]. The results indicated that, compared to treatment as usual, both CPT and Cognitive-Behavioral Therapy for Headache reduced PTSD symptoms on the PCL-5, but only Cognitive-Behavioral Therapy for Headache reduced headache disability symptoms [56].

Furthermore, one CAP study evaluated the sequencing of treatment for comorbid PTSD and insomnia [57] in military service members and veterans ($N = 94$). The RCT compared (1) 18 sessions of CPT alone, (2) 12 session of CPT followed by 6 sessions of Cognitive-Behavioral Therapy for Insomnia (CBT-I), or (3) 6 sessions of CBT-I followed by 12 sessions of CPT. The preliminary results [58] suggest that treatment sequencing matters and that there are greater reductions in PTSD symptoms when CPT is used first and is followed by CBT-I. Conversely, improved outcomes for insomnia occur when CBT-I is used first and followed by CPT.

3.2.3 Cognitive-Behavioral Conjoint Therapy

Cognitive-Behavioral Conjoint Therapy (CBCT) [59] is a couples-based, 15-session, weekly treatment program to address both PTSD symptoms and relationship functioning. Despite previous research to support the efficacy of CBCT in civilian and veteran couples, the first RCT with active duty military couples comparing CBCT to PE failed to replicate previous results [60]. One of the primary challenges in conducting CBCT with military couples was that the military work environment made it very difficult for both spouses to attend the proposed 15 treatment sessions, resulting in a high dropout rate. To address these challenges, the treatment protocol was redesigned as an abbreviated, intensive, multi-couple group version of CBCT in which the entire treatment protocol was delivered as a 2-day weekend retreat [61]. The results of a nonrandomized clinical trial (N = 24 couples) that included an active duty service member or veteran who had previously deployed found significant reductions in both clinician-rated and self-reported PTSD symptoms as well as significant improvements in relationship satisfaction. However, the results are limited by the nonrandomized design used for this pilot project. Additional research is needed comparing the abbreviated, intensive, multi-couple group version of CBCT to an active comparison intervention.

3.2.4 Written Exposure Therapy

One of the more recent developments to improve treatment efficacy and efficiency for PTSD and decrease dropout rates is a 5-session treatment called Written Exposure Therapy (WET) [62]. After almost 20 years of research with civilian and veteran populations to investigate imaginal exposure in a written form, the first RCT to treat service members in garrison was a 2-armed noninferiority RCT (N = 170) comparing WET to CPT [63]. The results indicated that the 5-session WET protocol was equally effective as the 12-session CPT protocol. However, drop-outs from treatment were significantly less for WET (24%) as compared to CPT (45%). The results demonstrate that WET is an efficient method to treat combat-related PTSD and results in fewer dropouts from treatment and may well represent an important treatment improvement from a public health perspective (i.e., fewer sessions needed and fewer dropouts).

The results of this initial WET study provided support for a follow-on study to evaluate a modified version of WET targeting co-morbid PTSD symptoms and suicidal ideations (WET-S) for service members hospitalized on a military psychiatric inpatient facility. Crisis Response Planning was added to the standard WET protocol to address the suicidal ideations. Recruitment is ongoing for this study, but preliminary results appear quite promising [64].

3.2.5 Medications and devices for the treatment of PTSD in military personnel

Although exposure-based cognitive-behavioral treatments have the largest number of studies supporting the efficacy in treating PTSD, other approaches exist and are promising. One CAP study was a double-blind RCT ($N = 119$) comparing 20 sessions of image-guided, robotically delivered transcranial magnetic stimulation (irTMS) to a sham TMS in service members and veterans hospitalized in a private psychiatric facility in San Antonio, Texas [65]. The treatment for PTSD was delivered to the right dorsolateral prefrontal cortex, an area related to the neural circuitry for stress and anxiety disorders. The preliminary results indicated that there were greater PCL-5 score reductions for active irTMS than for sham at every assessment time point.

Another CAP study was the largest RCT to date to evaluate ketamine for antidepressant-resistant PTSD in 156 service members and veterans randomized to 0.2 mg/kg ketamine, 0.5 mg/kg ketamine, or saline placebo delivered twice per week for 4 weeks [66]. The preliminary results indicated that there were no statisti-cally significant differences in reductions in PTSD among any of the treatment arms; however, there were significant reductions in depression with the higher dose of ketamine. More data analyses are ongoing to more fully understand the impact of ketamine treatment for combat-related PTSD.

4. Summary and conclusions

Over the past decade, the STRONG STAR Consortium and the Consortium to Alleviate PTSD successfully completed 20 clinical trials to evaluate various treatment interventions for combat-related PTSD in active duty military personnel. These studies documented that combat-related PTSD can be effectively treated in military personnel, with up to 80% having significant reductions in their PTSD symptoms and about one-half no longer meeting diagnostic criteria for PTSD at the end of treatment. Importantly, a clinical case series demonstrated that trauma-focused treatments to address combat operational stress reactions and combat-related PTSD can be successfully delivered in the military combat theater [33, 34]. Several studies presented above successfully adapted PE for military populations in various ways to improve access, reduce dropout, and enhance outcomes. These include shortening the time between sessions [39, 40], reducing the number of sessions [42–44], providing web-based treatment [46], reducing the length of sessions [47], and conducting intensive weekend retreats for couples [61]. Similarly, a variable length CPT protocol successfully treated active duty military with improved outcomes [51] and demonstrated efficacy in multiple in-person or telehealth settings [54]. A study showing individually delivered CPT to be more efficacious than CPT delivered in a group format [50] has important implications for health care delivery in both military and VA facilities. Studies of the treatment of comorbid posttraumatic headache [56] and insomnia [58] showed that CPT can be successfully paired with other treatments to improve outcomes. A pilot study of conjoint treatment for military couples using a weekend retreat format shows great promise for reducing PTSD symptoms as well as enhancing relationship satisfac-tion [59]. Finally, WET, a 5-session written exposure treatment, has been shown to treat service members in garrison as successfully as a 12-session CPT but with lower dropout [63]. Despite these important advances, there remains a critical need for research to further improve upon the assessment, diagnosis, treatment, and prevention of PTSD and comorbid conditions in service members and veterans.

Findings from multiple clinical trials have now demonstrated combat-related PTSD can be effectively treated in active duty service members and veterans, but there are additional challenges in the treatment of these populations as compared to many civilian traumas. The assessment and treatment approaches for these conditions must be adapted and tailored for the unique aspects of combat-related traumas and for PTSD that is complicated by one or more of the most common comorbid conditions including TBI, sleep disorders, substance use disorders, chronic pain, and risk for suicide. Clinical trials are also needed to further evaluate the combination of cognitive-behavioral therapies with medications and medical devices. In addition, brief interventions that can be administered soon after trauma exposure in far-forward combat locations need to be evaluated as methods to prevent the onset of chronic PTSD.

Funding

The authors' work on this chapter was supported by Consortium to Alleviate PTSD (CAP) award numbers W81XWH-13-2-0065 from the U.S. Department of Defense, Defense Health Program, Psychological Health and Traumatic Brain Injury Research Program (PH/TBI RP), and I01CX001136-01 from the U.S. Department of Veterans Affairs, Office of Research & Development, Clinical Science Research & Development Service.

Disclaimer

The views expressed herein are solely those of the authors and do not reflect an endorsement by or the official policy or position of the the Department of Defense, the Department of Veterans Affairs, or the U.S. Government.

Author details

Alan L. Peterson[1,2,3*], Barbara L. Niles[4,5], Stacey Young-McCaughan[1,2] and Terence M. Keane[4,5]

1 University of Texas Health Science Center at San Antonio, San Antonio, Texas, USA

2 South Texas Veterans Health Care System, San Antonio, Texas, USA

3 University of Texas at San Antonio, San Antonio, Texas, USA

4 National Center for PTSD, VA Boston Healthcare System, Boston, Massachusetts, USA

5 Boston University School of Medicine, Boston, Massachusetts, USA

*Address all correspondence to: petersona3@uthscsa.edu

References

[1] Kessler RC, Aguilar-Gaxiola S, Alonso J, et al. Trauma and PTSD in the WHO World Mental Health Surveys. *Eur J Psychotraumatol*. 2017;8(sup5):1353383. Published 2017 Oct 27.

[2] Kilpatrick DG, Resnick HS, Milanak ME, Miller MW, Keyes KM, Friedman MJ. National estimates of exposure to traumatic events and PTSD prevalence using DSM-IV and DSM-5 criteria. *J Trauma Stress*. 2013;26(5):537- 547. doi:10.1002/jts.21848

[3] Institute of Medicine. *Treatment of Posttraumatic Stress Disorder: An Assessment of the Evidence*. The National Academies Press; 2008.

[4] Institute of Medicine. *Treatment of Posttraumatic Stress Disorder in Military and Veteran Populations: Final Assessment*. The National Academies Press; 2014.

[5] Judkins JL, Moore BA, Collette TL, Hale WJ, Peterson AL, Morissette SB. Incidence Rates of Posttraumatic Stress Disorder Over a 17-Year Period in Active Duty Military Service Members. *J Trauma Stress*. 2020; 33(6):994-1006.

[6] Tanielian T, Jaycox, LH, eds. *Invisible Wounds of War: Psychological and Cognitive Injuries, Their Consequences, and Services to Assist Recovery*. RAND Corporation; 2008

[7] Bisson J, Andrew M. Psychological treatment of post-traumatic stress disorder (PTSD). *Cochrane Database Syst Rev*. 2007;(3):CD003388. Published 2007 Jul 18.

[8] Bisson JI, Ehlers A, Matthews R, Pilling S, Richards D, Turner S. Psychological treatments for chronic post-traumatic stress disorder. Systematic review and meta-analysis. *Br J Psychiatry*. 2007;190:97-104. doi:10.1192/bjp.bp.106.021402

[9] Foa EB, Keane TM, Friedman, MJ, eds. *Effective Treatments for PTSD: Practice Guidelines from the Intrnational Society for Traumatic Stress Studies*. Guilford Publications; 2000

[10] Hoge CW, Auchterlonie JL, Milliken CS. Mental health problems, use of mental health services, and attrition from military service after returning from deployment to Iraq or Afghanistan. *JAMA*. 2006;295(9):1023-1032. doi:10.1001/jama.295.9.1023

[11] Hoge CW, Terhakopian A, Castro CA, Messer SC, Engel CC. Association of posttraumatic stress disorder with somatic symptoms, health care visits, and absenteeism among Iraq war veterans. *Am J Psychiatry*. 2007; 164(1):150-153.

[12] Milliken CS, Auchterlonie JL, Hoge CW. Longitudinal assessment of mental health problems among active and reserve component soldiers returning from the Iraq war. *JAMA*. 2007;298(18):2141-2148. doi:10.1001/jama.298.18.2141

[13] Steenkamp MM, Litz BT, Hoge CW, Marmar CR. Psychotherapy for Military-Related PTSD: A Review of Randomized Clinical Trials. *JAMA*. 2015;314(5):489-500.

[14] Litz BT, Contractor AA, Rhodes C, et al. Distinct Trauma Types in Military Service Members Seeking Treatment for Posttraumatic Stress Disorder. *J Trauma Stress*. 2018;31(2):286-295. doi:10.1002/jts.22276

[15] Presseau C, Litz BT, Kline NK, et al. An epidemiological evaluation of

trauma types in a cohort of deployed service members. *Psychol Trauma*. 2019;11(8):877-885.

[16] Stein NR, Mills MA, Arditte K, et al. A scheme for categorizing traumatic military events. *Behav Modif*.2012;36(6):787-807.

[17] Weathers FW, Blake DD, Schnurr PP, et al. *The Clinician-Administered PTSD Scale for DSM-5 (CAPS-5)*. 2013. https://www. ptsd.va.gov.

[18] Weathers FW, Bovin MJ, Lee DJ, et al. The Clinician-Administered PTSD Scale for DSM-5 (CAPS-5): Development and initial psychometric evaluation in military veterans. *Psychol Assess*. 2018;30(3):383-395. doi:10.1037/pas0000486

[19] Barnes BJ, Presseau C, Jordan AH, et al. Common Data Elements in the Assessment of Military-Related PTSD Research Applied in the Consortium to Alleviate PTSD. *Mil Med*. 2019;184(5-6):e218-e226.

[20] Weathers FW, Litz BT, Keane TM, et al. *The PTSD Checklist for DSM-5 (PCL- 5)*. 2013. https://www.ptsd.va. gov/ professional/ assessment/adult-sr/ptsd-checklist.asp.

[21] Bovin MJ, Marx BP, Weathers FW, et al. Psychometric properties of the PTSD Checklist for Diagnostic and Statistical Manual of Mental Disorders-Fifth Edition (PCL-5) in veterans. *Psychol Assess*. 2016; 28(11):1379-1391

[22] Wortmann JH, Jordan AH, Weathers FW, et al. Psychometric analysis of the PTSD Checklist-5 (PCL-5) among treatment-seeking military service members. *Psychol Assess*. 2016; 28(11): 1392-1403. doi:10.1037/pas 0000260

[23] Prins A, Bovin MJ, Kimerling R, et al. Primary Care PTSD Screen for DSM-5 (PC-PTSD-5). 2015. https://www.ptsd.va.gov

[24] Kaloupek DG, Chard KM, Freed MC, et al. Common data elements for posttraumatic stress disorder research. *Arch Phys Med Rehabil*. 2010; 91(11):1684-1691.

[25] Foa EB, Dancu CV, Hembree EA, Jaycox LH, Meadows EA, Street GP. A comparison of exposure therapy, stress inoculation training, and their combination for reducing posttraumatic stress disorder in female assault victims. *J Consult Clin Psychol*. 1999;67(2):194-200. doi:10.1037//0022-006x.67.2.194

[26] Foa EB, Hembree EA, Cahill SP, et al. Randomized trial of prolonged exposure for posttraumatic stress disorder with and without cognitive restructuring: outcome at academic and community clinics. *J Consult Clin Psychol*. 2005;73(5):953-964.

[27] Monson CM, Fredman SJ, Adair KC. Cognitive-behavioral conjoint therapy for posttraumatic stress disorder: application to operation enduring and Iraqi Freedom veterans. *J Clin Psychol*. 2008;64(8):958-971.

[28] Resick PA, Nishith P, Weaver TL, Astin MC, Feuer CA. A comparison of cognitive-processing therapy with prolonged exposure and a waiting condition for the treatment of chronic posttraumatic stress disorder in female rape victims. *J Consult Clin Psychol*. 2002;70(4):867-879.

[29] Resick PA, Galovski TE, Uhlmansiek MO, Scher CD, Clum GA,

Young-Xu Y. A randomized clinical trial to dismantle components of cognitive processing therapy for posttraumatic stress disorder in female victims of interpersonal violence. *J Consult Clin Psychol*. 2008; 76(2):243-258.

[30] Foa EB, Hembree EA, Rothbaum BO. *Prolonged Exposure Therapy for PTSD: Emotional Processing Of Traumatic Experiences Therapist Guide;*Oxford University Press. 2007

[31] Peterson AL, Foa EB, Riggs DS. Prolonged exposure therapy. In Moore BA, Penk W, eds. *Treating PTSD in Military Personnel: A Clinical Handbook, 2nd ed.* Guilford; 2019: 46-62

[32] Resick PA, Monson CM, Chard KM. *Cognitive Processing Therapy for PTSD: Comprehensive Manual.* Guilford Press; 2017

[33] Cigrang JA, Peterson AL, Schobitz RP. Three American troops in Iraq: Evaluation of a brief exposure therapy treatment for the secondary prevention of combat-related PTSD. *Prag Case Stud Psychother. 2005;1*(2). doi. org/10.14713/pcsp.v1i2.857

[34] Peterson AL, Cigrang JA, Schobitz RP. Response to commentaries: the scientist-practitioner on the front line: development and formalization of evidenced-based interventions on the battlefield. *Prag Case Stud Psychother.* 2005;1,(2), Article 4;1-5.

[35] Peterson AL, Foa EB, Resick PA, et al. A Nonrandomized Trial of Prolonged Exposure and Cognitive Processing Therapy for Combat-Related Posttraumatic Stress Disorder in a Deployed Setting. *Behav Ther.* 2020;51(6):882-894. doi:10.1016/j.beth.2020.01.003

[36] Weathers FW, Litz BT, Herman DS, Huska JA, Keane TM. The PTSD Checklist (PCL): Reliability, validity, and diagnostic utility. Paper presented at the 9th annual meeting of the International Society for Traumatic Stress Studies; October 25, 1993; San Antonio, Texas.

[37] Bliese PD, Wright KM, Adler AB, Cabrera O, Castro CA, Hoge CW. Validating the primary care posttraumatic stress disorder screen and the posttraumatic stress disorder checklist with soldiers returning from combat. *J Consult Clin Psychol*. 2008;76(2):272-281.

[38] Peterson AL, Straud CL, Evans WR. Treating combat-related posttraumatic stress disorder during military deployments: importance, challenges, and special considerations. *The Behav Ther.* 2019;42:127-131. http://www.abct.org/Journals/?m=mJournal&fa=TBT

[39] Foa EB, McLean CP, Zang Y, et al. Effect of Prolonged Exposure Therapy Delivered Over 2 Weeks vs 8 Weeks vs Present-Centered Therapy on PTSD Symptom Severity in Military Personnel: A Randomized Clinical Trial [published correction appears in JAMA. 2018 Aug 21;320(7):724]. *JAMA*. 2018;319(4):354-364. doi:10.1001/jama.2017.21242

[40] Peterson AL, Foa EB, Blount TH, et al. Intensive prolonged exposure therapy for combat-related posttraumatic stress disorder: Design and methodology of a randomized clinical trial. *Contemp Clin Trials*. 2018; 72:126-136.

[41] Peterson AL, Blount TH, Foa EB, et al. Intensive prolonged exposure for combat-related PTSD: Results from a randomized clinical trial In Keane TM (chair), The Consortium to Alleviate Posttraumatic Stress Disorder Sympo-sium. Paper accepted for presentation at: 40th Annual Conference of the Anx-iety and Depression Association of America; March 20,

2020; San Antonio, TX. (Conference cancelled)

[42] Cigrang JA, Rauch SA, Avila LL, et al. Treatment of active-duty military with PTSD in primary care: early findings. *Psych Serv.* 2011; *8*(2):104-113.

[43] Cigrang JA, Rauch SA, Mintz J, et al. Treatment of active duty military with PTSD in primary care: A follow-up report. *J Anxiety Disord.* 2015;36:110-114. doi:10.1016/ j. janxdis.2015.10.003

[44] Cigrang JA, Rauch SA, Mintz J, et al. Moving effective treatment for posttraumatic stress disorder to primary care: A randomized controlled trial with active duty military. *Fam Syst Health.* 2017; 35(4):450-462.

[45] McLean CP, Rauch SAM, Foa EB, et al. Design of a randomized controlled trial examining the efficacy and biological mechanisms of web-prolonged exposure and present-centered therapy for PTSD among active-duty military personnel and veterans. *Contemp Clin Trials.* 2018; 64:41-48.

[46] McLean CP, Foa EB, Dondanville KA, et al. The effects of web-prolonged exposure among military personnel and veterans with posttraumatic stress disorder [published online ahead of print, 2020 Nov 19]. *Psychol Trauma.* 2020; 10.1037/tra0000978.

[47] Foa EB, Zandberg LJ, McLean CP, et al. The efficacy of 90-minute versus 60-minute sessions of prolonged exposure for posttraumatic stress disorder: Design of a randomized controlled trial in active duty military personnel. *Psychol Trauma.* 2019;11(3):307-313.

[48] Foa EB. 90-minute versus 60-minute sessions of prolonged exposure for the treatment of PTSD. Paper presented at: 5th Annual San Antonio Combat PTSD Conference; October 23, 2020; San Antonio, Texas.

[49] Resick PA, Wachen JS, Mintz J, et al. A randomized clinical trial of group cognitive processing therapy compared with group present-centered therapy for PTSD among active duty military personnel. *J Consult Clin Psychol.* 2015;83(6):1058-1068.

[50] Resick PA, Wachen JS, Dondanville KA, et al. Effect of Group vs Individual Cognitive Processing Therapy in Active-Duty Military Seeking Treatment for Posttraumatic Stress Disorder: A Randomized Clinical Trial [published correction appears in JAMA Psychiatry. 2017 Jun 1;74(6):655]. *JAMA Psychiatry.* 2017;74(1):28-36.

[51] Wachen JS, Dondanville KA, Young-McCaughan S, et al. Testing a variable-length Cognitive Processing Therapy intervention for posttraumatic stress disorder in active duty military: Design and methodology of a clinical trial. *Contemp Clin Trials Commun.* 2019;15:100381. Published 2019 May 23. doi:10.1016/j.conctc.2019.100381

[52] Wachen JS, Mintz J, Dondanville KA, et al. *Variable-length cognitive processing therapy: predicting length of treatment to good end state in an active duty military sample.* Poster presented at: Annual Meeting of the International Society for Traumatic Stress Studies; November 15, 2019; Boston, MA.

[53] Peterson AL, Resick PA, Mintz J, et al. Design of a clinical effectiveness trial of in-home cognitive processing therapy for combat-related PTSD. *Contemp Clin Trials.* 2018;73:27-35. doi:10.1016/j. cct.2018.08.005

[54] Peterson AL, Mintz J, Moring J, et al. In-office, in-home, and telebehavioral-health cognitive processing therapy for combat-related PTSD: preliminary results of a randomized clinical trial. Paper presented at: 4th Annual San Antonio Combat PTSD Conference; October 24, 2019; San Antonio, TX.

[55] McGeary DD, Penzien DB, Resick PA, et al. Study design for a randomized clinical trial of cognitive-behavioral therapy for posttraumatic headache. *Contemp Clin Trials*. 2021; 21.

[56] McGeary DD. Non-pharmacological management of posttraumatic headache in post-9/11 veterans: a Consortium to Alleviate PTSD study. In Keane TM (chair), *The Consortium to Alleviate Posttraumatic Stress Disorder Symposium*. Paper accepted for presentation at: 40th Annual Conference of the Anxiety and Depression Association of America; March 20, 2020; San Antonio, TX. (Conference cancelled)

[57] Taylor DJ, Pruiksma KE, Mintz J, et al. Treatment of comorbid sleep disorders and posttraumatic stress disorder in active duty military: Design and methodology of a randomized clinical trial. *Contemp Clin Trials*. 2020; 99:106186. doi:10.1016/j. cct.2020.106186

[58] Taylor DJ, Resick PA, Pruiksma KE, et al. Treatment of comorbid sleep disorders and PTSD. Paper presented at: Annual Meeting of the Inter-national Society for Traumatic Stress Studies; November 15, 2019; Boston, MA.

[59] Monson CM, Fredman SJ. *Cognitive-behavioral conjoint therapy for posttraumatic stress disorder: harnessing the healing power of relationships*. Guilford Press; 2012

[60] Monson CM. Cognitive-behavioral conjoint therapy versus prol-onged exposure for military-related PTSD: primary outcomes from a randomized controlled trial. Paper presented at: 2nd San Antonio Combat PTSD Conference; October 19, 2017; San Antonio, Texas.

[61] Fredman SJ, Macdonald A, Monson CM, et al. Intensive, Multi-Couple Group Therapy for PTSD: A Nonrandomized Pilot Study With Military and Veteran Dyads. *Behav Ther*. 2020;51(5):700-714. doi:10.1016/ j. beth.2019.10.003

[62] Sloan DM Marx BP. *Written Exposure Therapy for PTSD: A Brief Treatment Approach for Mental Health Professionals*. American Psychological Association; 2019.

[63] Sloan DM, Marx BP, Resick PA, et al. Study design comparing written exposure therapy to cognitive processing therapy for PTSD among military service members: A noninferiority trial. *Contemp Clin Trials Commun*. 2019;17:100507. Published 2019 Dec 10.

[64] Tyler HC, Fina BA, Marx BP, et al. (under review). Written Exposure Therapy for suicide in a psychiatric inpatient unit: a case series.

[65] Fox PT, Salinas F, Roache JD, et al. Image-guided, robotically delivered transcranial magnetic stimulation (irTMS) for combat-related PTSD: preliminary results of a randomized controlled trial. Paper presented at: 4th Annual San Antonio Combat PTSD Conference; October 24, 2019; San Antonio, Texas.

[66] Abdallah CG, Roache JD, Averill LA, et al. Repeated ketamine infusions for antidepressant-resistant PTSD: Methods of a multicenter, randomized, placebo-controlled clinical trial. *Contemp Clin Trials*. 2019; 81:11-18.

Permissions

All chapters in this book were first published by InTech Open; hereby published with permission under the Creative Commons Attribution License or equivalent. Every chapter published in this book has been scrutinized by our experts. Their significance has been extensively debated. The topics covered herein carry significant findings which will fuel the growth of the discipline. They may even be implemented as practical applications or may be referred to as a beginning point for another development.

The contributors of this book come from diverse backgrounds, making this book a truly international effort. This book will bring forth new frontiers with its revolutionizing research information and detailed analysis of the nascent developments around the world.

We would like to thank all the contributing authors for lending their expertise to make the book truly unique. They have played a crucial role in the development of this book. Without their invaluable contributions this book wouldn't have been possible. They have made vital efforts to compile up to date information on the varied aspects of this subject to make this book a valuable addition to the collection of many professionals and students.

This book was conceptualized with the vision of imparting up-to-date information and advanced data in this field. To ensure the same, a matchless editorial board was set up. Every individual on the board went through rigorous rounds of assessment to prove their worth. After which they invested a large part of their time researching and compiling the most relevant data for our readers.

The editorial board has been involved in producing this book since its inception. They have spent rigorous hours researching and exploring the diverse topics which have resulted in the successful publishing of this book. They have passed on their knowledge of decades through this book. To expedite this challenging task, the publisher supported the team at every step. A small team of assistant editors was also appointed to further simplify the editing procedure and attain best results for the readers.

Apart from the editorial board, the designing team has also invested a significant amount of their time in understanding the subject and creating the most relevant covers. They scrutinized every image to scout for the most suitable representation of the subject and create an appropriate cover for the book.

The publishing team has been an ardent support to the editorial, designing and production team. Their endless efforts to recruit the best for this project, has resulted in the accomplishment of this book. They are a veteran in the field of academics and their pool of knowledge is as vast as their experience in printing. Their expertise and guidance has proved useful at every step. Their uncompromising quality standards have made this book an exceptional effort. Their encouragement from time to time has been an inspiration for everyone.

The publisher and the editorial board hope that this book will prove to be a valuable piece of knowledge for researchers, students, practitioners and scholars across the globe.

List of Contributors

Manuel Mejías-Estévez
Primary Care District of Seville, Clinic Historical Round, Seville, Spain
University of Pablo de Olavide, Seville, Spain
Training and Research Department of the Sant Ángela Institute (ISA) for Chronic Disease and Palliative Care, Seville, Spain

Rocio Dominguez Álvarez
Internal Medicine Unit, Virgen Macarena University Hospital, Seville, Spain

Ignacio Jauregi Lobera
Department of Molecular Biology and Biochemical Engineering, University of Pablo de Olavide of Seville, Seville, Spain

Imre Lázár
Head of Medical Humanities Research Group, Institute of Behavioral Sciences, Semmelweis University, Budapest, Hungary
Faculty of Humanities and Social Sciences, Károli Gáspár University, Institution of Social and Communication Sciences, Budapest, Hungary

Ralf F. Tauber and Carola Nisch
Fachabteilung für Psychosomatik, Sachsenklinik, Bad Lausick, Germany

Mutahira M. Qureshi and Olivia Patsalos
Department of Psychological Medicine, Institute of Psychiatry, Psychology and Neuroscience, King's College London, London, UK

Hubertus Himmerich
Department of Psychological Medicine, Institute of Psychiatry, Psychology and Neuroscience, King's College London, London, UK
South London and Maudsley NHS Foundation Trust, London, UK

José Vicente Martínez-Quiñones
Department of Neurosurgery, Mutua de Accidentes de Zaragoza, Zaragoza, Spain

Ignacio Jáuregui-Lobera
Department of Molecular Biology and Biochemical Engineering, University of Pablo de Olavide of Seville, Seville, Spain

Yuanyuan Li, Xiaoyan Chen and Fang Fan
School of Psychology, Center for Studies of Psychological Application, and Key Laboratory of Mental Health and Cognitive Science of Guangdong Province, South China Normal University, Guangdong, China

Ya Zhou
Department of Psychology, Lund University, Lund, Sweden

George Musa and Christina Hoven
Department of Child and Adolescent Psychiatry, New York State Psychiatric Institute, Columbia University, New York, USA

Margaret Trey
Sibubooks; Center for Psychology and Mind Studies (Researcher & Author of two books on the effects of Falun Gong), New York, USA

Cirecie West-Olatunji
Center for Traumatic Stress Research, Xavier University of Louisiana, New Orleans, United States

Orla McDevitt-Petrovic and Karen Kirby
School of Psychology, Ulster University, United Kingdom

Ignacio Jáuregui-Lobera and Marian Montes-Martínez
Behavioral Sciences Institute, Seville, Spain

Ertuğrul Allahverdi
Department of Orthopedics and Traumatology, School of Medicine, Kafkas University, Kars, Turkey

Mar Martínez Gamarra
Storytelling Spanish Association (ASEST), Zaragoza, Spain

Emilija Stoimenova Canevska and Ena Canevska
European Accredited Psychotherapy Training Institute "Gestalt Institute" -Skopje (EAPTI GI-S), Skopje, R.N. Macedonia

Anne Iris Miriam Anders
Institute of Social and Cultural Anthropology, Ludwig Maximilians University Munich, Germany

Stacey Young-McCaughan
University of Texas Health Science Center at San Antonio, San Antonio, Texas, USA
South Texas Veterans Health Care System, San Antonio, Texas, USA

Alan L. Peterson
University of Texas Health Science Center at San Antonio, San Antonio, Texas, USA
South Texas Veterans Health Care System, San Antonio, Texas, USA
University of Texas at San Antonio, San Antonio, Texas, USA

Barbara L. Niles and Terence M. Keane
National Center for PTSD, VA Boston Healthcare System, Boston, Massachusetts, USA
Boston University School of Medicine, Boston, Massachusetts, USA

Index

O

P

Q

R

S

T

www.ingramcontent.com/pod-product-compliance
Lightning Source LLC
LaVergne TN
LVHW062129200926
848484LV00007B/1787